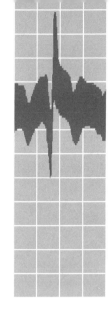

ECG Workout
Exercises in
Arrhythmia Interpretation

ECG Workout

Exercises in Arrhythmia Interpretation

Second Edition

Jane Huff, RN, CCRN

Nurse Manager, Critical Care Unit
Arrhythmia Instructor
Advanced Cardiac Life Support (ACLS) Instructor
Central Arkansas Hospital
Searcy, Arkansas

David P. Doernbach, MEd

President
Vital Signs Unlimited
Little Rock, Arkansas

Roger D. White, MD, FACC

Department of Anesthesiology
Mayo Clinic
Rochester, Minnesota

J.B. Lippincott Company
Philadelphia

Acquisitions Editor: David Carroll
Coordinating Editorial Assistant: Patty Shear
Project Editor: Jim Slade
Design Coordinator: Doug Smock
Interior Designer: Joan Jacobus
Cover Designer: Anne Bullen
Production Manager: Helen Ewan
Production Coordinator: Nannette Winski
Compositor: Bi-Comp, Incorporated
Printer/Binder: Courier Book Company/Kendallville

Second Edition

6 5 4 3

Huff, Jane.
    ECG workout : exercises in arrhythmia interpretation / Jane Huff,
David P. Doernbach, Roger D. White.—2nd ed.
        p.   cm.
    ISBN 0-397-55055-3
    1. Arrhythmia—Diagnosis—Problems, exercises, etc.
  2. Electrocardiography—Interpretation—Problems, exercises, etc.
  I. Doernbach, David P.   II. White, Roger D., 1939–   . III. Title.
    [DNLM: 1. Arrhythmia—diagnosis—problems.
  2. Electrocardiography—problems. WG 18 H889e 1993]
  RC685.A65H84 1993
  616.1′2807547—dc20
  DNLM/DLC
  for Library of Congress   93-12599
                                                                CIP

Any procedure or practice described in this book should be applied by the health care practitioner under appropriate supervision in accordance with professional standards of care used with regard to the unique circumstances that apply in each practice situation. Care has been taken to confirm the accuracy of information presented and to describe generally accepted practices. However, the authors, editors, and publisher cannot accept any responsibility for errors or omissions or for any consequences from application of the information in this book and make no warranty, express or implied, with respect to the contents of the book.

Every effort has been made to ensure drug selections and dosages are in accordance with current recommendations and practice. Because of ongoing research, changes in government regulations, and the constant flow of information on drug therapy, reactions, and interactions, the reader is cautioned to check the package insert for each drug for indications, dosages, warnings, and precautions, particularly if the drug is new or infrequently used.

The second edition of ECG Workout is dedicated to my children, Brandy and Scott, and to the critical care nurses and telemetry technicians at Central Arkansas Hospital who have given me their friendship, support, and encouragement and who over the years have collected many of the tracings seen in this book.

Jane Huff

To Donna and the elves.

David Doernbach

To my mother, and to the memory of my father, both of whom sacrificed much to enable me to acquire an education in medicine.

Roger White

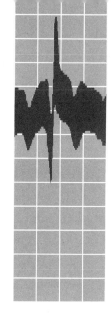

Contents

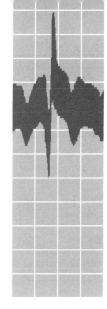

Introduction

As with the first edition, the primary goal of the second edition of *ECG Workout: Exercises in Arrhythmia Interpretation* is to provide a sufficient number of ECG practice strips so that the reader feels confident in arrhythmia interpretation. The text includes practice strips on each group of arrhythmias in addition to practice strips on pacemaker malfunctions and a two-part post-test. There are approximately 525 practice strips in all. Most of the ECG rhythm strips have been replaced and new ones added.

The second edition has been appreciably revised. New sections have been added on anatomy and physiology, electrophysiology; waveforms, intervals, segments, and complexes; and monitor equipment, lead placements, artifact, and steps in analyzing a rhythm strip. The four arrhythmia chapters include a discussion of each specific rhythm along with examples and treatment protocols if appropriate. The pacemaker section has been expanded to include a discussion of pacemaker terminology, pacemaker malfunctions, malfunction examples, and steps in analyzing a pacemaker rhythm strip.

The ECG tracings included in the text are actual strips from patients. Above each rhythm strip are 3- and 6-second indicators for rapid rate calculation. For more precise rate calculation an electrocardiographic conversion table is provided on the inside back cover. The rates listed in the answer keys were determined by as precise measurement as possible and will not always agree exactly with the rapid method of rate calculation.

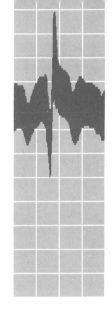

ECG Workout
Exercises in
Arrhythmia Interpretation

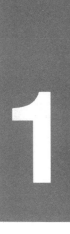

Anatomy and Physiology of the Heart

DESCRIPTION

The heart is a hollow, four-chambered, muscular organ whose primary function is to pump blood throughout the body via a closed circuit of vessels. It lies in the center of the chest between two lungs; it is contained between the second and sixth ribs; and it lies behind the sternum and in front of the spine (Figure 1-1). The lower border of the heart, which forms a blunt point known as the apex, lies on the diaphragm and points to the left. The average adult heart is 5 inches long and 3½ inches wide, and it corresponds to an average sized man's fist.

HEART SURFACES

There are four main heart surfaces to consider when discussing the heart: anterior, posterior, inferior, and lateral (Figure 1-2). A simplified concept of the heart surfaces is listed below.

Anterior: the front
Posterior: the back
Inferior: the bottom
Lateral: the side

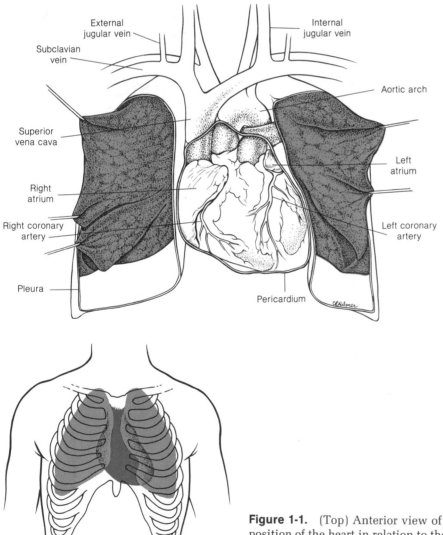

Figure 1-1. (Top) Anterior view of the heart and great vessels; (bottom) position of the heart in relation to the skeletal structures of the chest cage. (From Porth CM. Pathophysiology, 3rd ed. Philadelphia: JB Lippincott, 1990.)

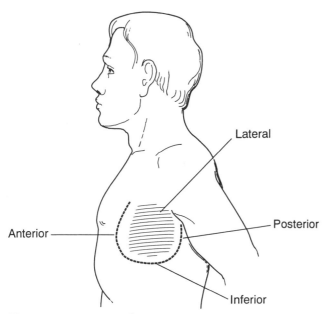

Figure 1-2. Heart surfaces.

HEART STRUCTURE

The heart is enclosed in a loose-fitting sac called the pericardium. The pericardium consists of two parts: a fibrous portion and a serous portion. The outermost portion (fibrous pericardium) is tough, inelastic, and helps support the heart inside the chest cavity. The inner portion (serous pericardium) is divided into the parietal layer, which lines the fibrous sac, and the visceral layer, which lines the outer surface of the heart muscle. Between the parietal and visceral layers is a small space, the pericardial space, which contains serous fluid. This well-lubricated, loose-fitting sac prevents friction during heart contraction and relaxation.

The muscular portion of the heart is called the myocardium. It makes up the bulk of the heart wall (Figure 1-3).

The endocardium is the inner surface of the heart. It is a membranous covering that lines the heart chambers and valves. Papillary muscles originate in the endocardium, which lines the ventricles.

HEART CHAMBERS

The interior of the heart is divided by a septum into a left side and a right side and into four chambers: two upper and two lower. The two upper chambers are called the atria, and the two lower chambers are called the ventricles (Figure 1-4).

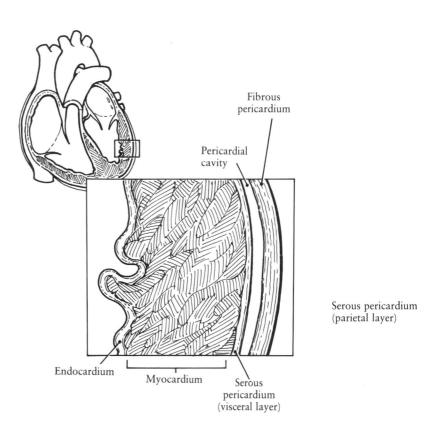

Figure 1-3. Heart wall. (From Bullock BL, Rosendahl PP: Pathophysiology, 3rd ed. Philadelphia: JB Lippincott, 1992.)

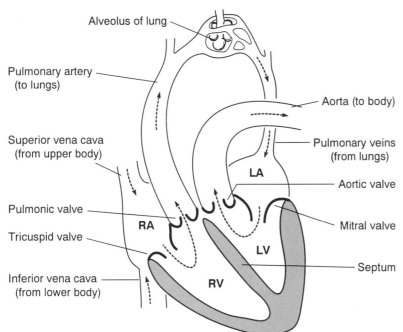

Figure 1-4. Chambers, valves, blood flow. *RA,* right atrium; *RV,* right ventricle; *LA,* left atrium; *LV,* left ventricle.

The two atria are thin-walled, low-pressure chambers that act as reservoirs of blood for their respective ventricle. The two ventricles are thick-walled and act as pumps to eject blood into the pulmonary and systemic circulation.

The heart acts as a double pump, pumping oxygenated blood and nutrients (arterial blood) from the left side of the heart to the body tissues and organs and pumping deoxygenated blood with carbon dioxide and cellular waste products (venous blood) from the right side of the heart to the lungs for removal.

HEART VALVES

There are four valves in the heart: the mitral valve, separating the left atrium from the left ventricle; the tricuspid valve, separating the right atrium from the right ventricle; the aortic valve, separating the left ventricle from the aorta; and the pulmonic valve, separating the right ventricle from the pulmonary artery (see Figure 1-4). The primary function of the valves is to permit the flow of blood in one direction only, thereby preventing a backflow of blood.

The mitral and tricuspid valves are sometimes referred to as atrioventricular valves. The atrioventricular valves have cusps or leaflets, which are connected to fingerlike projections (papillary muscles) in the ventricles by thin cords called chordae tendineae (Figure 1-5). The chordae tendineae prevent backflow of blood into the atria during ventricular contraction. Closure of the atrioventricular valves constitutes the first heart sound (S_1).

The aortic and pulmonic valves are sometimes referred to as semilunar valves. These semilunar valves have half-moon–shaped cusps, which lie flat against the vessel walls during ventricular ejection. Following ventricular ejection, a small amount of blood flows back down the vessel walls into the valve cusps, pushing them away from the vessel walls and causing them to shut. The construction of the valves prevents backflow of blood into the ventricles. Closure of the semilunar valves constitutes the second heart sound (S_2).

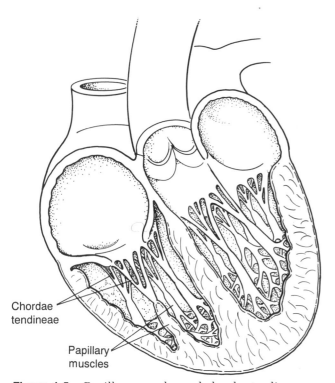

Figure 1-5. Papillary muscles and chordae tendineae.

Figure 1-6. Coronary blood supply. (From Porth CM: Pathophysiology, 3rd ed. Philadelphia: JB Lippincott, 1990.)

BLOOD FLOW THROUGH THE HEART AND LUNGS

Blood flow through the heart and lungs is regulated by the heart valves and is dependent on pressure changes within the system (see Figure 1-4). Venous blood is returned to the right side of the heart via the superior and inferior venae cavae and coronary sinus and collected in the right atrium. As the right atrium fills with blood, the pressure in the chamber increases. When the pressure in the right atrium exceeds that of the right ventricle, the tricuspid valve opens, allowing blood to enter the right ventricle. When right ventricular pressure exceeds that of the pulmonary artery, the ventricle contracts, closing the tricuspid valve and forcing blood through the pulmonic valve to the pulmonary artery into the pulmonary capillaries of the lungs.

Oxygenated blood from the lungs is returned to the left side of the heart via four pulmonary veins and collected in the left atrium. When left atrial pressure exceeds that of the left ventricle, the mitral valve opens, allowing blood to enter the left ventricle. When left ventricular pressure exceeds aortic pressure, the left ventricle contracts, closing the mitral valve and forcing blood through the aortic valve to the aorta, the systemic arteries, and all parts of the body.

CORONARY BLOOD SUPPLY

The blood supply to the heart is provided by the left and right coronary arteries, which arise from the aorta just above the aortic valve (Figure 1-6). The right coronary artery travels down the right side of the heart, curves around the bottom of the heart, and supplies blood to the back via the posterior descending branch. It supplies blood to the right atrium, the right ventricle, the sinoatrial node, the atrioventricular node, and the inferior and posterior walls of the left ventricle. Occlusion of the right coronary artery can result in a posterior or inferior myocardial infarction.

The left coronary artery has two branches: the anterior descending branch, which courses down the front of the heart, and the circumflex, which travels down the side. The left coronary artery supplies blood to the anterior and lateral walls of the left ventricle. Occlusion of either branch of the left coronary artery can result in an anterior or lateral myocardial infarction.

Variations in blood distribution of the coronary arteries are common. Left or right coronary artery dominance denotes which artery supplies the greater amount of blood to the left ventricle. Sometimes the blood distribution is balanced between the right and left coronary artery systems, and neither one is considered dominant.

2

Electrophysiology

CARDIAC CELLS

The heart consists of electrical cells and mechanical cells. The electrical cells are responsible for impulse formation and conduction whereas the mechanical cells are responsible for muscular contraction.

The electrical cells are distributed in an orderly fashion along the conduction system of the heart. These cells possess three specific properties:

1. *Automaticity:* the ability of the cell to spontaneously generate and discharge an electrical impulse

2. *Excitability:* the ability of the cell to respond to an electrical impulse

3. *Conductivity:* the ability of the cell to transmit an electrical impulse from one cell to another

The heart not only contains an orderly arrangement of electrical cells, it also includes an organized arrangement of mechanical or working cells. The mechanical cells possess two specific properties. These properties are:

1. *Contractility:* the ability of the cell to shorten and lengthen its muscle fibers

2. *Extensibility:* the ability of a cell to stretch

DEPOLARIZATION AND REPOLARIZATION

To understand the interrelationship between the electrical cells and the mechanical cells, one must consider a single cardiac cell (Figure 2-1). Each cell is surrounded by and filled with a solution that contains positively charged ions and negatively charged ions. At rest, K^+ is found in greater quantities inside the cell while Na^+ and Ca^{++} are found in greater quantities outside the cell. The cell membrane is influenced the most by Na^{++} and K^+ ions. There is a continual movement of these ions across the cell membrane.

As ionic concentrations change between the intercellular and extracellular compartments, an electrical difference exists between the inside and the outside of the cell. Although positively and negatively charged ions are found on both sides of the cell membrane, the concentration is such that there is a net negative charge inside the cell and a net positive charge outside the cell. The cell maintains this state until stimulated.

When the cell is stimulated, the cell membrane becomes more permeable, allowing an influx of Na^+

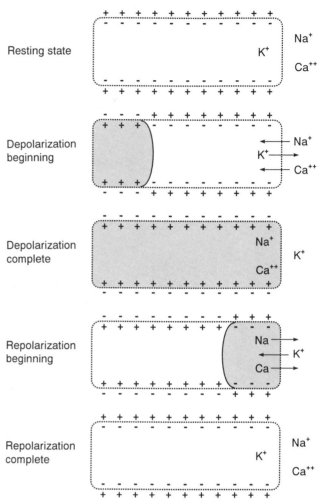

Figure 2-1. Depolarization and repolarization of a cardiac cell.

and Ca^{++} to enter the cell and causing K^+ to move outside the cell. The inside cell becomes electropositive, and the outside cell becomes electronegative. Movement of these ions across the cell membrane generates an electrical current, which results in muscle contraction called depolarization. Following depolarization, the cell returns to its resting ionic state. This process is called repolarization or recovery. During repolarization, K^+ is returned in greater concentrations to the inside of the cell and Na^+ and Ca^{++} is pumped in greater concentration to the outside of the cell.

ELECTRICAL CONDUCTION SYSTEM OF THE HEART

The heart is endowed with a special system that generates and conducts electrical impulses along a conducting pathway to the heart muscle, resulting in

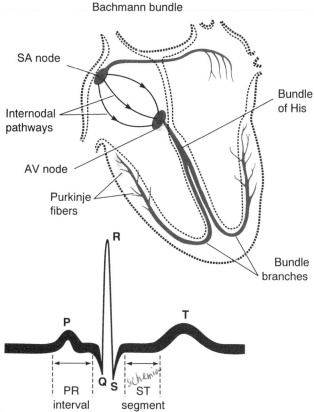

Bachmann bundle

SA node

Internodal pathways

AV node

Purkinje fibers

Bundle of His

Bundle branches

R

P

T

PR interval

Q S

ischemic

ST segment

Figure 2-2. Relationship of the electrical conduction system to the ECG.

The electrical activity during the cardiac cycle is transmitted to the surface of the body, where it can be picked up by the skin electrodes and recorded on an electrocardiograph. The electrical activity is characterized by five separate waves or deflections designated as P, Q, R, S, and T. As the impulse leaves the SA node it travels though the atria by way of the internodal pathways and the Bachmann bundle, causing the atria to contract simultaneously. Atrial depolarization is represented as the P wave on the electrocardiogram (ECG). The impulse reaches the AV node, where it is momentarily slowed. Next, the impulse travels rapidly through the bundle of His and the left and right bundle branches, terminating in a network of Purkinje fibers deeply embedded in the ventricular myocardium. The PR interval on the ECG depicts the impulse from the time it leaves the SA node through the delay at the AV node and its arrival at the terminal Purkinje fibers. The impulse then activates the ventricles to contract. Ventricular depolarization is represented as the QRS on the ECG. Following depolarization, the ventricles rest (represented as the ST segment) and repolarize (represented by the T wave).

CARDIAC CYCLE

The term cardiac cycle means a complete heart beat, consisting of contraction (systole) and relaxation (diastole) of both atria plus contraction and relaxation of both ventricles. During atrial systole both atria contract, pumping blood into the ventricles while the ventricles relax and fill with blood (diastole). During ventricular systole both ventricles contract, pumping blood to the lungs and body while the atria are in diastole. The combined phases of systole and diastole constitute one cardiac cycle.

The ECG can be correlated with the systolic and diastolic phases of ventricular action, as shown in Figure 2-3. Ventricular systole begins at the peak of

muscular contraction (Figure 2-2). The system consists of the sinoatrial (SA) node, internodal pathways, Bachmann bundle, atrioventricular (AV) node, bundle of His, left and right bundle branches, and Purkinje fibers.

The electrical impulse originates in the SA node, located in the upper wall of the right atrium. Specialized electrical cells, called pacemaker cells (p-cells) in the SA node discharge impulses at a rate of 60 to 100 times per minute in rhythmic fashion. These cells have the ability to initiate impulses on their own (automaticity), a property inherent to cardiac tissue. Because the SA node normally controls the heart rate, it is designated as the pacemaker.

Other areas of the heart (AV node and ventricles) contain a scattering of p-cells and have the potential to serve as pacemaker, although they assume this role only under abnormal circumstances. Pacemakers other than the SA node are called ectopic pacemakers. Although ectopic pacemakers fire rhythmically, their rate of discharge is much slower than the SA node (40 to 60 per minute for AV node and 30 to 40 per minute for ventricles). Therefore, they do not serve as the dominant pacemaker.

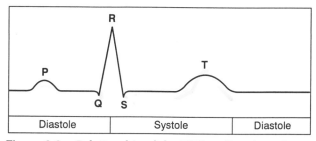

R

P

T

Q S

Diastole | Systole | Diastole

Figure 2-3. Relationship of the ECG to diastole and systole.

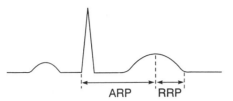

Figure 2-4. The refractory period: *ARP*, absolute refractory period; *RRP*, relative refractory period.

the QRS complex and ends near the completion of the T wave. Diastole begins at this time and continues until the next R wave.

REFRACTORINESS

The refractory period of the cardiac cycle refers to a state of unresponsiveness following excitation of the cardiac muscle cell (Figure 2-4). When stimulated, the muscle cell will respond completely or not at all. This is known as the all-or-none principle. After excitation, the cardiac muscle cell becomes completely unresponsive to any stimulus. This period is called the refractory period and is divided into two portions:

1. *Absolute refractory period:* No stimulus (no matter how powerful) can excite the tissue. If the cell is stimulated during this period, the stimulus is rejected.

2. *Relative refractory period:* Some of the cells have returned to their original state (repolarized) and a strong stimulus can excite the tissue. This period is also referred to as the "vulnerable period" because an impulse striking at this time can initiate life-threatening dysrhythmias (ventricular tachycardia and ventricular fibrillation).

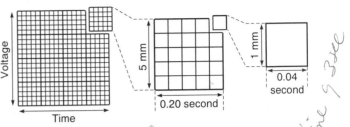

Figure 2-6. Electrocardiographic paper.

TIME AND VOLTAGE MEASUREMENTS

A point of reference on the ECG is the isoelectric line or baseline (Figure 2-5). This is the flat line between the T wave and the P wave. Any deflection above the isoelectric line is considered positive and any wave deflection below this line is considered negative. Waveforms that are both positive and negative are called biphasic.

ELECTROCARDIOGRAPHIC PAPER

The ECG graph paper (Figure 2-6) is made up of horizontal and vertical lines. The horizontal lines measure time in seconds. Each small square measured horizontally represents 0.04 seconds in time. The width of the R wave deflection in Figure 2-7 extends across for 2 squares and represents 0.08 seconds (0.04 seconds × 2 squares). The vertical lines measure voltage (or height) in millimeters. Each small square measured vertically represents 1 mm in height. The height of the R wave deflection in Figure 2-7 extends upward 16 small squares and represents 16 mm (1 mm × 16 squares). Voltage is always measured upward or downward from the isoelectric line.

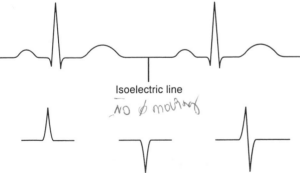

Figure 2-5. Relationship between waveforms and the isoelectric line.

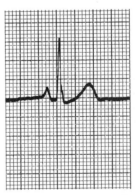

Figure 2-7. QRS width: 0.08 seconds; QRS height: 16 mm

3

Waveforms, Intervals, Segments, and Complexes

Huff J, Doernbach DP, White RD: *ECG WORKOUT: EXERCISES IN ARRHYTHMIA INTERPRETATION*, 2nd ed. © 1993 J.B. Lippincott Company.

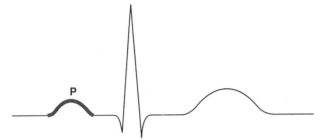

Figure 3-1. The P wave.

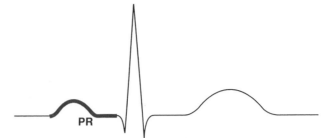

Figure 3-3. The PR interval.

P WAVE

The P wave is the first waveform on the electrocardiogram tracing (Figure 3-1). The P wave is normally small, smooth, and slightly rounded in shape, upright in the most common monitoring leads (I, II, V_6), and inverted or biphasic in lead V_1. There should be one P wave before each QRS.

The P wave represents atrial depolarization. The duration of the P wave denotes the time required for the impulse to travel through the atrial muscle and cause atrial contraction.

If P waves are present and are of normal size, shape, and position, it is likely that the impulse originated in the sinoatrial node. If these waves are absent or abnormally positioned, it implies that the impulse originated outside the sinoatrial node.

Identification of P waves is the most important factor in differentiating sinus rhythms from ectopic rhythms. Several P wave examples are shown in Figure 3-2.

PR INTERVAL

The period from the beginning of the P wave to the beginning of the QRS complex is designated as the PR interval (Figure 3-3). This interval represents the time taken for the original impulse to leave the

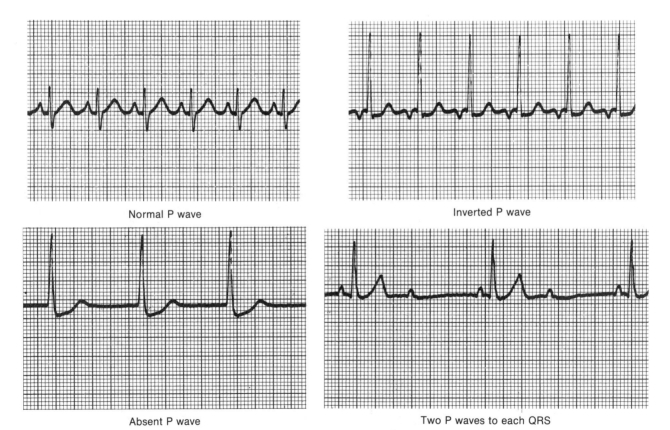

Normal P wave

Inverted P wave

Absent P wave

Two P waves to each QRS

Figure 3-2. P wave examples.

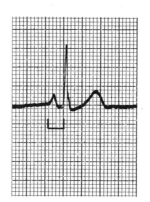

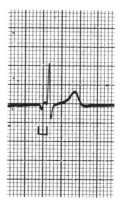

Normal PR interval of 0.16 seconds (0.04 seconds × 4 squares)

Short PR interval of 0.08 seconds (0.04 seconds × 2 squares)

Long PR interval of 0.38 seconds (0.04 seconds × 9½ squares)

Figure 3-4. PR interval examples.

sinoatrial node and travel through the atria, the atrioventricular node, the bundle branches, and the Purkinje fibers. The flat line between the P wave and QRS represents the delay at the atrioventricular node.

The PR interval is measured from the beginning of the P wave as it leaves the isoelectric line to the beginning of the QRS; it is normally 0.12 to 0.20 seconds in duration.

PR intervals shorter than 0.12 seconds imply accelerated conduction of the impulse to the ventricles either through a shorter than normal pathway (Wolff-Parkinson-White syndrome and Lown-Ganong-Levine syndrome) or through a pacemaker site located close to the ventricles (atrioventricular node). PR intervals longer than 0.20 seconds imply delayed conduction of the impulse to the ventricles. Long PR intervals are seen in heart blocks. Examples of PR intervals are shown in Figure 3-4.

QRS COMPLEX

The QRS complex represents ventricular depolarization (Figure 3-5). The duration of the QRS represents the time required for the electrical impulse to

travel through the right and left ventricles, resulting in ventricular contraction.

The QRS complex is composed of three waveforms: Q, R, and S waves. Many variations exist in the shape of the QRS (Figure 3-6). A QRS complex may contain only one or two or all three waveforms. Whatever the variation, the complex is still termed the QRS complex.

The first negative deflection of the QRS complex is always termed the Q wave. The first positive deflection is always called the R wave. The negative deflection after the R wave is always termed an S wave. It is possible to have more than one R wave or S wave in a QRS complex. The second R wave is labeled R prime (R') and the second S wave is labeled S prime (S').

The normal QRS duration is less than 0.12 seconds. The QRS complex is measured from the beginning of the QRS as it leaves the isoelectric line until the end of the QRS when it returns to the isoelectric line.

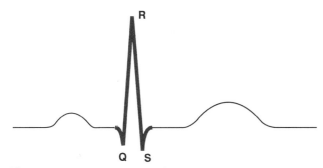

Figure 3-5. The QRS complex.

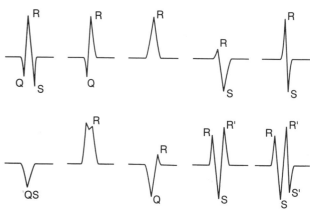

Figure 3-6. QRS variations: An R wave is a positive deflection; a Q wave is a negative deflection before an R wave; an S wave is a negative deflection after an R wave.

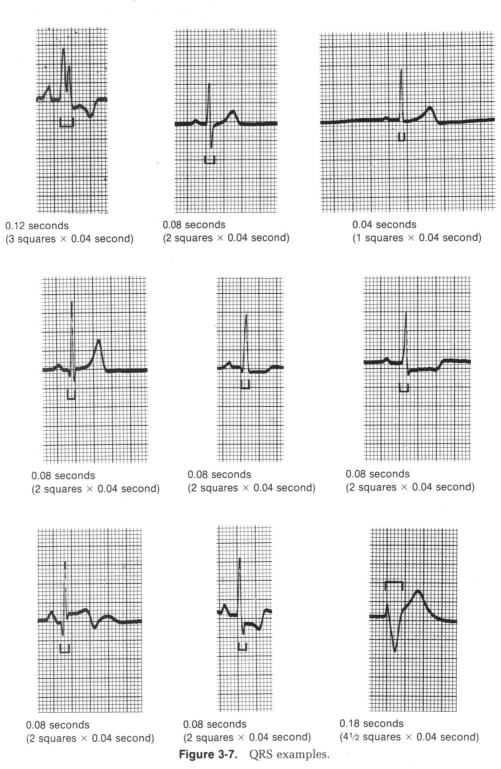

0.12 seconds
(3 squares × 0.04 second)

0.08 seconds
(2 squares × 0.04 second)

0.04 seconds
(1 squares × 0.04 second)

0.08 seconds
(2 squares × 0.04 second)

0.08 seconds
(2 squares × 0.04 second)

0.08 seconds
(2 squares × 0.04 second)

0.08 seconds
(2 squares × 0.04 second)

0.08 seconds
(2 squares × 0.04 second)

0.18 seconds
(4½ squares × 0.04 second)

Figure 3-7. QRS examples.

In some instances, the flat line following the QRS (ST segment) is elevated or depressed. This makes ending the QRS measurement more difficult. The QRS ends as soon as the straight line of the ST segment begins, even though the straight line may be above or below baseline. Examples of some QRS measurements are shown in Figure 3-7.

ST SEGMENT

The ST segment is the straight line between the QRS and the T wave (Figure 3-8). It represents the time between the completion of ventricular depolarization and the beginning of repolarization (T wave) and is sometimes referred to as the resting phase of

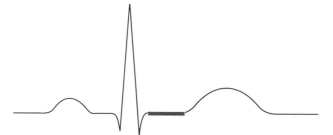

Figure 3-8. The ST segment.

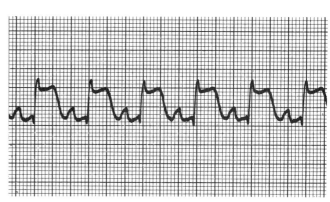

Figure 3-10. The T wave.

the cardiac cycle. Normally this segment is isoelectric, meaning it is neither elevated or depressed. Elevation or depression of the ST segment is abnormal.

ST segment elevation indicates myocardial injury. The ST segments associated with injury are elevated above baseline, usually in an upward curving manner. ST segment depression indicates myocardial ischemia. The ST segments associated with ischemia are depressed below baseline in a horizontal line, or they sag downward like a sagging clothesline. Examples of ST segments are shown in Figure 3-9.

T WAVE

The T wave is a rounded waveform, taller and wider than the P wave, which follows the QRS complex and the ST segment. Normal T waves are upright in the most common monitoring leads (I, II, V_6) and may be upright or inverted in lead V_1 (Figure 3-10).

Myocardial ischemia produces T wave changes. Typically, the T waves of ischemia are inverted and sharply pointed (resembling an arrowhead). Examples of T waves are shown in Figure 3-11.

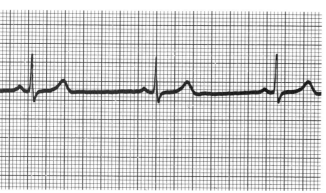

Normal ST segment

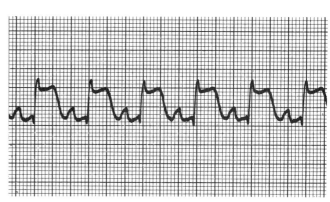

Elevated ST segments

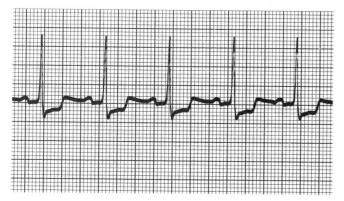

Horizontal depression

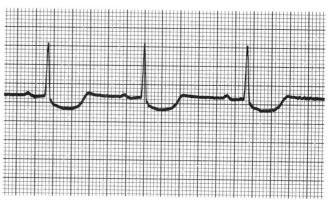

Sagging depression   ISCHEMIA

Figure 3-9. ST segment examples.

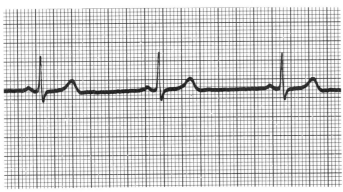

Normal T wave

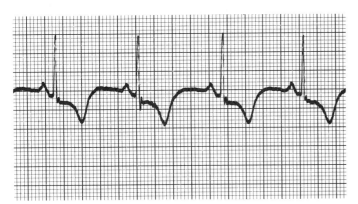

T wave of ischemia

Figure 3-11. T wave examples.

U WAVE

The U wave is a small, rounded, low-amplitude deflection occurring just after the T wave and before the next P wave. It normally goes unnoticed because of its low voltage (Figure 3-12). It is normally in the same direction as the T wave.

The appearance of the U wave has been related to late repolarization of the ventricles and low serum potassium levels. A U wave that is opposite in direction to the T wave is diagnostic of cardiac disease, especially of coronary artery or hypertensive origin. Examples of U waves are shown in Figure 3-13.

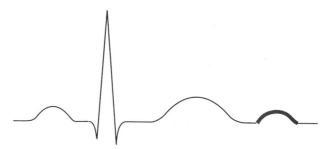

Figure 3-12. The U wave.

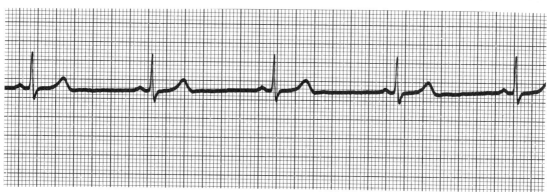

ECG without U wave

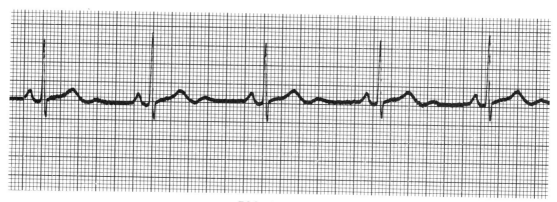

ECG with U wave

Figure 3-13. U wave example.

P wave depolarization of the atria   .12 to .20

PQR

T wave repolarization

↑ U is ↓ in K⁺

↓ U = cardiac disease

atrial fib

P wave is a sinus rythm

def ∴ premature AC & PAT (150 to 250)

if P is there is a block & sinus arrest

Waveform Practice—Labeling Waves

Directions: For each of the following rhythms strips (Strips 3-1 through 3-11), label the P, Q, R, S, T, and U waves. Some of the strips may not have all of these waveforms. Check your answers with the answer keys in the Appendix.

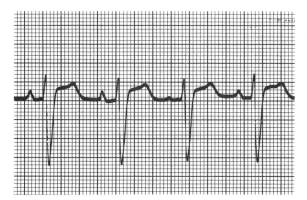

Strip 3-1.

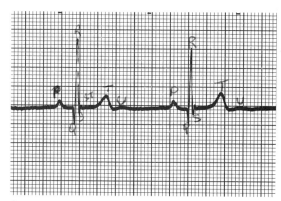

Strip 3-2.

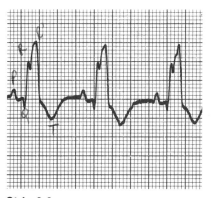

Strip 3-3.

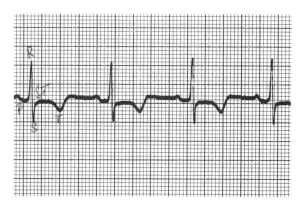

Strip 3-4.

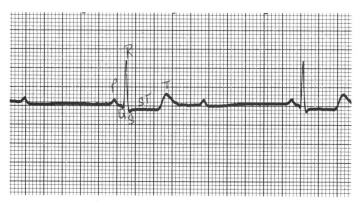

Strip 3-5.

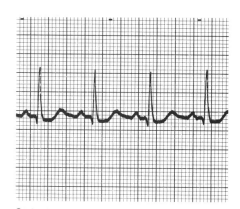

Strip 3-6.

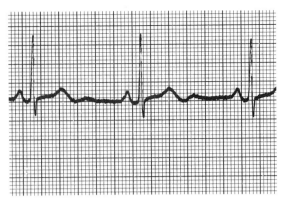

Strip 3-7.

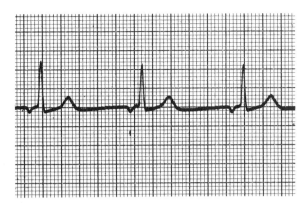

Strip 3-8.

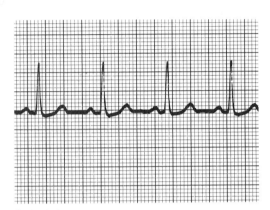

Strip 3-9.

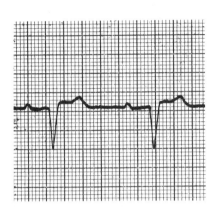

Strip 3-10.

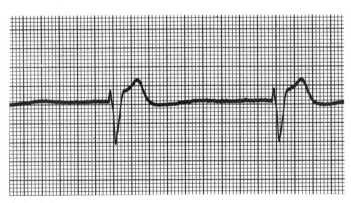

Strip 3-11.

4

Cardiac Monitors

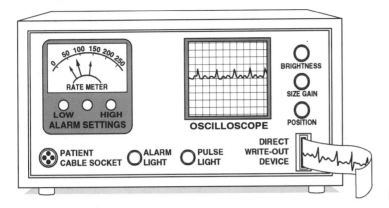

Figure 4-1. A basic cardiac monitor.

PURPOSE OF CARDIAC MONITORING

Each heart beat is the result of an electrical stimulus. This impulse, which originates in a specialized area of the right atrium called the sinoatrial node, is conducted along a conduction pathway to the ventricles, which are stimulated to contract. The electrical force spreads outward from the heart to the surface of the body, where it can be detected with monitoring electrodes attached to the skin. The cardiac monitor picks up these electrical signals and displays them as waveforms on a monitor screen (oscilloscope). The oscilloscope provides a continuous visual picture of a person's heartbeat. By analyzing the waveforms, changes in heart rate, rhythm, or conduction can be identified.

EQUIPMENT

There are many types of cardiac monitors currently available (Figure 4-1). Although these monitoring systems vary according to size, shape, dependability, accessory devices, and cost, all monitor systems have these basic capabilities:

1. Ability to pick up electrical signals from the skin electrodes and display the waveforms on an oscilloscope screen.

2. Ability to adjust the size, position, and brightness of the cardiac tracing to obtain a clear picture.

3. Ability to detect, count, and display the heart rate; most systems have a light that flashes and a beep that sounds with each heartbeat.

4. Ability to trigger an alarm if the patient's heartbeat falls below a preset level or raises above a preset level.

5. Ability to provide a printed record on graph paper of the cardiac tracing seen on the oscilloscope.

The printed record (rhythm strip) provides documentation of heart pattern changes and is also useful for comparing electrocardiogram (ECG) changes over time.

ELECTRODE AND LEAD POSITIONS

In the early 1960s, when the first coronary care units were established, the main goals of monitoring included heart rate surveillance and identifying ventricular ectopics, ventricular fibrillation, and ventricular tachycardia. Recently, the goals of monitoring have become more complex and involve monitoring for ST segment changes after thrombolytic therapy or balloon angioplasty and distinguishing ventricular tachycardia from supraventricular tachycardia with bundle branch block or aberrant conduction. Such situations require observation of criteria from specific leads. Accuracy in cardiac

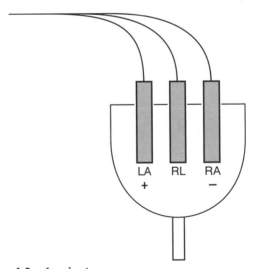

Figure 4-2. Lead wires.

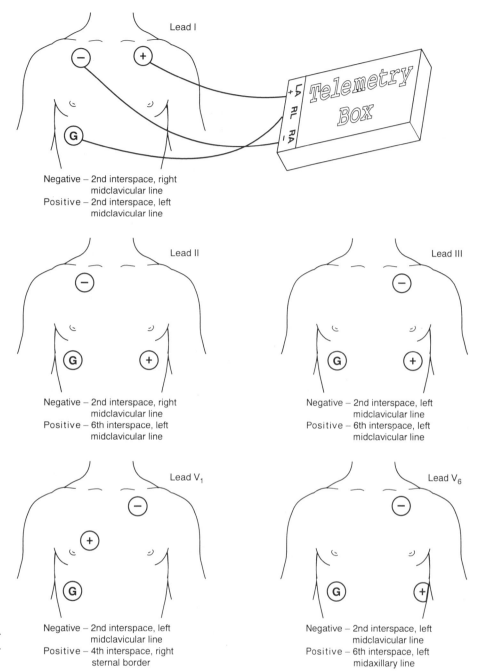

Lead I

Negative – 2nd interspace, right midclavicular line
Positive – 2nd interspace, left midclavicular line

Lead II

Negative – 2nd interspace, right midclavicular line
Positive – 6th interspace, left midclavicular line

Lead III

Negative – 2nd interspace, left midclavicular line
Positive – 6th interspace, left midclavicular line

Lead V₁

Negative – 2nd interspace, left midclavicular line
Positive – 4th interspace, right sternal border

Lead V₆

Negative – 2nd interspace, left midclavicular line
Positive – 6th interspace, left midaxillary line

Figure 4-3. Telemetry monitoring: electrode and lead positions.

monitoring depends on appropriate electrode and lead placement.

Most monitoring systems use a 3-lead system: one lead is positive, one is negative, and one acts as a ground lead. The lead wires are labeled as follows (Figure 4-2):

RA (right arm): designated as negative lead
LA (left arm): designated as positive lead
RL (right leg): designated as ground lead

Most monitor systems also have a color code designating certain colors for positive, negative, and ground leads. Be aware that color codes vary with different monitoring systems, and caution should be used in relying on color codes alone, especially if several varieties of monitors are in use.

Electrode placement positions and lead wire attachments for telemetry monitoring are shown in Figure 4-3. Figure 4-4 shows positions and attachments for bedside monitors using a lead selector switch.

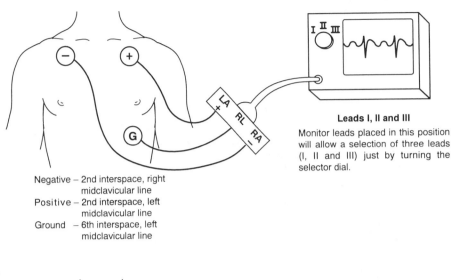

Leads I, II and III

Monitor leads placed in this position will allow a selection of three leads (I, II and III) just by turning the selector dial.

Negative – 2nd interspace, right
           midclavicular line
Positive – 2nd interspace, left
           midclavicular line
Ground   – 6th interspace, left
           midclavicular line

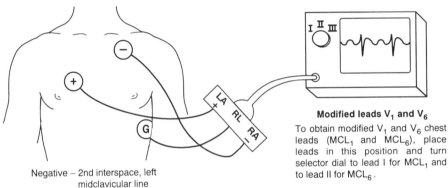

Negative – 2nd interspace, left
           midclavicular line
Positive – 4th interspace, right
           sternal border
Ground   – 6th interspace, left
           midaxillary line

Modified leads V$_1$ and V$_6$

To obtain modified V$_1$ and V$_6$ chest leads (MCL$_1$ and MCL$_6$), place leads in this position and turn selector dial to lead I for MCL$_1$ and to lead II for MCL$_6$.

Figure 4-4. Bedside monitoring with lead selector: electrode and lead positions.

ELECTRODE ATTACHMENT

Proper attachment of the electrodes to the skin is the most important step in obtaining a good quality ECG tracing. Unless there is good contact between the skin and the electrode pad, distortions (artifacts) may appear in the tracing. An artifact is anything on the ECG tracing that is not generated by the heart. The procedure for attaching the electrodes is as follows:

1. *Choose lead placement*. It is helpful to assess the 12-lead ECG to ascertain which leads provide the best QRS voltage and P wave identification. Avoid placing pads over bony areas, such as the clavicles, or prominent rib markings.
2. *Prepare the skin*.
   a. Shave the sites, if necessary, with a razor.
   b. Wipe sites with alcohol pad to remove skin oil; allow to dry.
   c. If the patient is perspiring, apply a thin coat of tincture of benzoin and allow to dry.
3. *Attach electrode pads*.
   a. Remove pads from packaging; check disk for sufficient, moist gel. Dried conductive gel can cause loss of ECG signal.
   b. Place electrode pad to prepared sites, pressing firmly around the periphery of the disk.
4. Connect the positive, negative, and ground lead wires to electrode pads according to established electrode-lead positions.

MONITOR PROBLEMS: TROUBLESHOOTING

Many problems may be encountered during cardiac monitoring. Some of these problems are related to the patient and some to the monitor or

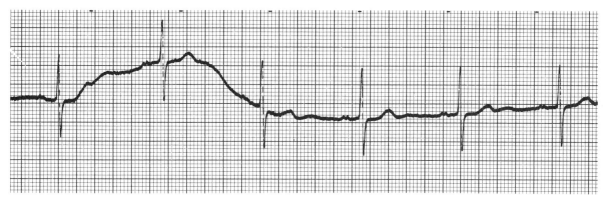

Figure 4-5. *Cause:* patient movement—patient turning in bed; *Solution:* transient problem—will correct itself.

other equipment in the room. However, the majority of problems are caused by improper technique related to skin preparation and electrode-lead attachments.

Monitor problems can cause artifacts on the ECG tracing, making identification of arrhythmias difficult, or they can trigger false monitor alarms. Some problems are potentially serious and require intervention, whereas others are transient, non–life-threatening occurrences that will correct themselves.

The nurse or monitor technician needs to develop troubleshooting skills sufficient to recognize the monitoring problem, identify probable causes, and seek solutions to correct the problem. The most common monitoring difficulties are discussed here.

False High Rate Alarms

The monitor is designed to detect and count the number of ventricular complexes occurring each minute and display this information as a heart rate on a rate meter. Unfortunately, the monitor is unable to distinguish high-voltage artifact potentials from QRS complexes. If a patient turns in bed, moves his or her extremities, or has muscle tremors, the rate meter may misinterpret these deflections as heartbeats and cause a false high rate alarm (Figures 4-5 through 4-8).

False Low Rate Alarms

Any disturbance in the transmission of the electrical signal from the skin electrode to the monitoring system can activate a false low rate alarm. This problem is usually caused by ineffective contact between the skin and the electrode or lead wire due to dried conductive gel, a loose electrode, or a disconnected lead wire. The low rate alarm also can be activated by low voltage QRS complexes. If the ventricular waveforms are not tall enough, the monitor detects no electrical activity and will sound the low rate alarm (Figures 4-9 through 4-12).

(text continues on page 28)

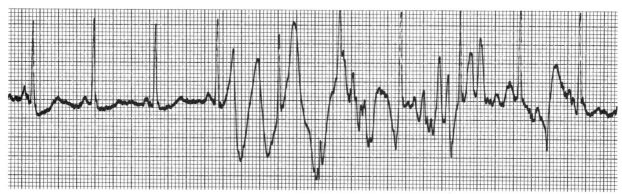

Figure 4-6. *Cause:* patient movement—moving upper extremities; *Solution:* avoid placing electrode pad over bony areas such as the clavicles.

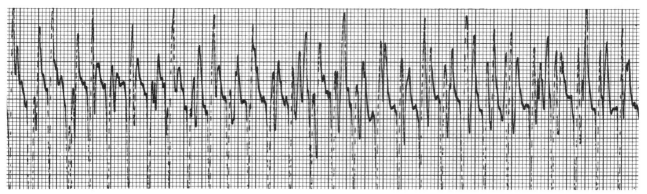

Figure 4-7. *Cause:* muscle tremors (extreme)—seizure activity; *Solution:* treat seizure.

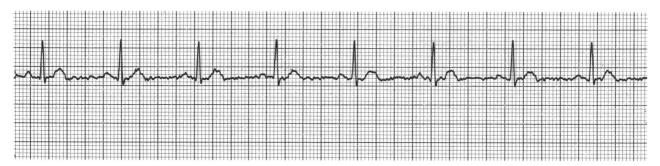

Figure 4-8. *Cause:* muscle tremors (mild)—shivering/tense muscles; *Solution:* treat fever or anxiety.

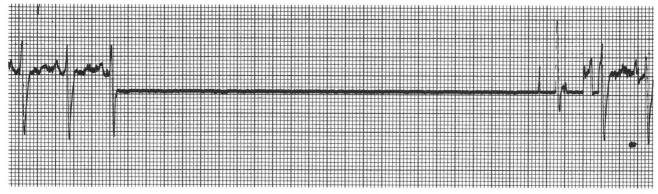

Figure 4-9. *Cause:* loose electrode pad; *Solution:* re-prep and attach new electrode pad.

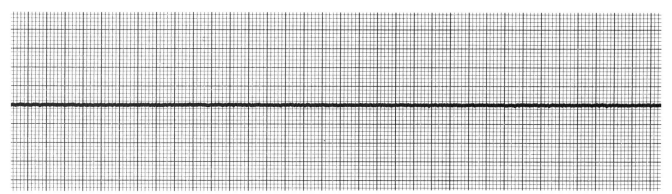

Figure 4-10. *Cause:* dried conductive gel, disconnected lead wire, or disconnected electrode pad; *Solution:* check electrode–lead system; re-prep and attach as necessary.

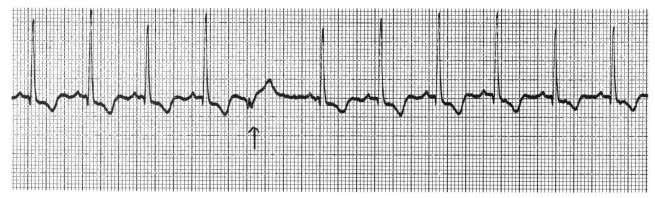

Figure 4-11. *Cause:* low waveform voltage (single beat); *Solution:* If problem is frequent, change lead positions.

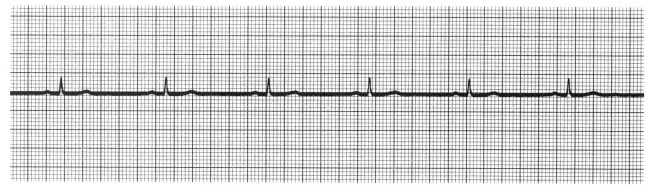

Figure 4-12. *Cause:* low waveform voltage (continuous); *Solution:* turn up amplitude (gain) knob or change lead positions.

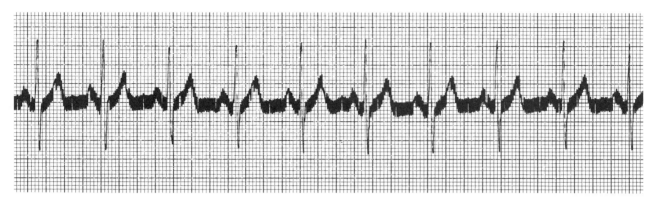

Figure 4-13. *Cause:* patient using electrical equipment (shaver or hair dryer); multiple electrical equipment in use; improperly grounded equipment; loose electrical connections. *Solution:* 1. If patient is using electrical equipment, problem is transient and will correct itself. 2. If patient not using electrical equipment: a. unplug all equipment not in continuous use; b. remove from service and report any equipment with breaks or wires showing; and c. ask electrical engineer to check wiring.

Electrical Interference

Electrical interference produces distortion of the baseline. It appears on the oscilloscope or monitor tracing as a wide baseline with a series of fine, rapid spikes (60/sec). It is sometimes referred to as 60 cycle or AC interference. Electrical interference is caused by the use of or problems with electrical equipment (Figure 4-13).

Wandering Baseline

A monitor pattern that wanders up and down on the oscilloscope screen or monitor tracing is called a wandering baseline. It is usually caused by respiratory movements and is common in patients with respiratory distress (chronic obstructive pulmonary disease) (Figure 4-14).

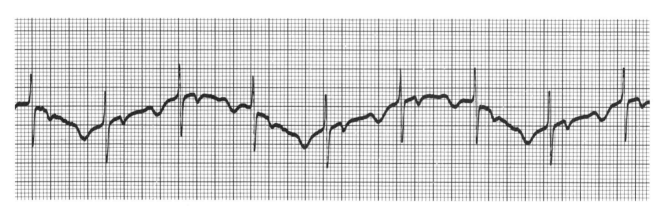

Figure 4-14. *Cause:* respiratory movements; *Solution:* avoid placing electrode pads over ribs; the upper back or top of the shoulders can be used if necessary.

5

Analyzing a Rhythm Strip

Huff J, Doernbach DP, White RD: *ECG WORKOUT: EXERCISES IN ARRHYTHMIA INTERPRETATION, 2nd ed.* © 1993 J.B. Lippincott Company.

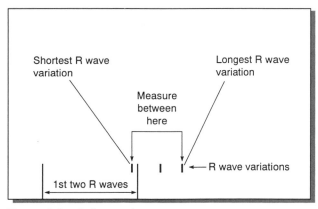

Figure 5-1. Index card.

There are five basic steps to be followed in analyzing a rhythm strip. Each step should be followed in sequence. Eventually, this will become a habit and will enable one to identify a strip quickly and accurately.

Step 1: Determine the regularity (rhythm) of the R waves. Starting at the left side of the rhythm strip, place an index card above the first two QRS complexes (Figure 5-1). Mark on the index card the top of the two R waves. Measure from R wave to R wave across the rhythm strip, marking on the index card any variation in R wave regularity. If the rhythm varies by 0.12 seconds (3 squares) or more between the shortest and longest R wave variations marked on the index card, the rhythm is irregular. If the rhythm does not vary or varies by less than 0.12 seconds, the rhythm is considered regular (Figures 5-2 through 5-4).

Step 2: Calculate the heart rate. This measurement will always refer to the ventricular rate unless the atrial and ventricular rates differ, in which case, both will be given. The ventricular rate is the number of QRS complexes in a 6-second rhythm strip. The top of the electrocardiogram paper is marked at 3-second intervals; two intervals equals 6 seconds

(Figure 5-5). There are several ways to calculate heart rate. One is given to use with regular rhythms and one to use with irregular rhythms.

Regular rhythms: Count the number of small squares between two R waves, and refer to the conversion table printed on the back inside cover (Figure 5-6). If a conversion table is not at hand, divide the number of squares between two R waves into 1500.

Irregular rhythms: Count the number of R waves in a 6-second strip and multiply by 10, or count the number of R waves in a 3-second strip and multiply by 20 (Figure 5-7).

The following are other hints:

When rhythm strips have premature beats (Figure 5-8), the premature beats are not included in the calculation of the rate. Count the rate in the uninterrupted section; this is the underlying rhythm. In this example, the uninterrupted section is regular, and the heart rate is 56 (27 squares between R waves = 56).

When rhythm strips have more than one rhythm on a 6-second strip (Figure 5-9), rates must be calculated for each rhythm. This will aid in the identification of each rhythm. In the example below, the first rhythm is irregular and the heart rate is 180 (nine R waves in 3 seconds × 20 = 180). The second rhythm is regular, and the heart rate is 214 (7 squares between R waves = 214).

When a rhythm covers less than 3 seconds on a rhythm strip (Figure 5-10), rate calculation is difficult but not impossible. In the example below, the first rhythm takes up half of a 3-second interval. There are only two R waves; therefore, you cannot determine if the rhythm is regular or irregular. In this situation, multiply the two R waves by 40 to obtain an ap-

(text continues on page 33)

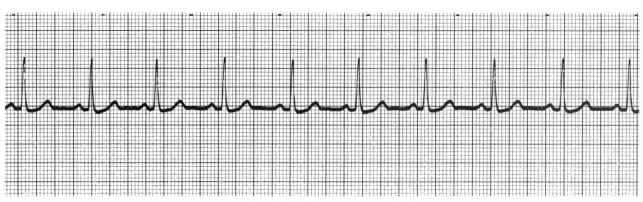

Figure 5-2. Regular rhythm; RR intervals do not vary.

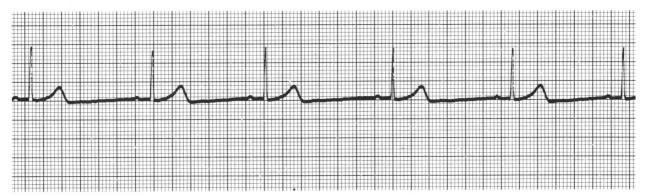

Figure 5-3. Irregular rhythm; RR intervals vary by 0.20 seconds.

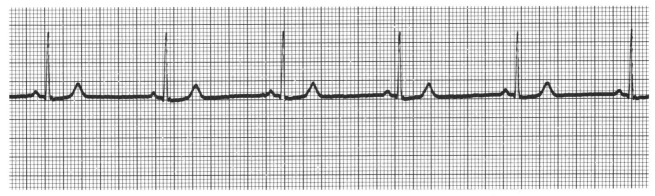

Figure 5-4. Regular rhythm; RR intervals vary by 0.08 seconds.

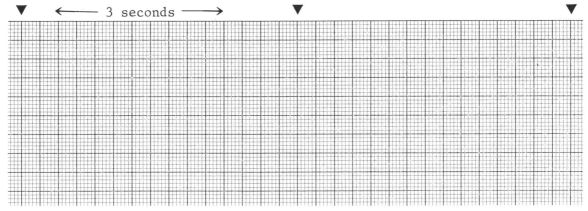

Figure 5-5. ECG graph paper.

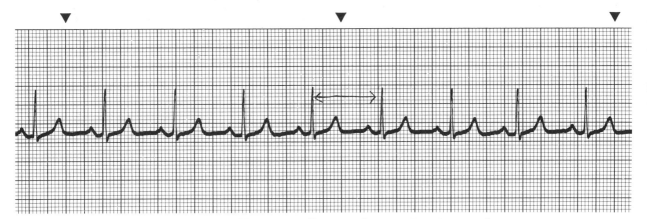

Figure 5-6. Regular rhythm; 19 small squares between R waves = 79 heart rate.

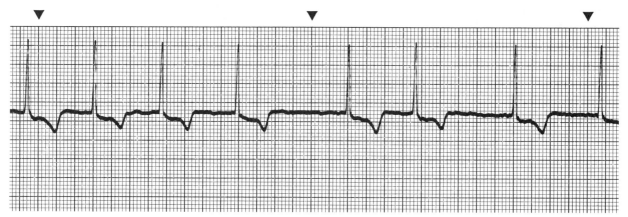

Figure 5-7. Irregular rhythm; 6 R waves × 10 = 60 heart rate.

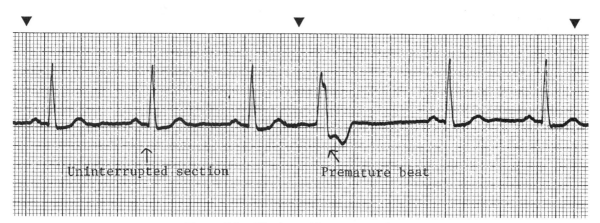

Figure 5-8. Rhythm with premature beat.

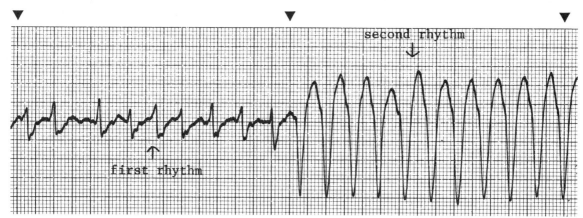

Figure 5-9. Rhythm strip with two different rhythms.

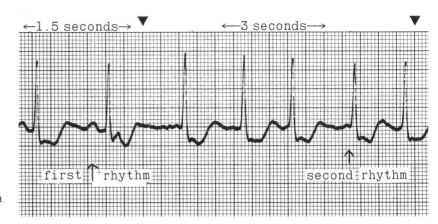

Figure 5-10. Calculating rate when a rhythm covers less than 3 seconds.

proximate rate of 80. The second rhythm is irregular, with a heart rate of 100 (five R waves × 20 = 100).

Step 3: Identify and examine P waves. Analyze the P waves; one P wave should precede each QRS complex. All P waves should be identical (or near identical) in size, shape, and position. In Figure 5-11, there is one P wave to each QRS; all P waves are identical in size, shape, and position. In Figure 5-12, there is one P wave to each QRS, but the P waves vary in size, shape, and position.

Step 4: Measure the PR interval. Measure from the beginning of the P wave as it leaves baseline to the beginning of the QRS complex. Count the number of squares contained in this interval and multiply by 0.04 seconds. In Figure 5-13, the PR interval is 0.16 seconds (4 squares × 0.04 seconds = 0.16 seconds).

Step 5: Measure the QRS. Measure from the beginning of the QRS as it leaves baseline until the end of the QRS, when it returns to baseline. Count the number of squares contained in this interval and multiply by 0.04 seconds. In Figure 5-14, the QRS takes up 3 squares and represents 0.12 seconds (3 squares × 0.04 seconds = 0.12 seconds). In Figure 5-15, the QRS takes up 2½ squares and represents 0.10 seconds (2½ squares × 0.04 seconds = 0.10 seconds) (Box 5-1).

Box 5-1. Summary: Rhythm Strip Analysis

1. Determine regularity (rhythm)
2. Calculate rate
3. Examine P waves
4. Measure PR interval
5. Measure QRS complex

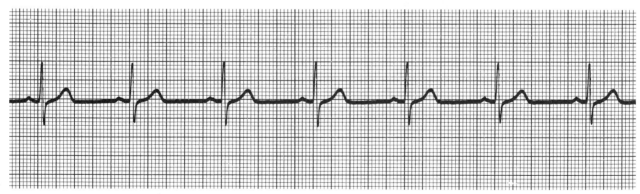

Figure 5-11. Normal P waves.

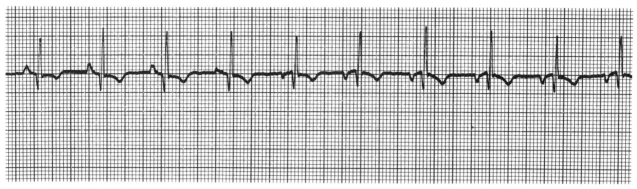

Figure 5-12. Abnormal P waves.

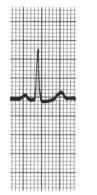

Figure 5-13. PR 0.16 seconds.

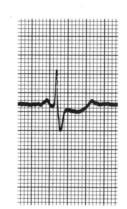

Figure 5-14. QRS 0.12 seconds.

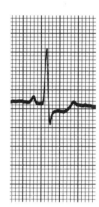

Figure 5-15. QRS 0.10 seconds.

Waveform Practice—
Analyzing Rhythm Strips

Directions: Analyze the following rhythm strips using the 5-step process discussed in this chapter. Check your answers with the answer keys in the appendix.

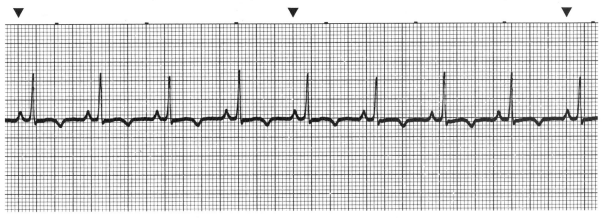

Strip 5-1. Rhythm: _Regular_   Rate: _80 BPM_   P wave: _SINUS_
PR interval: _.14 - .16_   QRS: _.06 - .08_

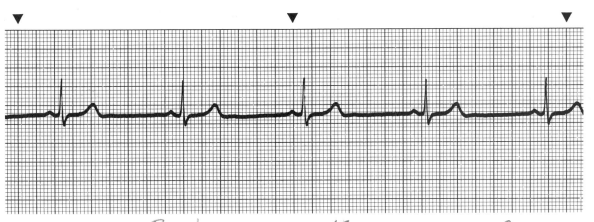

Strip 5-2. Rhythm: _Regular_   Rate: _45_   P wave: _Sinus_
PR interval: _.16_   QRS: _.04 - 0.6_

2   .14   2
34)1500
        140
          04

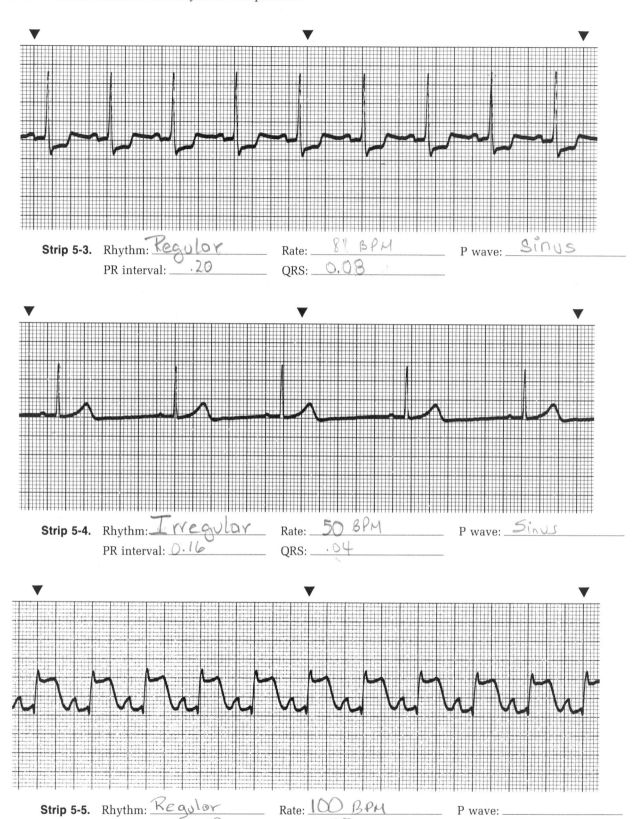

Strip 5-3. Rhythm: *Regular*   Rate: *84 BPM*   P wave: *sinus*

PR interval: *.20*   QRS: *0.08*

Strip 5-4. Rhythm: *Irregular*   Rate: *50 BPM*   P wave: *Sinus*

PR interval: *0.16*   QRS: *.04*

Strip 5-5. Rhythm: *Regular*   Rate: *100 BPM*   P wave: _____

PR interval: *0.20*   QRS: *0.08*

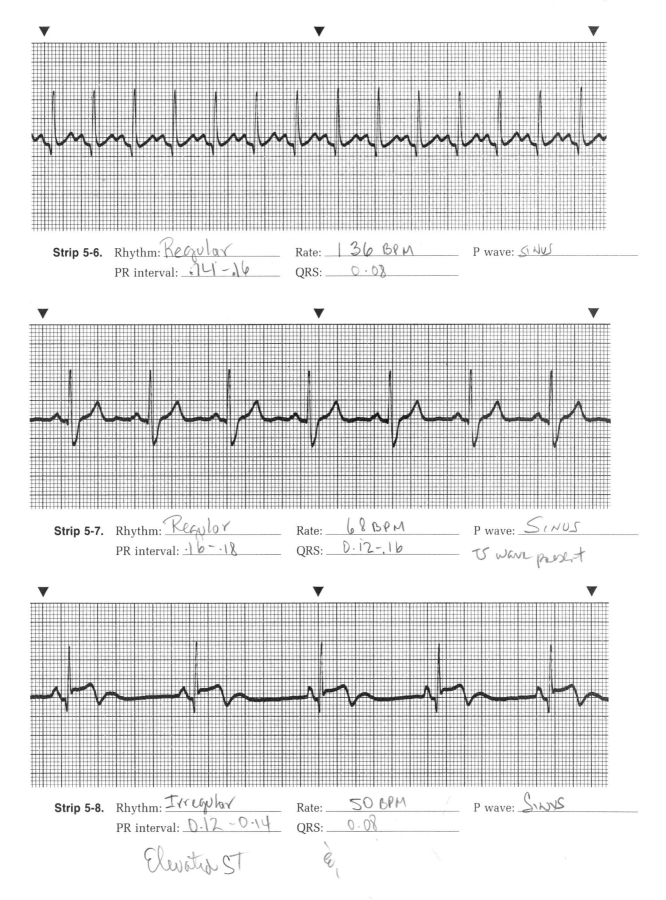

Strip 5-6. Rhythm: _Regular_   Rate: _136 BPM_   P wave: _SINUS_
PR interval: _.14-.16_   QRS: _0.08_

Strip 5-7. Rhythm: _Regular_   Rate: _68 BPM_   P wave: _SINUS_
PR interval: _.16-.18_   QRS: _0.12-.16_   U wave present

Strip 5-8. Rhythm: _Irregular_   Rate: _50 BPM_   P wave: _Sinus_
PR interval: _0.12 - 0.14_   QRS: _0.08_
Elevated ST

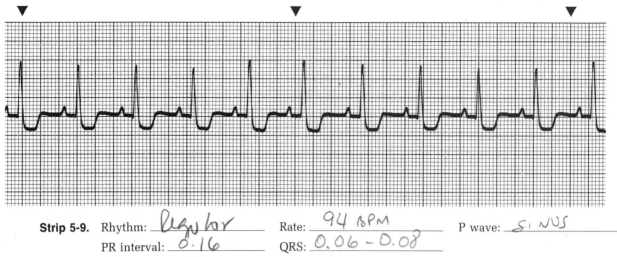

Strip 5-9. Rhythm: _Regular_ Rate: _94 BPM_ P wave: _SINUS_

PR interval: _0.16_ QRS: _0.06 – 0.08_

Depress ST wave

6

Sinus Rhythms

Huff J, Doernbach DP, White RD: *ECG WORKOUT: EXERCISES IN ARRHYTHMIA INTERPRETATION, 2nd ed.* © 1993 J.B. Lippincott Company.

Normal sinus rhythm

Sinus bradycardia

Sinus tachycardia

Sinus arrhythmia

Sinus arrest

Sinus block

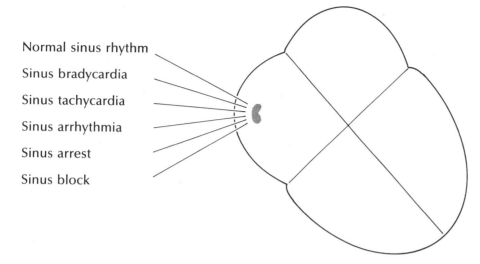

Figure 6-1. Sinus rhythms.

Sinus rhythms result from disturbances in impulse formation in the sinus node (Figure 6-1). The sinus node retains its role as pacemaker but discharges impulses too fast (sinus tachycardia) or too slow (sinus bradycardia), discharges impulses irregularly (sinus arrhythmia), fails to discharge an impulse (sinus arrest), or the impulses discharged are blocked (sinus block).

Impulse formation is under the control of the sympathetic and the parasympathetic nervous systems. The sympathetic system is responsible for speeding up the heart rate, whereas the parasympathetic system (vagal influence) slows down the heart rate. Normally, these systems are balanced, maintaining a heart rate between 60 and 100 beats per minute.

NORMAL SINUS RHYTHM

A normal sinus rhythm occurs when the impulse originates in the sinus node and impulses are discharged regularly at a rate of 60 to 100 beats per

Box 6-1.	**Normal Sinus Rhythm—Identifying ECG Features**
Rhythm:	Regular
Rate:	60 to 100
P waves:	Normal in configuration; precede each QRS
PR:	Normal (0.12 to 0.20 seconds)
QRS:	Normal (less than 0.12 seconds)

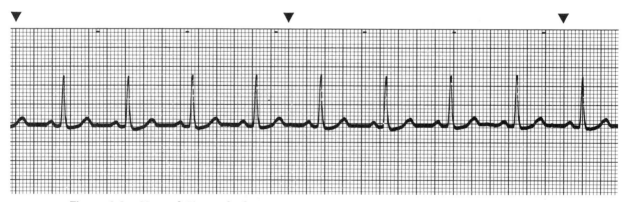

Figure 6-2. Normal Sinus Rhythm.

Rhythm: Regular

Rate: 84

P waves: Normal and precede each QRS

PR: 0.14 to 0.16 seconds

QRS: 0.06 to 0.08 seconds.

minute. The P waves are normal in configuration and precede each QRS complex. The PR interval and QRS duration are within normal limits (Box 6-1) (Figure 6-2).

SINUS TACHYCARDIA

Sinus tachycardia occurs when the sinus node discharges impulses at a rate faster than 100 beats per minute. The P waves are normal in configuration and precede each QRS complex. The PR interval and QRS duration are within normal limits. Sinus tachycardia begins and ends gradually in contrast to other tachycardias, which begin and end abruptly.

The acceleration in heart rate reflects overactivity of the sympathetic nervous system and is a normal reaction to fever, anxiety, physical exertion, anemia, hypovolemia, or hypotension. The heart rate also may increase to compensate for a failing left ventricle (heart failure). Treatment should focus on the cause of the sinus tachycardia (Box 6-2) (Figure 6-3).

Box 6-2. Sinus Tachycardia—Identifying ECG Features

Rhythm:	Regular
Rate:	100 to 150
P waves:	Normal in configuration; precede each QRS
PR:	Normal (0.12 to 0.20 seconds)
QRS:	Normal (less than 0.12 seconds)

SINUS BRADYCARDIA

Sinus bradycardia occurs when the sinus node discharges impulses at a rate below 60 beats per minute. The P waves are normal in configuration and precede each QRS complex. The PR interval and QRS duration are within normal limits. (Box 6-3) (Figure 6-4).

Box 6-3. Sinus Bradycardia—Identifying ECG Features

Rhythm:	Regular
Rate:	40 to 60 usually (may be slower)
P waves:	Normal in configuration; precede each QRS complex
PR:	Normal (0.12 to 0.20 seconds)
QRS:	Normal (less than 0.12 seconds)

Sinus bradycardia frequently occurs in healthy young adults, particularly well-trained athletes. During sleep the normal heart rate can fall between 35 and 40 beats per minute, especially in young adults and adolescents. Sinus bradycardia also occurs during vomiting or vasovagal syncope. Sinus bradycardia occurs in 10% to 15% of patients with acute myocardial infarction. It usually is transient and occurs more commonly during inferior than anterior infarction; it has been noted during reperfusion with thrombolytic agents

Treatment of sinus bradycardia usually is not necessary. If the patient with an acute myocardial

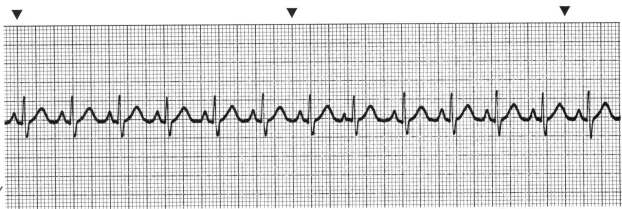

Figure 6-3. Sinus Tachycardia.

Rhythm:	Regular
Rate:	115
P waves:	Normal in configuration; precede each QRS
PR:	0.12 seconds
QRS:	0.08 seconds

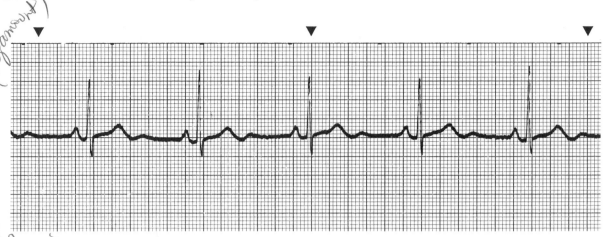

Figure 6-4. Sinus Bradycardia with U Wave.

Rhythm:	Regular
Rate:	50
P waves:	Normal in configuration; precede each QRS
PR:	0.16 to 0.20 seconds
QRS:	0.06 to 0.08 seconds.

infarction is asymptomatic, it is best not to speed up the heart rate. If cardiac output is inadequate or if arrhythmias are associated with the slow rate, atropine (0.5 mg intravenously, repeated if necessary up to 3 mg) is usually effective. Lower doses of atropine can exert an initial bradycardic effect and are not recommended. When atropine is ineffective and the patient is symptomatic or hypotensive, or both, transcutaneous (external) or transvenous pacing is indicated.

SINUS ARRHYTHMIA

Sinus arrhythmia occurs when the sinus node discharges impulses irregularly. The P waves are normal in configuration and precede each QRS complex. The PR interval and QRS duration are within normal limits.

Sinus arrhythmia is the most frequent form of arrhythmia, and it is considered to be a normal event. In most instances, the irregularity is related to the phases of respiration, with the rate increasing

during inspiration and decreasing during expiration. Sinus arrhythmia commonly occurs in the young, especially with slower heart rates or following enhanced vagal tone, and decreases with age or with autonomic dysfunction. Treatment is usually unnecessary (Box 6-4) (Figure 6-5).

SINUS ARREST AND SINUS BLOCK

Both sinus arrest and sinus block are recognized by a pause in the sinus rhythm in which one or more beats (cardiac cycles) are missing. Involvement of the sinus node by acute myocardial infarction, fibrosis involving the atrium, and excessive vagal stimulation as well as drugs such as digitalis, quinidine, and procainamide can produce sinus arrest or sinus block.

In sinus arrest, the SA node fails to discharge an impulse. This interrupts the normal regularity of the sinus node discharge, and the rhythm will not resume on time (the pause will not be an exact multiple of the other RR intervals). In sinus block, the SA node discharges the impulse, but the impulse is blocked as it exits the SA node. The impulse discharge is not interrupted (just blocked); therefore, the rhythm will resume on time (the pause will be an exact multiple of the other RR intervals).

The above criteria may be used to differentiate SA arrest from SA block if the basic underlying rhythm is regular. If the underlying rhythm is irregular, as in sinus arrhythmia, it is often impossible to distinguish one from the other without direct record-

Box 6-4.	Sinus Arrhythmia—Identifying ECG Features
Rhythm:	Irregular
Rate:	60 to 100 usually but is fairly common with sinus bradycardia
P waves:	Normal in configuration; precede each QRS
PR:	Normal (0.12 to 0.20 seconds)
QRS:	Normal (less than 0.12 seconds)

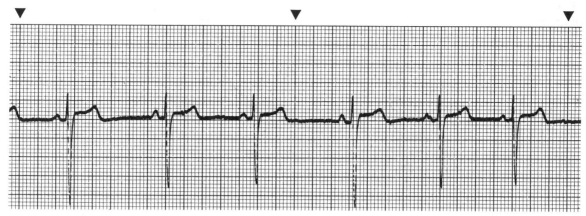

Figure 6-5. Sinus Arrhythmia.

Rhythm: Irregular

Rate: 60

P waves: Normal in configuration; precede each QRS

PR: 0.14 to 0.16 seconds

QRS: 0.08 seconds

ings of sinus node discharge. In areas where sinus node electrograms are unavailable, the rhythm may be interpreted as sinus arrest–block.

Treatment is as outlined for sinus bradycardia.

In patients with a chronic form of sinus node disease characterized by marked bradycardia, sinus arrest, or sinus block, permanent pacing is often necessary (Boxes 6-5 and 6-6) (Figures 6-6 through 6-8).

Box 6-5.	Sinus Arrest—Identifying ECG Features
Rhythm:	Irregular during pause
Rate:	Usually slow (40 to 60) but may be normal
P waves:	Absent during pause
PR:	Absent during pause
QRS:	Absent during pause

Note: The duration of the pause *is not* an exact multiple of the other RR intervals.

Box 6-6.	Sinus Block—Identifying ECG Features
Rhythm:	Irregular during pause
Rate:	Usually slow (40 to 60) but may be normal
P waves:	Absent during pause
PR:	Absent during pause
QRS:	Absent during pause

Note: The duration of the pause *will be* an exact multiple of the other RR intervals.

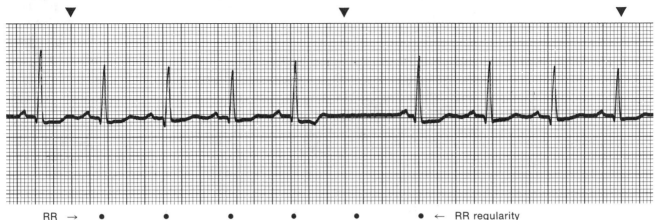

RR → • • • • • • ← RR regularity
regularity not interrupted;
rhythm resumes on time
after pause

Figure 6-6. Normal Sinus Rhythm with Sinus Block.

Rhythm: Basic rhythm regular, irregular during pause

Rate: Basic rhythm 84

P waves: Normal in basic rhythm, absent during pause

PR: 0.16 to 0.18 seconds in basic rhythm, absent during pause

QRS: 0.08 to 0.10 seconds in basic rhythm, absent during pause

Comment: ST segment depression is present

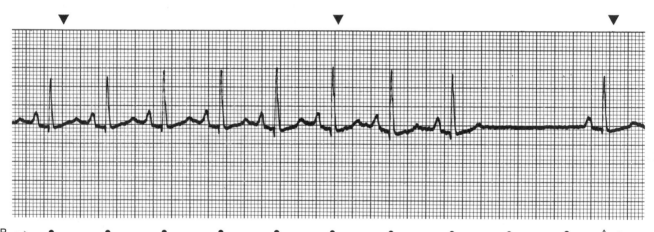

RR → • • • • • • • • • •   • ↑ •
regularity

                                        RR regularity is
                                        interrupted; rhythm
                                        does not resume on
                                        time after pause

Figure 6-7. Normal Sinus Rhythm with Sinus Arrest.

Rhythm: Basic rhythm regular, irregular during pause

Rate: Basic rhythm 94

P waves: Normal in basic rhythm, absent during pause

PR: 0.16 to 0.18 seconds in basic rhythm, absent during pause

QRS: 0.06 to 0.08 seconds in basic rhythm, absent during pause

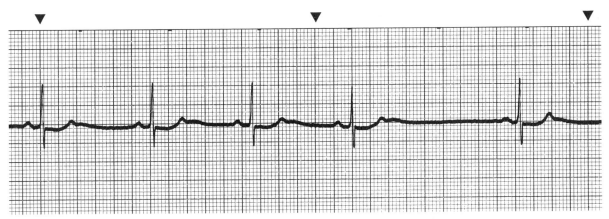

Figure 6-8. **Sinus Arrhythmia with Sinus Arrest-Block**

Rhythm: Basic rhythm irregular

Rate: Basic rhythm 60

P waves: Normal in basic rhythm, absent during pause

PR: 0.16 to 0.18 seconds in basic rhythm, absent during pause

QRS: 0.06 seconds in basic rhythm, absent during pause

Comment: Owing to the irregularity of the basic rhythm, sinus arrest cannot be differenti-
              ated from sinus block, and the rhythm is interpreted as sinus arrest-block.

Comment: ST segment depression and a U wave are present.

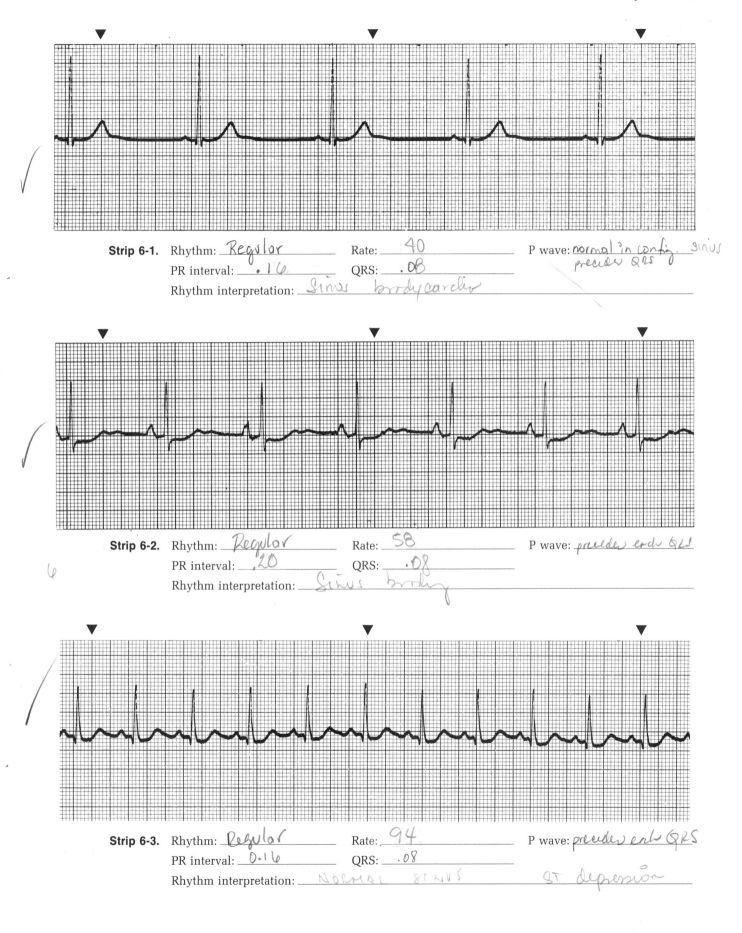

Strip 6-1. Rhythm: _Regular_   Rate: _40_   P wave: _normal in config. sinus precedes QRS_
PR interval: _.16_   QRS: _.08_
Rhythm interpretation: _Sinus brodycardia_

Strip 6-2. Rhythm: _Regular_   Rate: _58_   P wave: _precedes each QRS_
PR interval: _.20_   QRS: _.08_
Rhythm interpretation: _Sinus brody_

Strip 6-3. Rhythm: _Regular_   Rate: _94_   P wave: _precedes each QRS_
PR interval: _0.16_   QRS: _.08_   _ST depression_
Rhythm interpretation: _NORMAL SINUS_

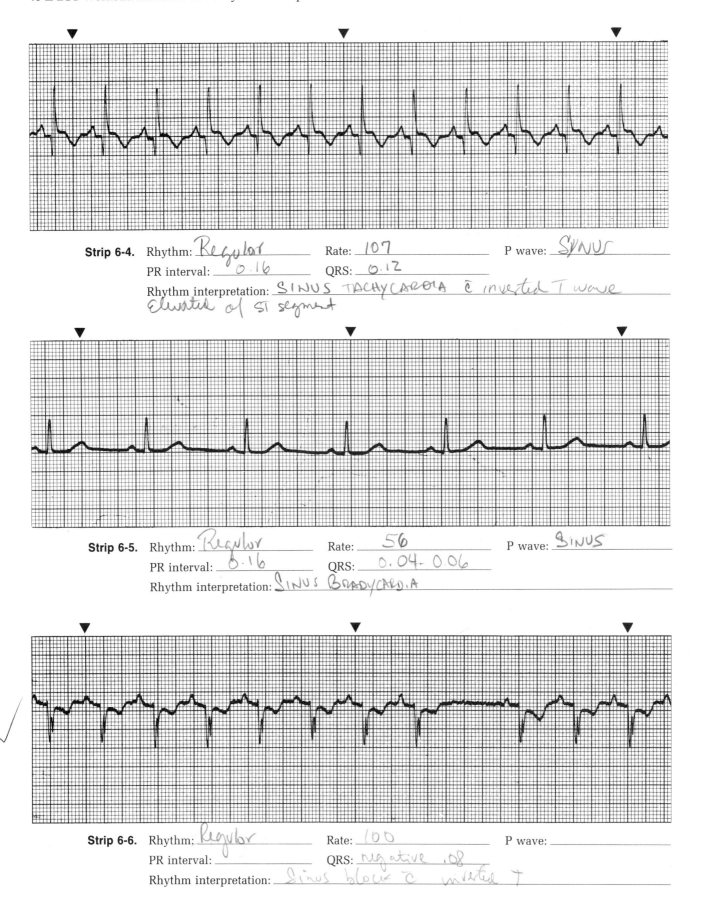

Strip 6-4. Rhythm: _Regular_   Rate: _107_   P wave: _Sinus_
PR interval: _0.16_   QRS: _0.12_
Rhythm interpretation: _SINUS TACHYCARDIA c̄ inverted T wave_
Elevated of ST segment

Strip 6-5. Rhythm: _Regular_   Rate: _56_   P wave: _Sinus_
PR interval: _0.16_   QRS: _0.04- 0.06_
Rhythm interpretation: _SINUS BRADYCARDIA_

Strip 6-6. Rhythm: _Regular_   Rate: _100_   P wave: _____
PR interval: _____   QRS: _negative .08_
Rhythm interpretation: _Sinus block c̄ inverted T_

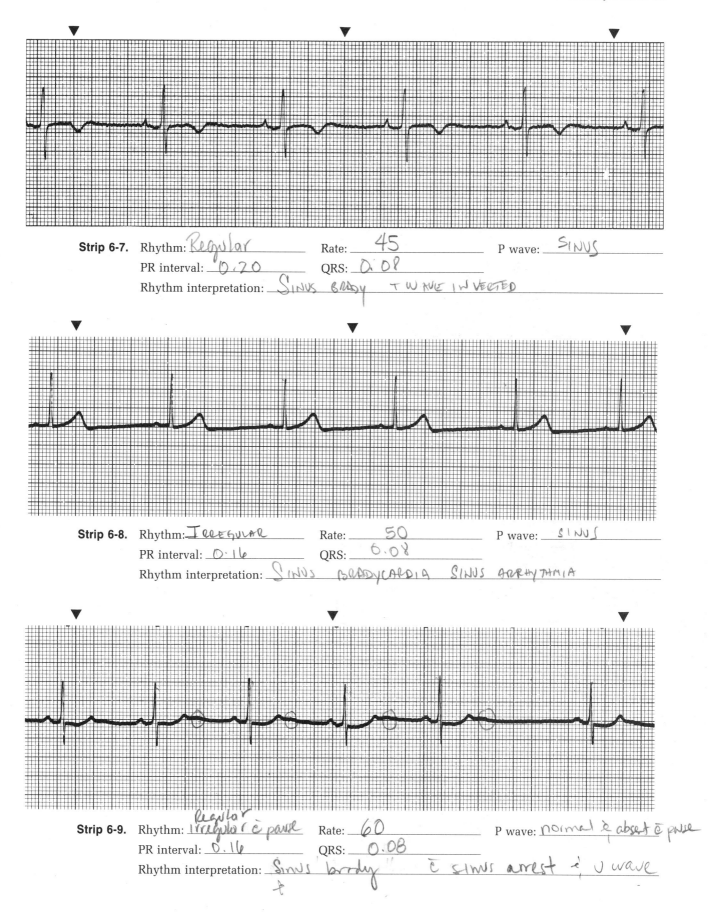

Strip 6-7. Rhythm: _Regular_ Rate: _45_ P wave: _SINUS_
PR interval: _0.20_ QRS: _0.08_
Rhythm interpretation: _Sinus brady T WAVE INVERTED_

Strip 6-8. Rhythm: _Irregular_ Rate: _50_ P wave: _SINUS_
PR interval: _0.16_ QRS: _0.08_
Rhythm interpretation: _Sinus BRADYCARDIA SINUS ARRHYTHMIA_

Strip 6-9. Rhythm: _Regular Irregular c pause_ Rate: _60_ P wave: _normal c absent c pause_
PR interval: _0.16_ QRS: _0.08_
Rhythm interpretation: _Sinus brady c sinus arrest c u wave_

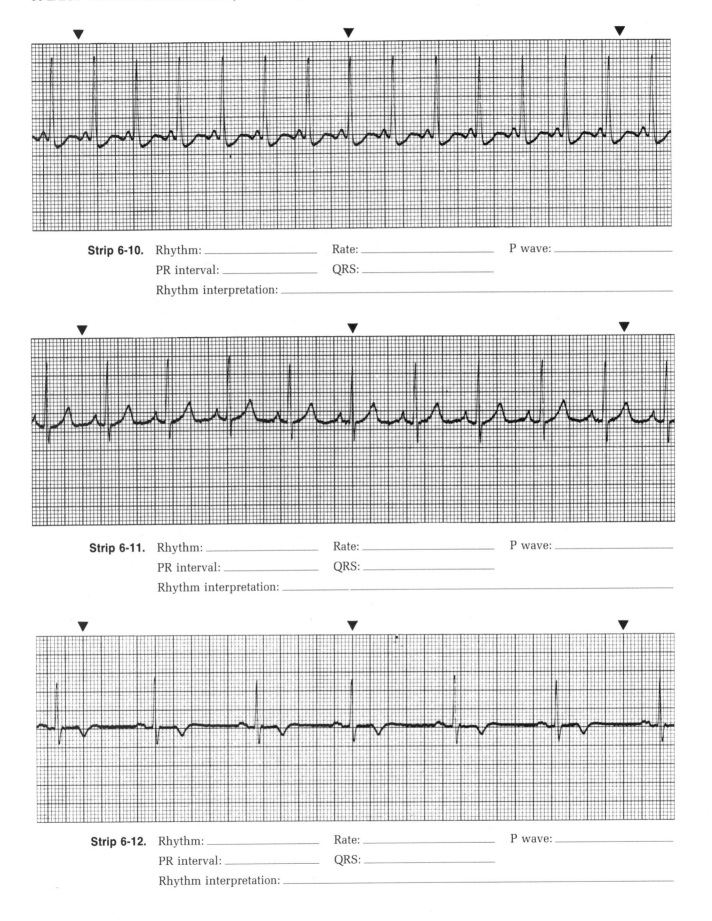

Strip 6-10. Rhythm: _____ Rate: _____ P wave: _____

PR interval: _____ QRS: _____

Rhythm interpretation: _____

Strip 6-11. Rhythm: _____ Rate: _____ P wave: _____

PR interval: _____ QRS: _____

Rhythm interpretation: _____

Strip 6-12. Rhythm: _____ Rate: _____ P wave: _____

PR interval: _____ QRS: _____

Rhythm interpretation: _____

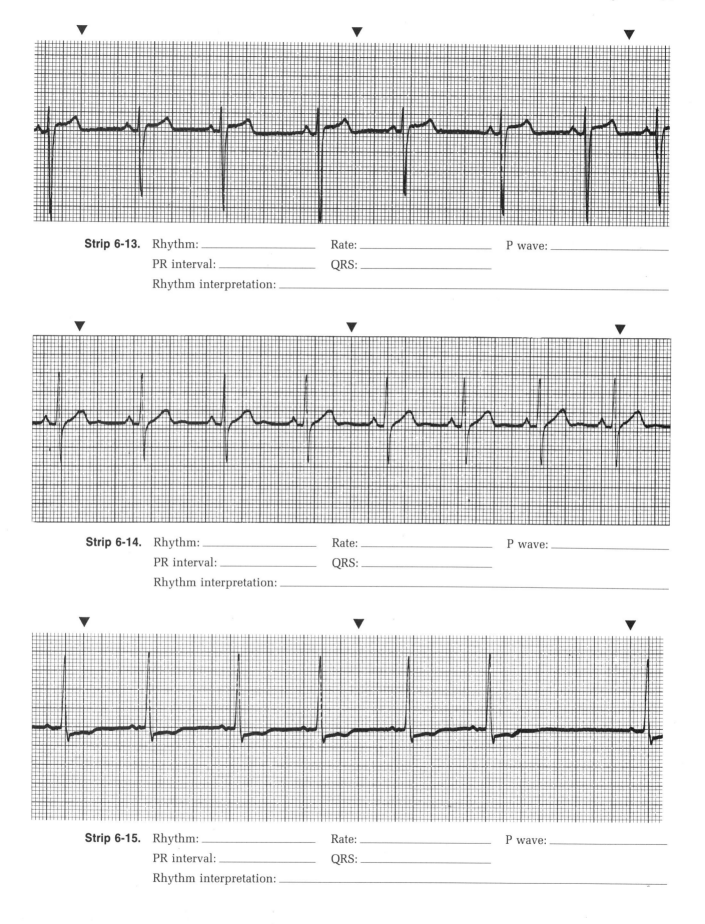

Strip 6-13. Rhythm: _____ Rate: _____ P wave: _____

PR interval: _____ QRS: _____

Rhythm interpretation: _____

Strip 6-14. Rhythm: _____ Rate: _____ P wave: _____

PR interval: _____ QRS: _____

Rhythm interpretation: _____

Strip 6-15. Rhythm: _____ Rate: _____ P wave: _____

PR interval: _____ QRS: _____

Rhythm interpretation: _____

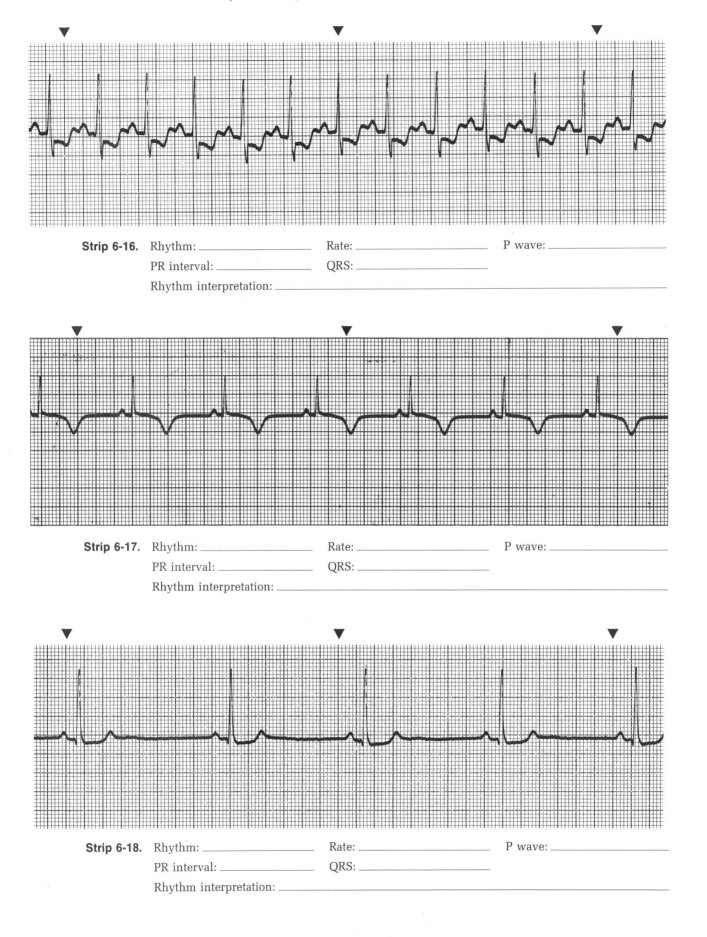

Strip 6-16. Rhythm: _____ Rate: _____ P wave: _____

PR interval: _____ QRS: _____

Rhythm interpretation: _____

Strip 6-17. Rhythm: _____ Rate: _____ P wave: _____

PR interval: _____ QRS: _____

Rhythm interpretation: _____

Strip 6-18. Rhythm: _____ Rate: _____ P wave: _____

PR interval: _____ QRS: _____

Rhythm interpretation: _____

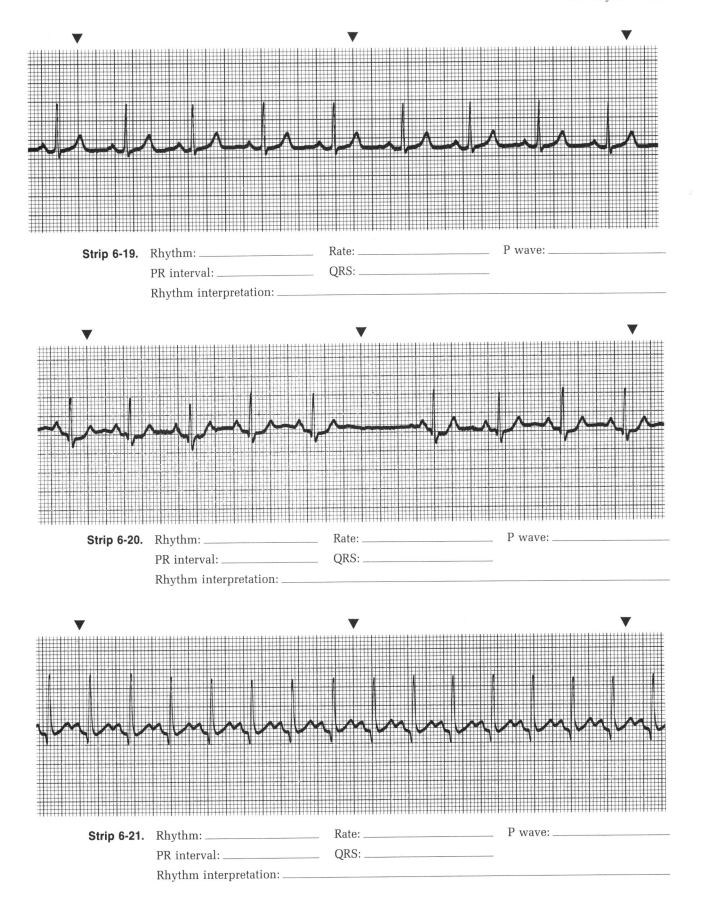

Strip 6-19. Rhythm: _____ Rate: _____ P wave: _____

PR interval: _____ QRS: _____

Rhythm interpretation: _____

Strip 6-20. Rhythm: _____ Rate: _____ P wave: _____

PR interval: _____ QRS: _____

Rhythm interpretation: _____

Strip 6-21. Rhythm: _____ Rate: _____ P wave: _____

PR interval: _____ QRS: _____

Rhythm interpretation: _____

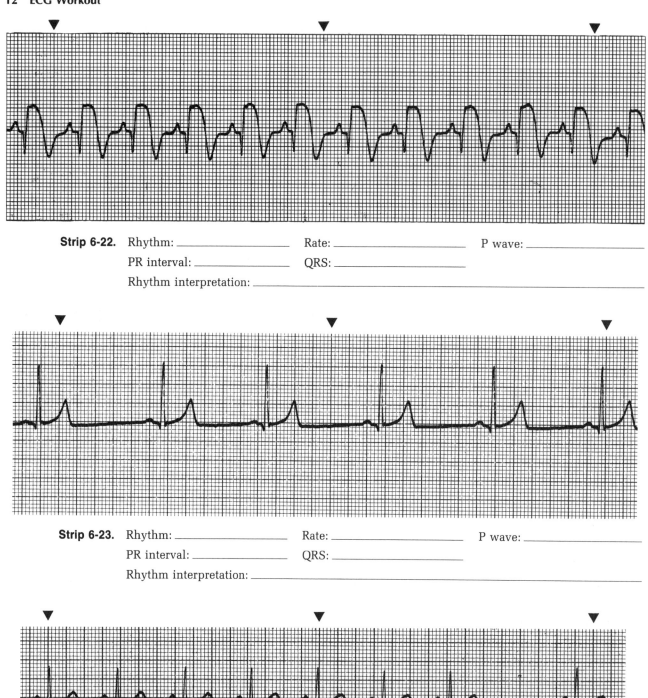

Strip 6-22. Rhythm: _____   Rate: _____   P wave: _____

PR interval: _____   QRS: _____

Rhythm interpretation: _____

Strip 6-23. Rhythm: _____   Rate: _____   P wave: _____

PR interval: _____   QRS: _____

Rhythm interpretation: _____

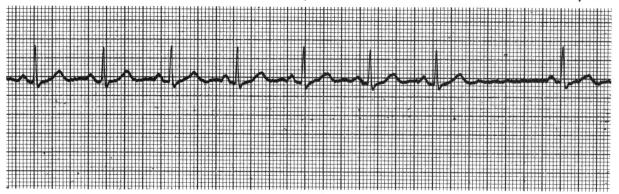

Strip 6-24. Rhythm: _____   Rate: _____   P wave: _____

PR interval: _____   QRS: _____

Rhythm interpretation: _____

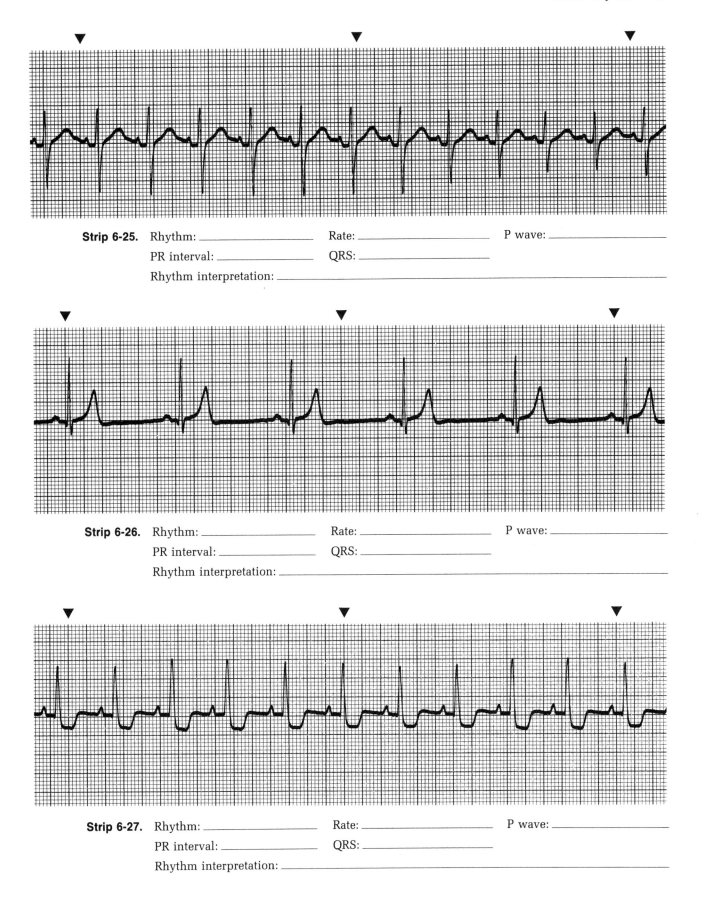

Strip 6-25. Rhythm: _____ Rate: _____ P wave: _____

PR interval: _____ QRS: _____

Rhythm interpretation: _____

Strip 6-26. Rhythm: _____ Rate: _____ P wave: _____

PR interval: _____ QRS: _____

Rhythm interpretation: _____

Strip 6-27. Rhythm: _____ Rate: _____ P wave: _____

PR interval: _____ QRS: _____

Rhythm interpretation: _____

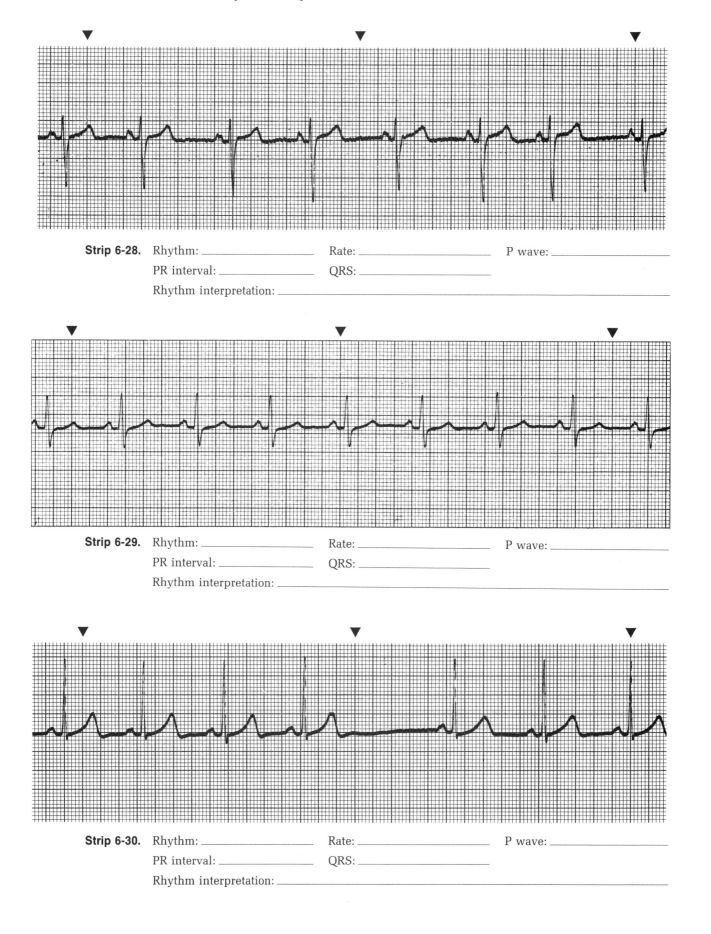

Strip 6-28. Rhythm: _____ Rate: _____ P wave: _____

PR interval: _____ QRS: _____

Rhythm interpretation: _____

Strip 6-29. Rhythm: _____ Rate: _____ P wave: _____

PR interval: _____ QRS: _____

Rhythm interpretation: _____

Strip 6-30. Rhythm: _____ Rate: _____ P wave: _____

PR interval: _____ QRS: _____

Rhythm interpretation: _____

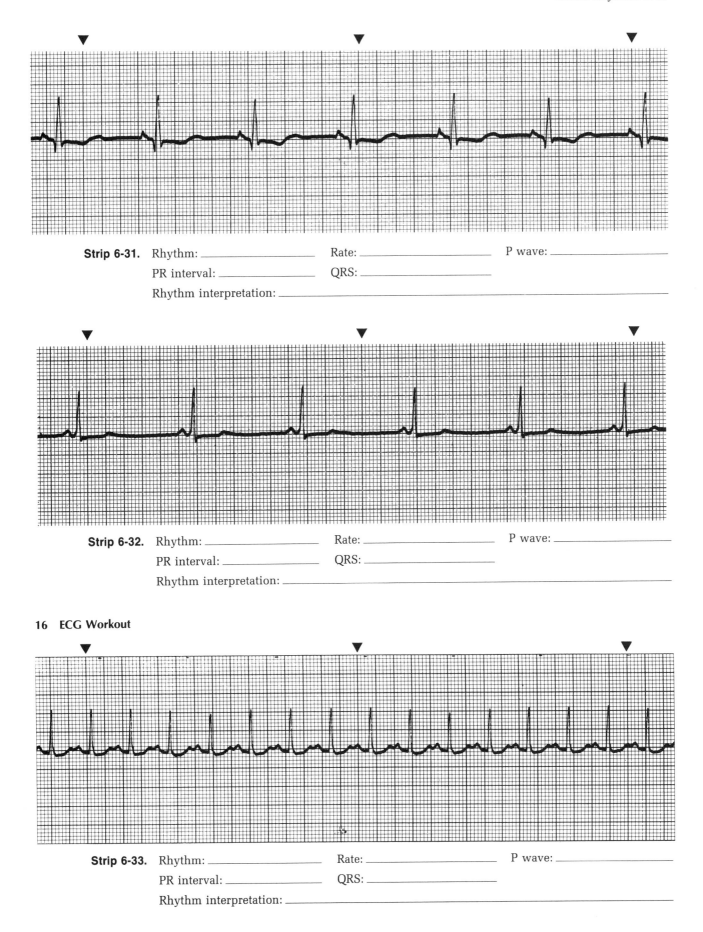

Strip 6-31. Rhythm: _____ Rate: _____ P wave: _____

PR interval: _____ QRS: _____

Rhythm interpretation: _____

Strip 6-32. Rhythm: _____ Rate: _____ P wave: _____

PR interval: _____ QRS: _____

Rhythm interpretation: _____

16 ECG Workout

Strip 6-33. Rhythm: _____ Rate: _____ P wave: _____

PR interval: _____ QRS: _____

Rhythm interpretation: _____

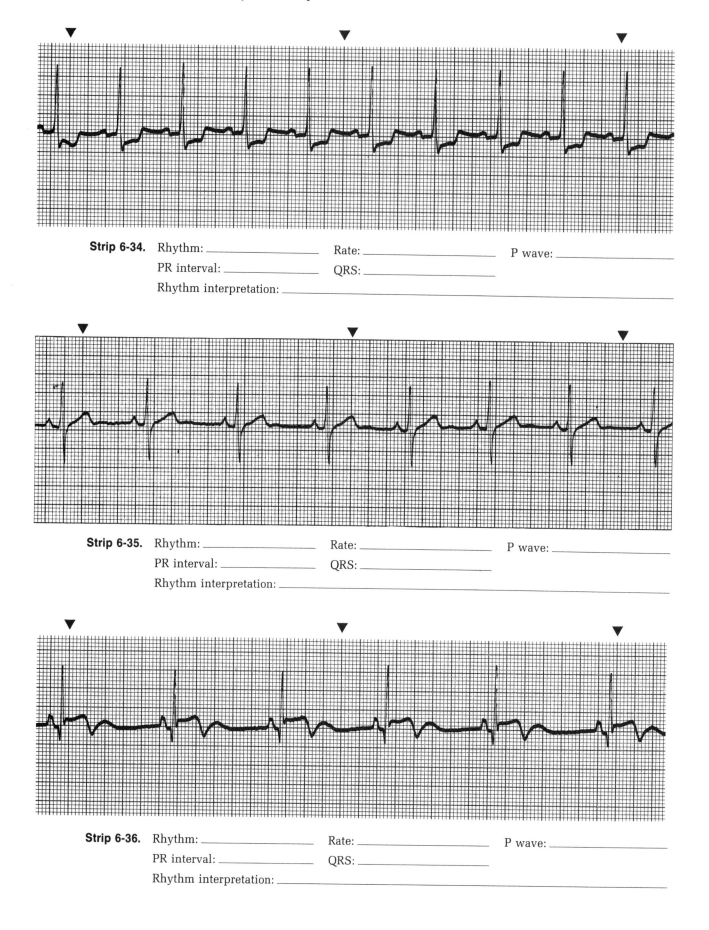

Strip 6-34. Rhythm: _____ Rate: _____ P wave: _____

PR interval: _____ QRS: _____

Rhythm interpretation: _____

Strip 6-35. Rhythm: _____ Rate: _____ P wave: _____

PR interval: _____ QRS: _____

Rhythm interpretation: _____

Strip 6-36. Rhythm: _____ Rate: _____ P wave: _____

PR interval: _____ QRS: _____

Rhythm interpretation: _____

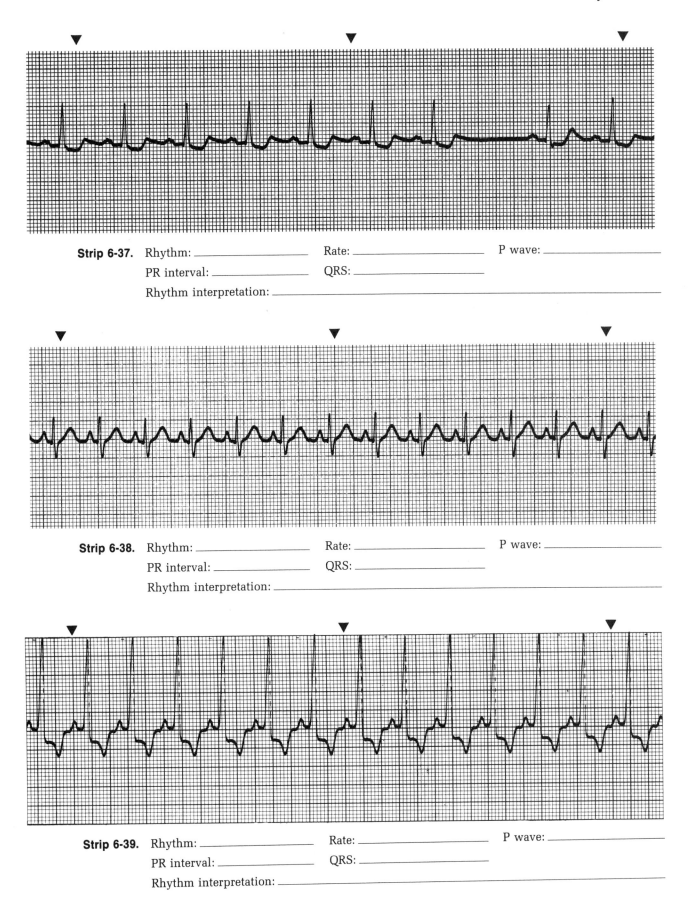

Strip 6-37. Rhythm: _____ Rate: _____ P wave: _____

PR interval: _____ QRS: _____

Rhythm interpretation: _____

Strip 6-38. Rhythm: _____ Rate: _____ P wave: _____

PR interval: _____ QRS: _____

Rhythm interpretation: _____

Strip 6-39. Rhythm: _____ Rate: _____ P wave: _____

PR interval: _____ QRS: _____

Rhythm interpretation: _____

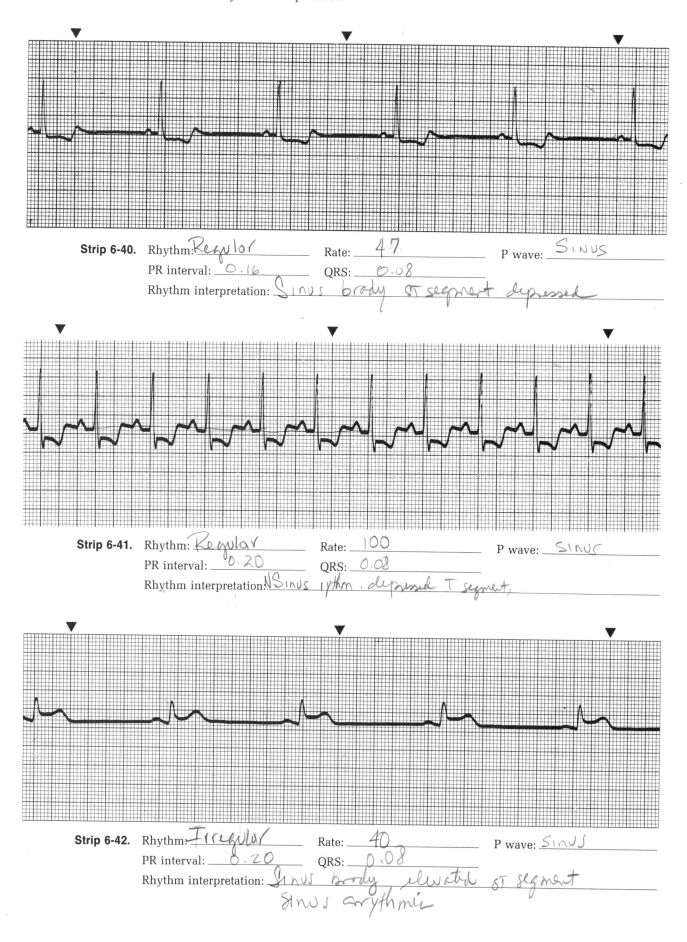

Strip 6-40. Rhythm: Regular   Rate: 47   P wave: Sinus

PR interval: 0.16   QRS: 0.08

Rhythm interpretation: Sinus brady ST segment depressed

Strip 6-41. Rhythm: Regular   Rate: 100   P wave: Sinus

PR interval: 0.20   QRS: 0.08

Rhythm interpretation: NSinus rythm. depressed T segment,

Strip 6-42. Rhythm: Irregular   Rate: 40   P wave: Sinus

PR interval: 0.20   QRS: 0.08

Rhythm interpretation: Sinus brody elevated ST segment
Sinus arrythmia

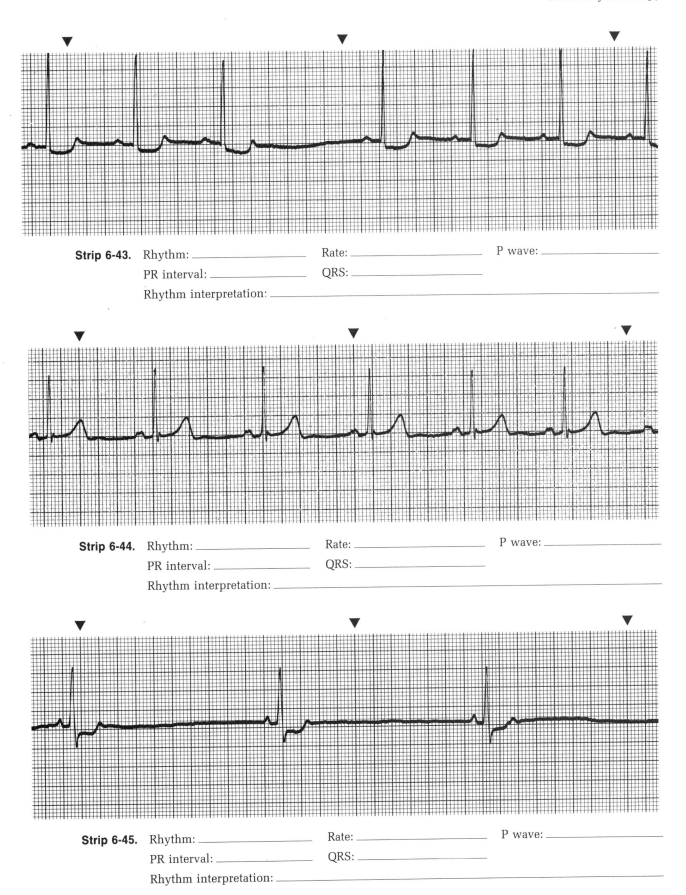

Strip 6-43. Rhythm: _____ Rate: _____ P wave: _____

PR interval: _____ QRS: _____

Rhythm interpretation: _____

Strip 6-44. Rhythm: _____ Rate: _____ P wave: _____

PR interval: _____ QRS: _____

Rhythm interpretation: _____

Strip 6-45. Rhythm: _____ Rate: _____ P wave: _____

PR interval: _____ QRS: _____

Rhythm interpretation: _____

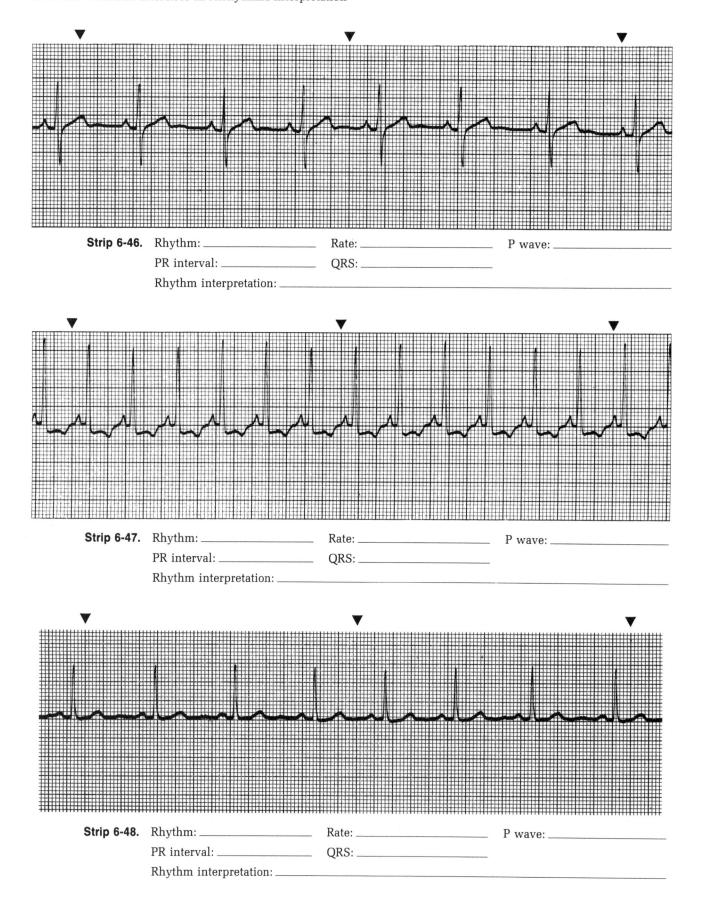

Strip 6-46. Rhythm: _____ Rate: _____ P wave: _____

PR interval: _____ QRS: _____

Rhythm interpretation: _____

Strip 6-47. Rhythm: _____ Rate: _____ P wave: _____

PR interval: _____ QRS: _____

Rhythm interpretation: _____

Strip 6-48. Rhythm: _____ Rate: _____ P wave: _____

PR interval: _____ QRS: _____

Rhythm interpretation: _____

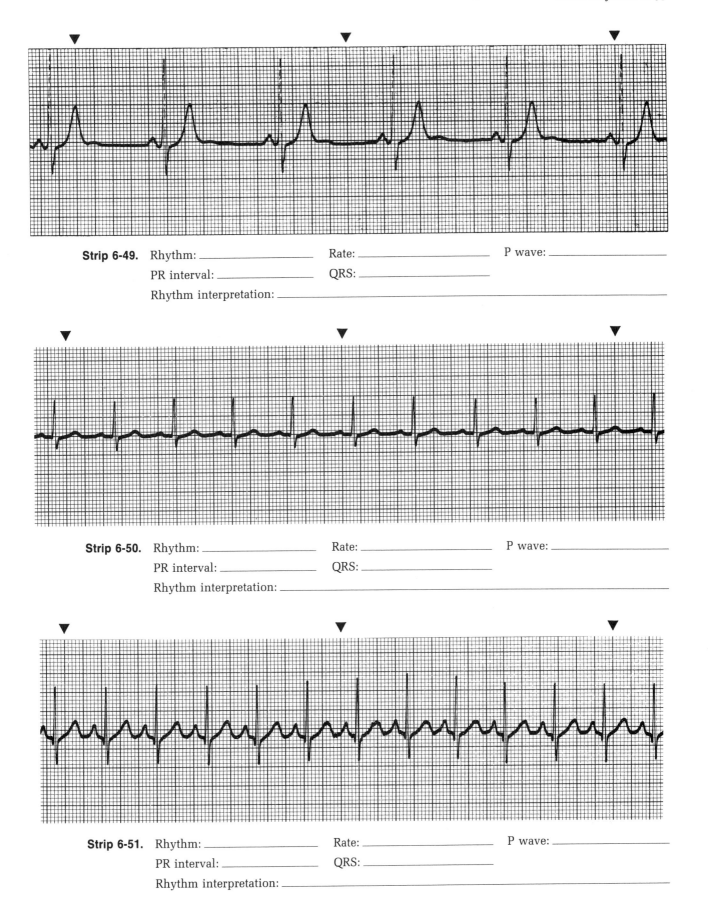

Strip 6-49. Rhythm: _____ Rate: _____ P wave: _____

PR interval: _____ QRS: _____

Rhythm interpretation: _____

Strip 6-50. Rhythm: _____ Rate: _____ P wave: _____

PR interval: _____ QRS: _____

Rhythm interpretation: _____

Strip 6-51. Rhythm: _____ Rate: _____ P wave: _____

PR interval: _____ QRS: _____

Rhythm interpretation: _____

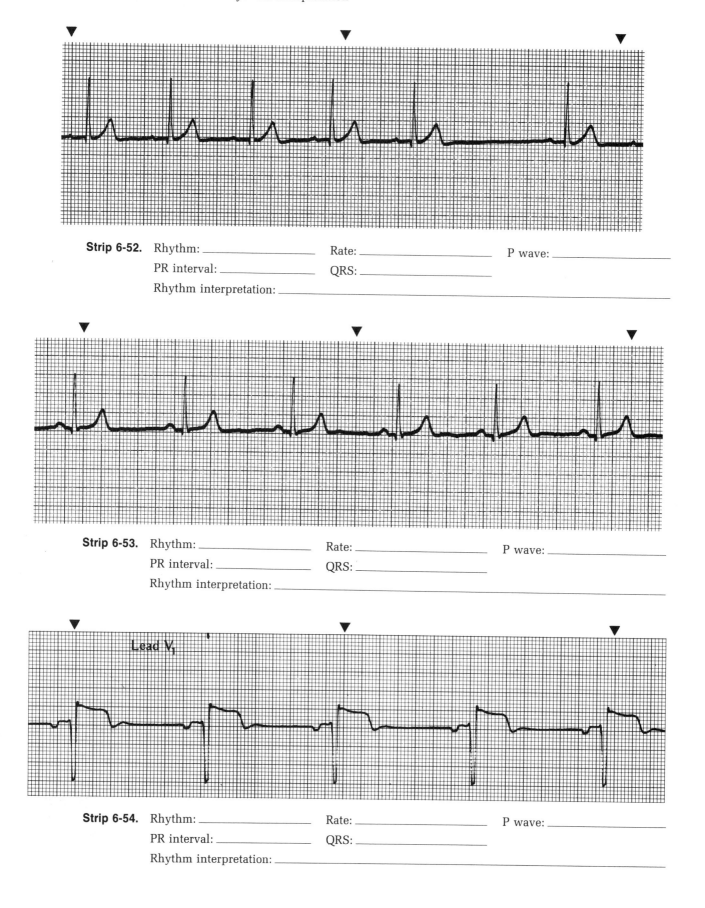

Strip 6-52. Rhythm: _____ Rate: _____ P wave: _____

PR interval: _____ QRS: _____

Rhythm interpretation: _____

Strip 6-53. Rhythm: _____ Rate: _____ P wave: _____

PR interval: _____ QRS: _____

Rhythm interpretation: _____

Lead V₁

Strip 6-54. Rhythm: _____ Rate: _____ P wave: _____

PR interval: _____ QRS: _____

Rhythm interpretation: _____

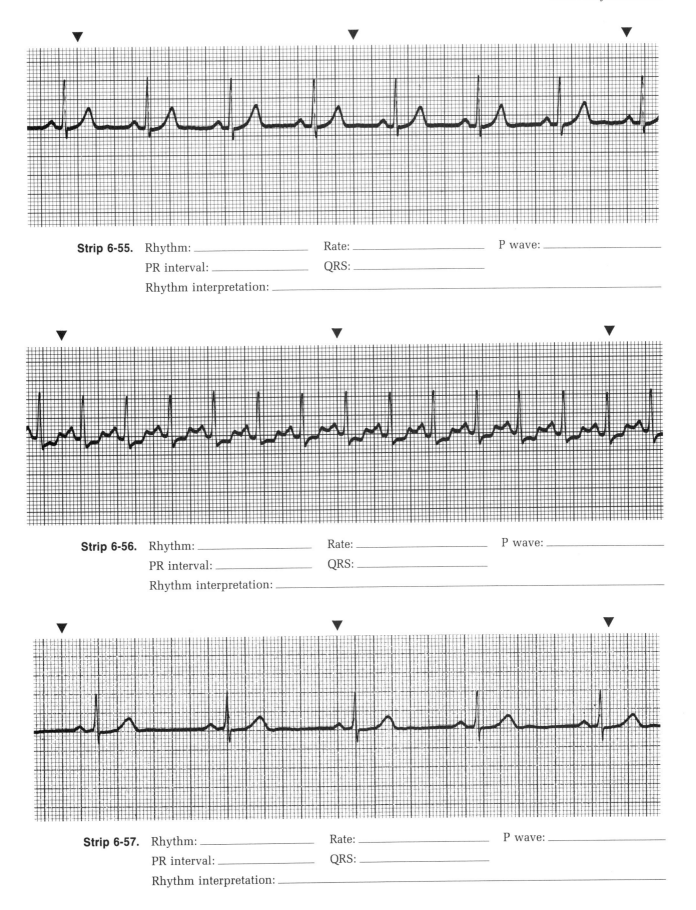

Strip 6-55. Rhythm: _____ Rate: _____ P wave: _____

PR interval: _____ QRS: _____

Rhythm interpretation: _____

Strip 6-56. Rhythm: _____ Rate: _____ P wave: _____

PR interval: _____ QRS: _____

Rhythm interpretation: _____

Strip 6-57. Rhythm: _____ Rate: _____ P wave: _____

PR interval: _____ QRS: _____

Rhythm interpretation: _____

PVC

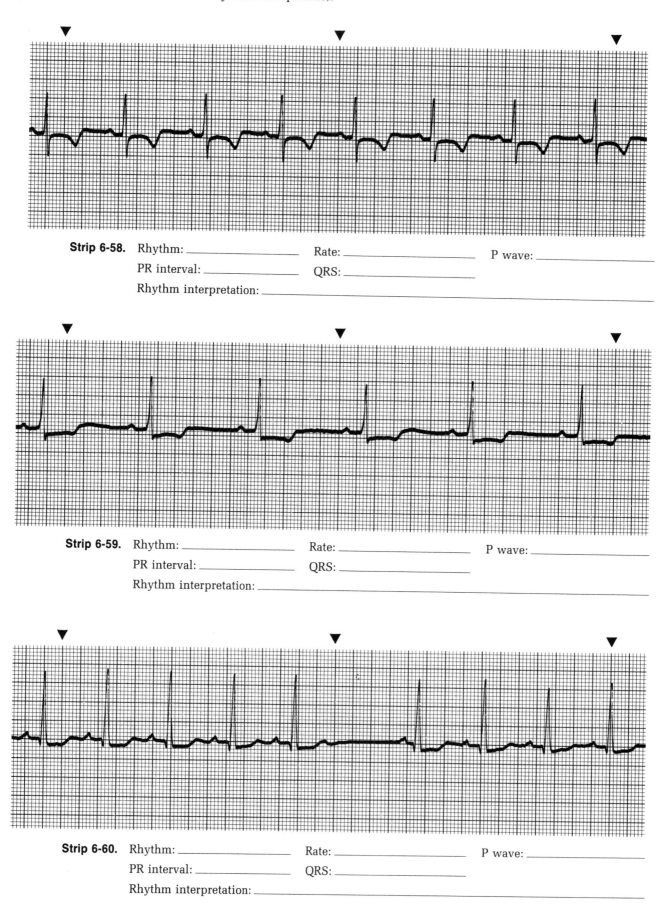

Strip 6-58. Rhythm: _____ Rate: _____ P wave: _____

PR interval: _____ QRS: _____

Rhythm interpretation: _____

Strip 6-59. Rhythm: _____ Rate: _____ P wave: _____

PR interval: _____ QRS: _____

Rhythm interpretation: _____

Strip 6-60. Rhythm: _____ Rate: _____ P wave: _____

PR interval: _____ QRS: _____

Rhythm interpretation: _____

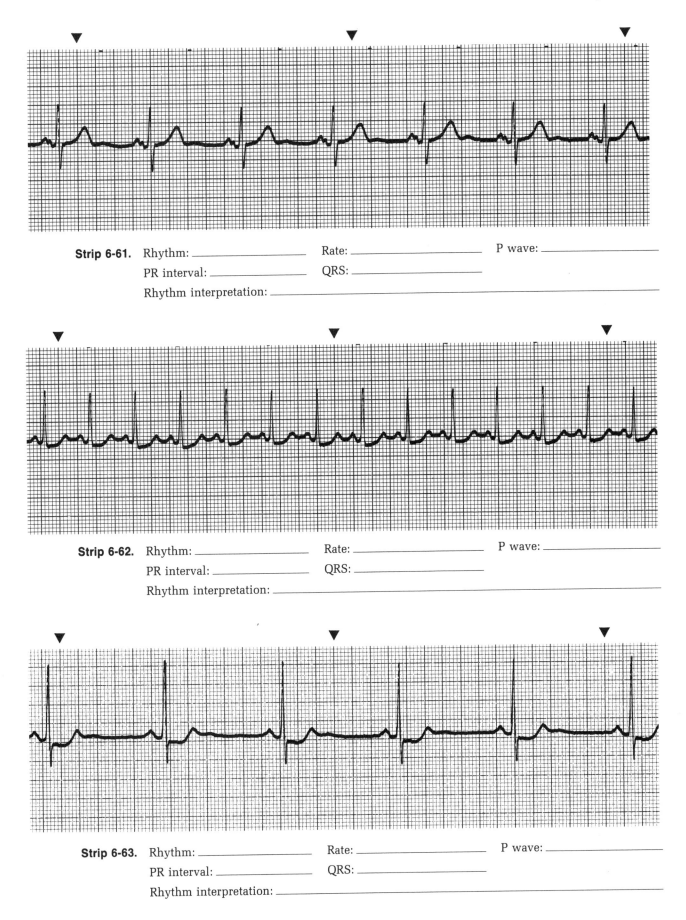

Strip 6-61. Rhythm: _____ Rate: _____ P wave: _____

PR interval: _____ QRS: _____

Rhythm interpretation: _____

Strip 6-62. Rhythm: _____ Rate: _____ P wave: _____

PR interval: _____ QRS: _____

Rhythm interpretation: _____

Strip 6-63. Rhythm: _____ Rate: _____ P wave: _____

PR interval: _____ QRS: _____

Rhythm interpretation: _____

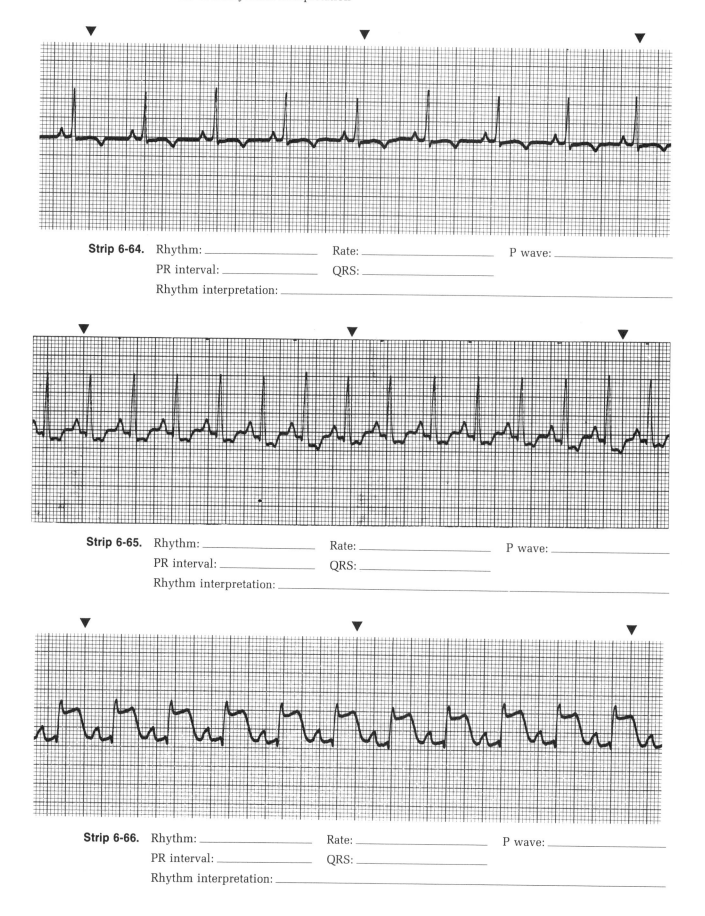

Strip 6-64. Rhythm: _____ Rate: _____ P wave: _____

PR interval: _____ QRS: _____

Rhythm interpretation: _____

Strip 6-65. Rhythm: _____ Rate: _____ P wave: _____

PR interval: _____ QRS: _____

Rhythm interpretation: _____

Strip 6-66. Rhythm: _____ Rate: _____ P wave: _____

PR interval: _____ QRS: _____

Rhythm interpretation: _____

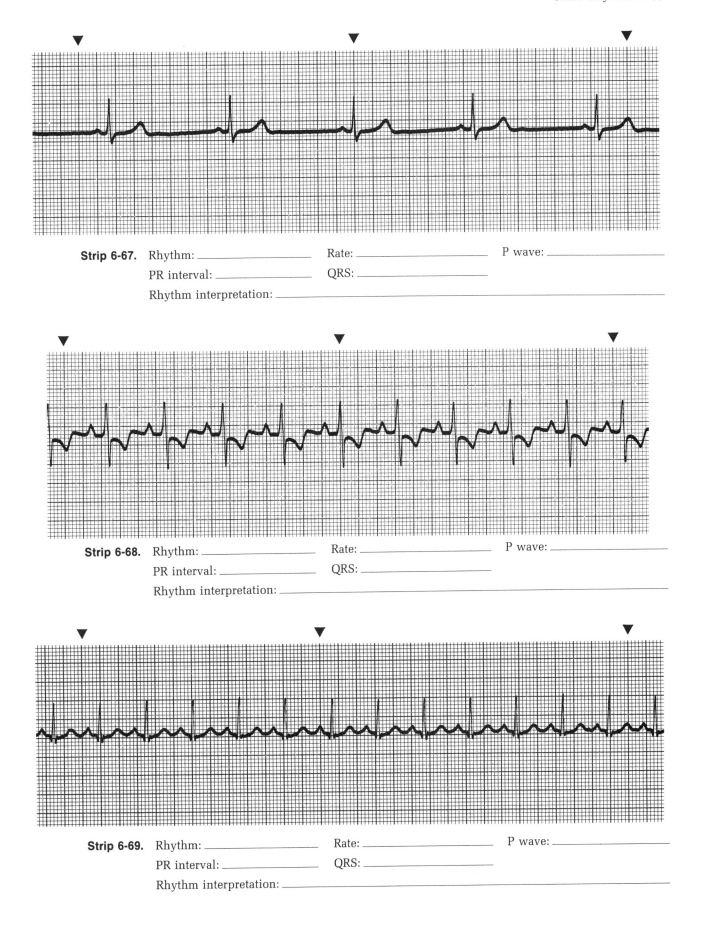

Strip 6-67. Rhythm: _____ Rate: _____ P wave: _____

PR interval: _____ QRS: _____

Rhythm interpretation: _____

Strip 6-68. Rhythm: _____ Rate: _____ P wave: _____

PR interval: _____ QRS: _____

Rhythm interpretation: _____

Strip 6-69. Rhythm: _____ Rate: _____ P wave: _____

PR interval: _____ QRS: _____

Rhythm interpretation: _____

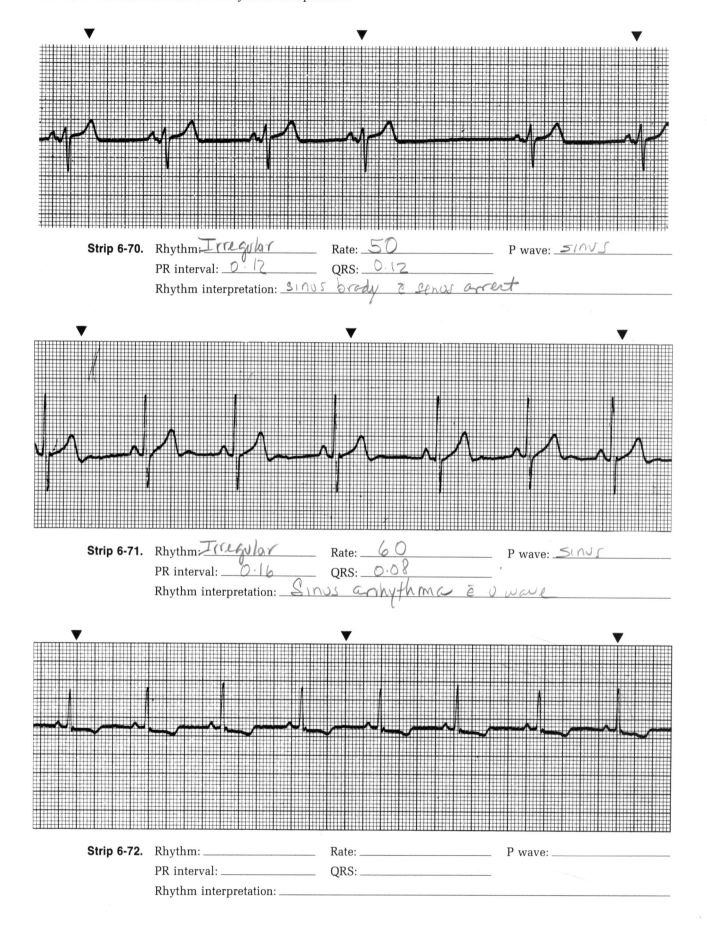

Strip 6-70. Rhythm: Irregular   Rate: 50   P wave: sinus
PR interval: 0.12   QRS: 0.12
Rhythm interpretation: sinus brady c̄ sinus arrest

Strip 6-71. Rhythm: Irregular   Rate: 60   P wave: sinus
PR interval: 0.16   QRS: 0.08
Rhythm interpretation: Sinus arrhythma c̄ u wave

Strip 6-72. Rhythm: _____   Rate: _____   P wave: _____
PR interval: _____   QRS: _____
Rhythm interpretation: _____

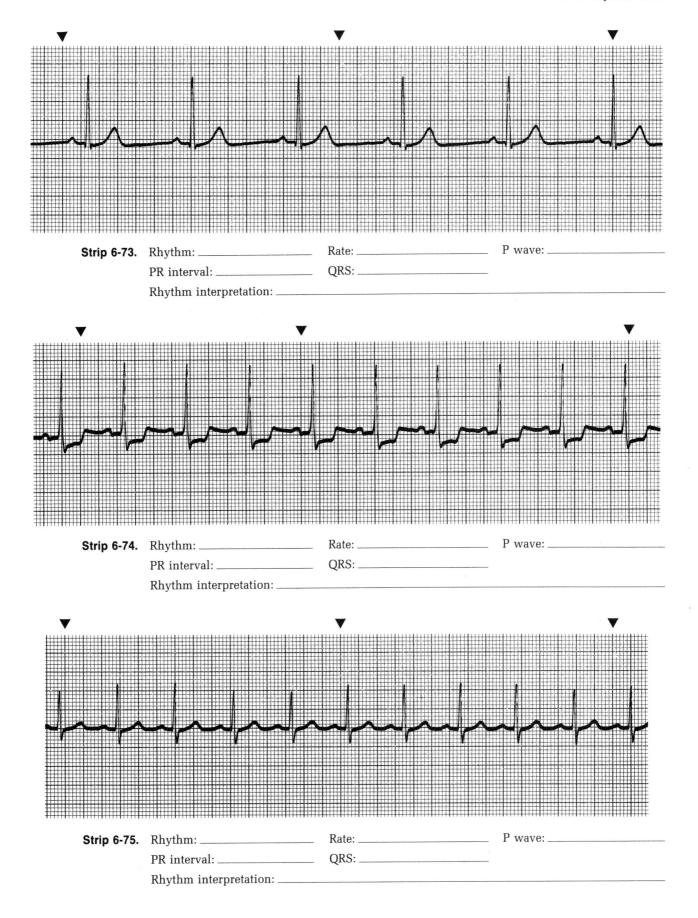

Strip 6-73. Rhythm: _____ Rate: _____ P wave: _____

PR interval: _____ QRS: _____

Rhythm interpretation: _____

Strip 6-74. Rhythm: _____ Rate: _____ P wave: _____

PR interval: _____ QRS: _____

Rhythm interpretation: _____

Strip 6-75. Rhythm: _____ Rate: _____ P wave: _____

PR interval: _____ QRS: _____

Rhythm interpretation: _____

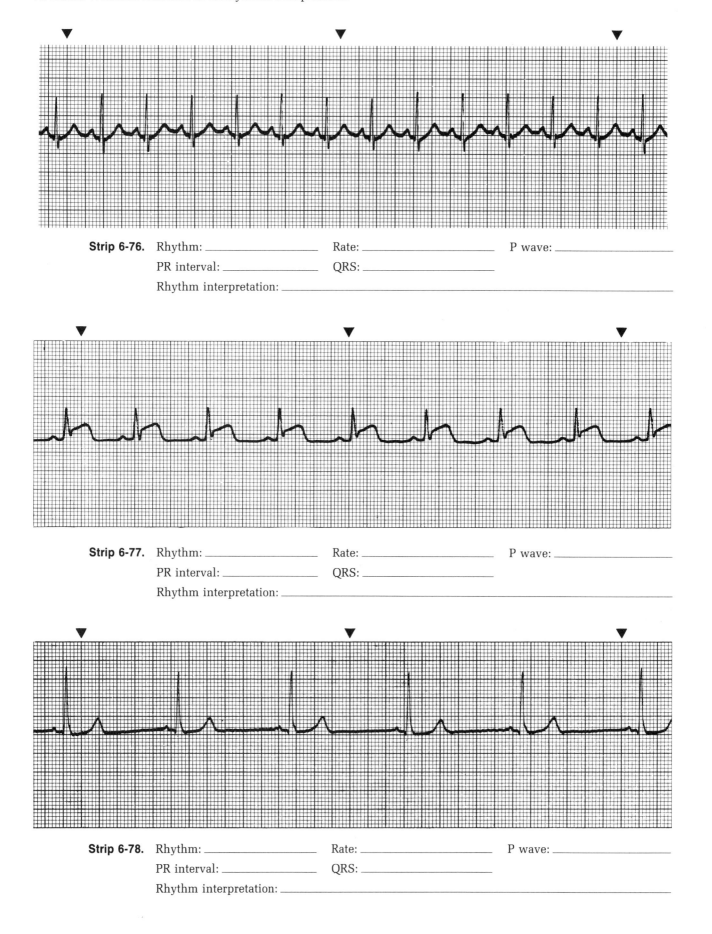

Strip 6-76. Rhythm: _____ Rate: _____ P wave: _____

PR interval: _____ QRS: _____

Rhythm interpretation: _____

Strip 6-77. Rhythm: _____ Rate: _____ P wave: _____

PR interval: _____ QRS: _____

Rhythm interpretation: _____

Strip 6-78. Rhythm: _____ Rate: _____ P wave: _____

PR interval: _____ QRS: _____

Rhythm interpretation: _____

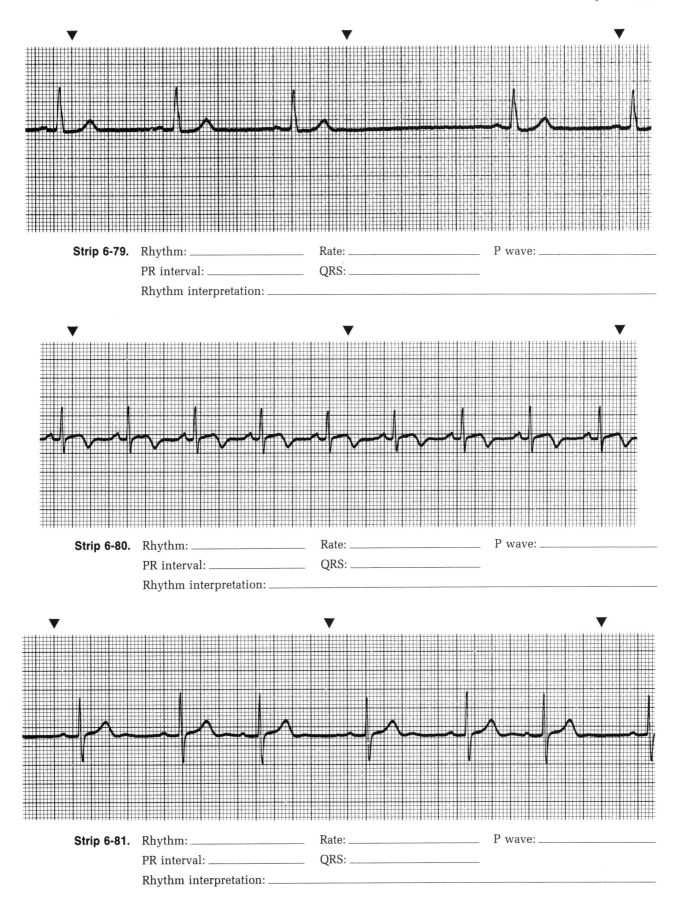

Strip 6-79. Rhythm: _____ Rate: _____ P wave: _____

PR interval: _____ QRS: _____

Rhythm interpretation: _____

Strip 6-80. Rhythm: _____ Rate: _____ P wave: _____

PR interval: _____ QRS: _____

Rhythm interpretation: _____

Strip 6-81. Rhythm: _____ Rate: _____ P wave: _____

PR interval: _____ QRS: _____

Rhythm interpretation: _____

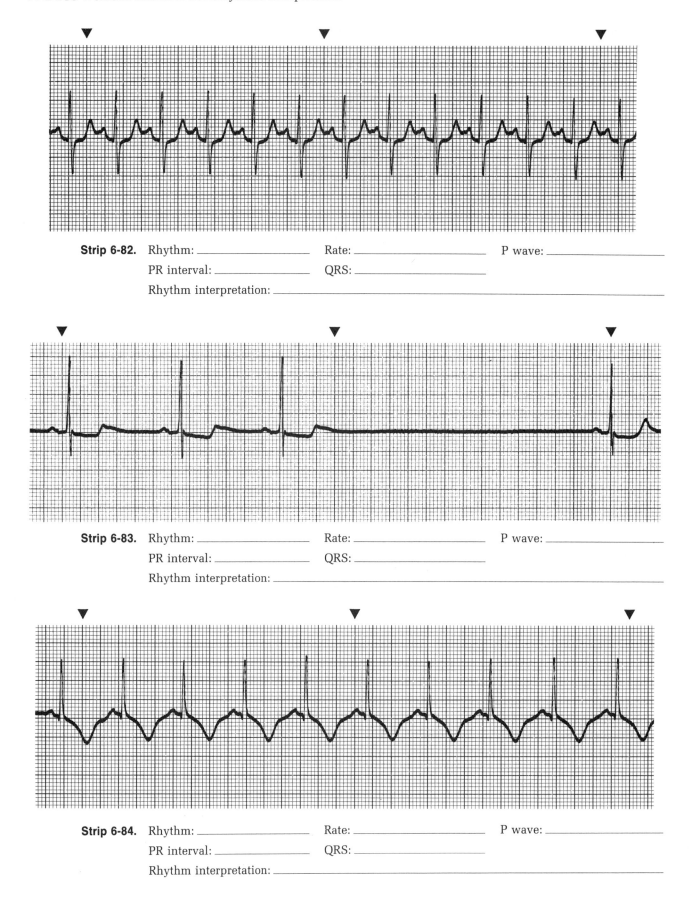

Strip 6-82. Rhythm: _____ Rate: _____ P wave: _____

PR interval: _____ QRS: _____

Rhythm interpretation: _____

Strip 6-83. Rhythm: _____ Rate: _____ P wave: _____

PR interval: _____ QRS: _____

Rhythm interpretation: _____

Strip 6-84. Rhythm: _____ Rate: _____ P wave: _____

PR interval: _____ QRS: _____

Rhythm interpretation: _____

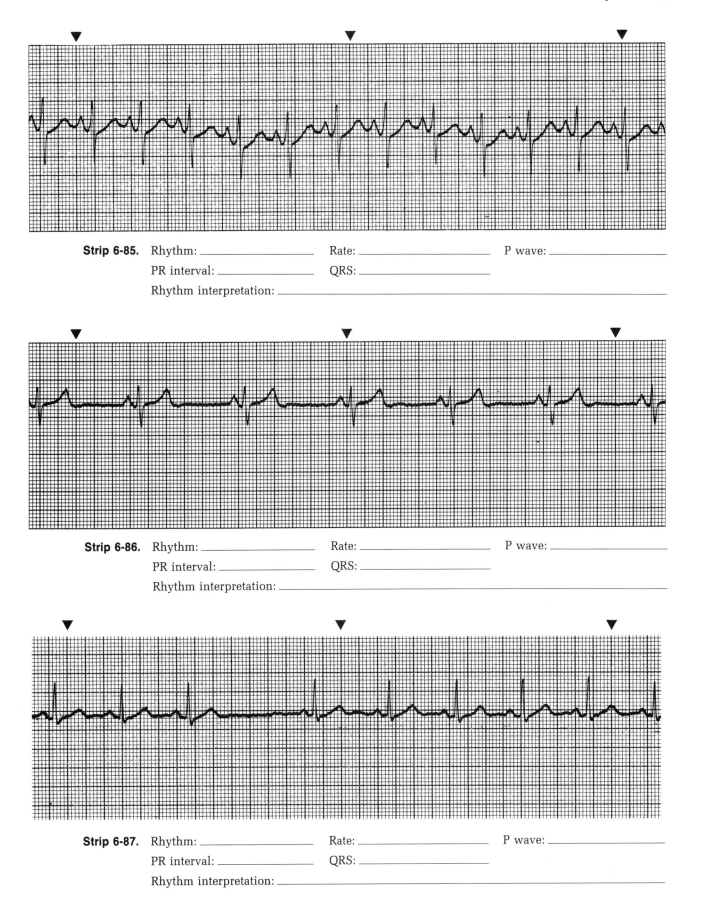

Strip 6-85. Rhythm: _____ Rate: _____ P wave: _____

PR interval: _____ QRS: _____

Rhythm interpretation: _____

Strip 6-86. Rhythm: _____ Rate: _____ P wave: _____

PR interval: _____ QRS: _____

Rhythm interpretation: _____

Strip 6-87. Rhythm: _____ Rate: _____ P wave: _____

PR interval: _____ QRS: _____

Rhythm interpretation: _____

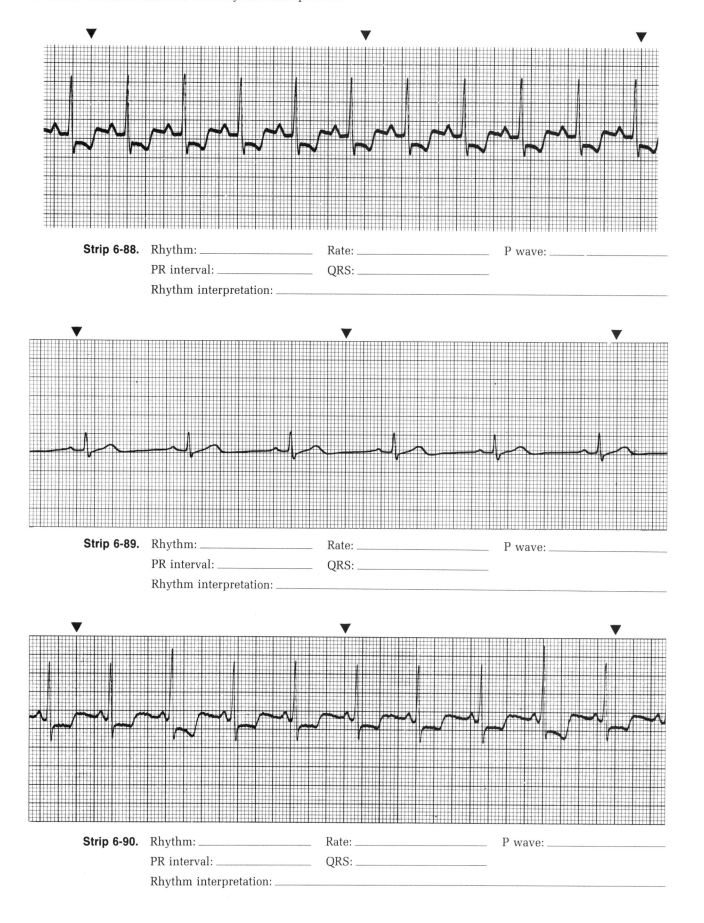

Strip 6-88. Rhythm: _____ Rate: _____ P wave: _____

PR interval: _____ QRS: _____

Rhythm interpretation: _____

Strip 6-89. Rhythm: _____ Rate: _____ P wave: _____

PR interval: _____ QRS: _____

Rhythm interpretation: _____

Strip 6-90. Rhythm: _____ Rate: _____ P wave: _____

PR interval: _____ QRS: _____

Rhythm interpretation: _____

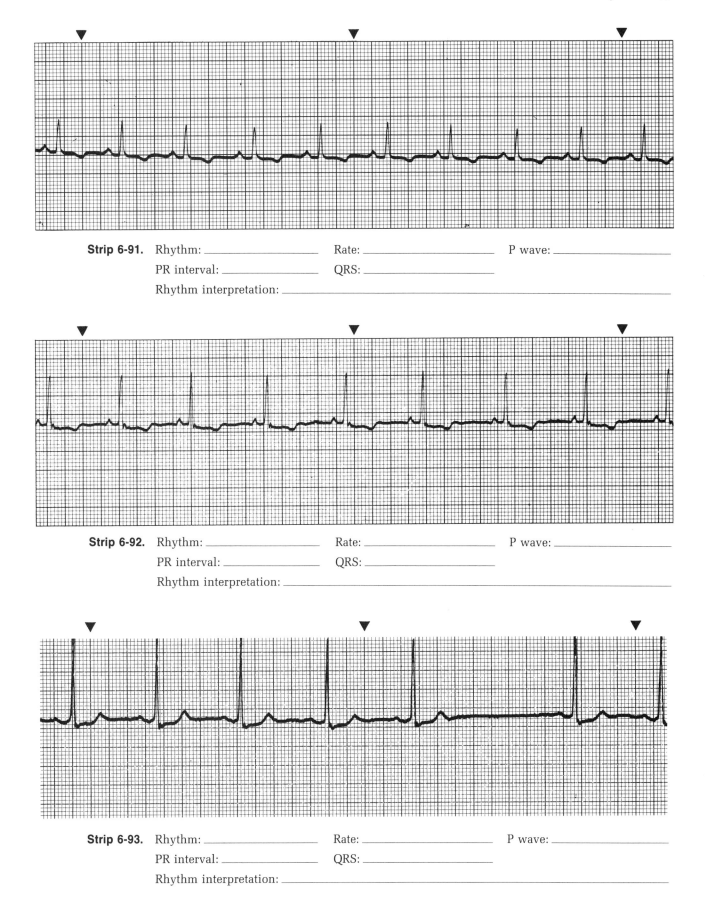

Strip 6-91. Rhythm: _____ Rate: _____ P wave: _____

PR interval: _____ QRS: _____

Rhythm interpretation: _____

Strip 6-92. Rhythm: _____ Rate: _____ P wave: _____

PR interval: _____ QRS: _____

Rhythm interpretation: _____

Strip 6-93. Rhythm: _____ Rate: _____ P wave: _____

PR interval: _____ QRS: _____

Rhythm interpretation: _____

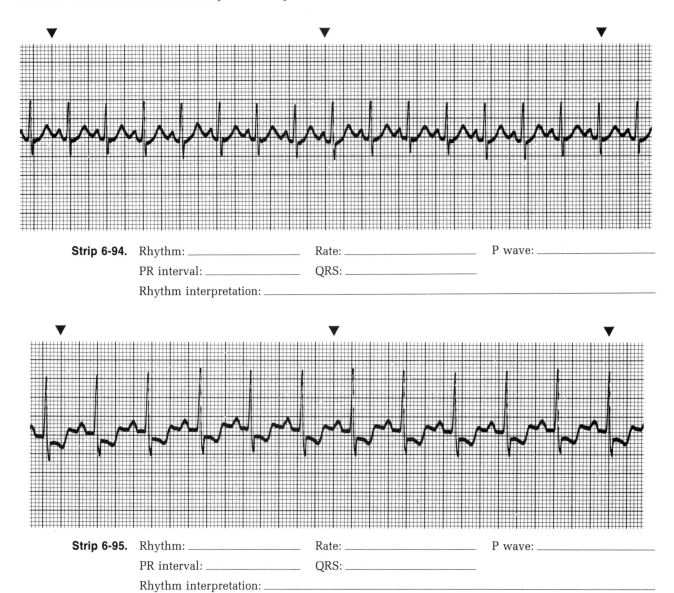

Strip 6-94. Rhythm: _____ Rate: _____ P wave: _____

PR interval: _____ QRS: _____

Rhythm interpretation: _____

Strip 6-95. Rhythm: _____ Rate: _____ P wave: _____

PR interval: _____ QRS: _____

Rhythm interpretation: _____

7

Atrial Rhythms

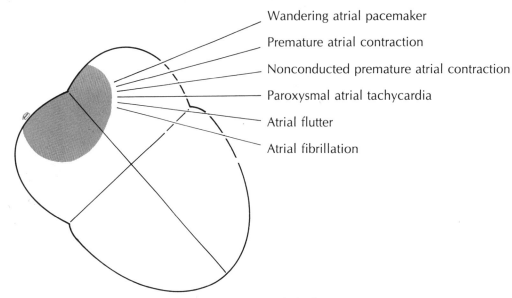

Wandering atrial pacemaker

Premature atrial contraction

Nonconducted premature atrial contraction

Paroxysmal atrial tachycardia

Atrial flutter

Atrial fibrillation

Figure 7-1. Atrial rhythms.

In atrial rhythms, a focus in the atrium initiates impulses more rapidly than those arising in the sinoatrial (SA) node (Figure 7-1). The ectopic site in the atria replaces the SA node as pacemaker. This may occur for 1 beat (premature atrial contraction) or continuously (paroxysmal atrial tachycardia, atrial flutter, or atrial fibrillation).

Because the impulse originates outside the SA node, the P waves are different in configuration (morphology) from the sinus P waves. In slower atrial rhythms (less than 200 per minute), the P wave may be visible and is often small and pointed (Figure 7-2A) in configuration. In faster atrial rhythms, the P wave contour changes to a sawtooth (see Figure 7-2B) or a wavy (see Figure 7-2C) baseline.

With slower atrial rates, the atrioventricular (AV) node accepts and conducts each impulse to the ventricles. The atrial and ventricular rates remain the same. With faster atrial rates, the AV node is unable to accept each impulse and blocks many of the impulses. The atrial and ventricular rates will be different. The impulses that pass the AV node are conducted normally to the ventricles and result in a normal QRS complex.

Atrial rhythms associated with rapid rates increase myocardial oxygen demand and reduce cardiac output because the amount of blood ejected with each contraction is decreased as a result of short ventricular filling times between beats.

WANDERING ATRIAL PACEMAKER

A wandering atrial pacemaker occurs when the pacemaker site shifts back and forth between the SA node, other atrial sites, or the AV junctional tissue while maintaining essentially the same rhythm and rate. The main characteristic of this rhythm is the constantly changing P wave morphology across the rhythm strip. The PR interval may vary slightly depending on the changing pacemaker location.

A wandering atrial pacemaker is usually caused by increased parasympathetic (vagal) influence. With an increase in vagal tone, the SA node slows, allowing another pacemaker site in the atrium to take control briefly. As soon as vagal tone decreases, the SA node regains control of the heart beat again.

A $\left(\sim \Lambda \sim \right)$

B $\left(\wedge \wedge \wedge \wedge \wedge \right)$

C $\left(\sim \sim \sim \sim \sim \right)$

Figure 7-2. Atrial P waves: **A**, pointed P wave; **B**, sawtooth P wave; and **C**, wavy P waves.

Box 7-1.	Wandering Atrial Pacemaker— Identifying ECG Features
Rhythm:	Usually regular
Rate:	Usually normal (60 to 100) but may be slow
P waves:	Vary in size, shape, and position across the rhythm strip
PR:	May vary slightly depending on the changing pacemaker location
QRS:	Normal (less than 0.12 seconds)

Atrial quick
↓ digitalis too slow then P̄
quinidine

inverted P
∅ tx

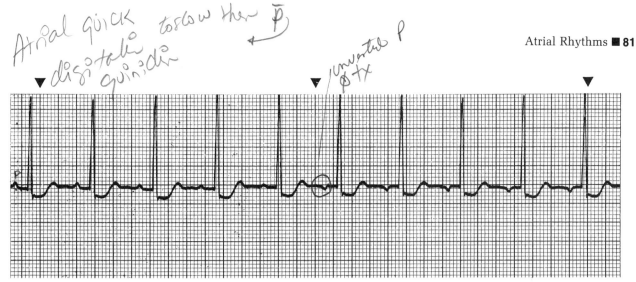

Figure 7-3. **Wandering Atrial Pacemaker**

Rhythm:	Regular
Rate:	88
P wave:	Vary in size, shape, and position
PR:	0.16 to 0.18 seconds
QRS:	0.06 seconds
Comment:	ST segment depression is present.

is supraventricular
b/c QRS NORMAL

Wandering atrial pacemaker is a normal phenomenon that occurs in the young, particularly athletes. Generally, there is no risk to this rhythm, and no treatment is necessary (Box 7-1) (Figure 7-3).

PREMATURE ATRIAL CONTRACTION

A premature atrial contraction (PAC) results from the premature discharge of an ectopic atrial focus. The PAC is characterized by a premature, abnormal P wave accompanied by a normal QRS and followed by a pause.

The shape of the P wave depends on the ectopic focus site. If the ectopic focus is in the vicinity of the sinus node, the P wave may closely resemble the normal sinus P wave. Its sole distinguishing feature may be that it is premature. If the ectopic focus is located away from the sinus node, the P wave will be abnormal in configuration. It is usually small, pointed, and upright, although the P wave may be inverted. If the premature beat occurs early, the P wave can be found hidden in the preceding T wave, causing a distortion of the T wave contour (Figure 7-4). The PR interval of the PAC is usually normal but can be short or prolonged. The impulse is conducted normally to the ventricles, resulting in a normal QRS. The early beat is followed by a pause. The pause is usually less than two RR intervals and is called a noncompensatory pause (Figure 7-5), in contrast to the compensatory pause occurring with the premature ventricular contraction.

PACs do not constitute a basic rhythm but occur in conjunction with the sinus rhythms (normal sinus rhythm, sinus bradycardia, or sinus tachycardia). PACs may occur as a single premature beat, every other beat (bigeminal PACs), every third beat (trigeminal PACs), in pairs, or in runs. When PACs occur in runs of three or more, the rhythm is called paroxysmal atrial tachycardia (PAT).

PACs can occur in myocardial ischemia and are often provoked by anxiety, smoking, or ingestion of caffeine or alcohol. PACs generally do not require therapy. When PACs induce tachycardias, treatment with digitalis; a beta-blocker, such as Inderal; or a calcium antagonist, such as verapamil, can be tried (Box 7-2).

Box 7-2.	Premature Atrial Contraction—Identifying ECG Features
Rhythm:	Irregular owing to premature beat and pause
Rate:	Usually normal but can occur with sinus bradycardia or sinus tachycardia
P wave:	P wave of PAC is premature and abnormal in size, shape, or position (usually small, pointed, and upright but can be inverted); P wave is often found hidden in preceding T wave distorting the T wave contour
PR:	Usually normal but can be short or prolonged
QRS:	Normal (less than 0.12 seconds)

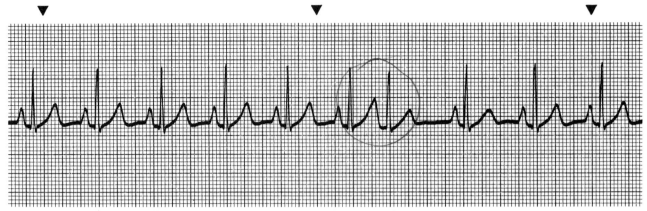

Figure 7-4. Normal Sinus Rhythm with Premature Atrial Contraction

Rhythm: Basic rhythm regular, irregular with PAC

Rate: Basic rhythm rate 84

P wave: Sinus P waves with basic rhythm; premature, abnormal P wave with PAC. The P wave of the PAC is hidden in the preceding T wave distorting the T wave contour (T wave is taller and more pointed.)

PR: 0.12 to 0.14 seconds (basic rhythm)

QRS: 0.06 to 0.08 seconds

On some occasions an atrial beat may occur late instead of early. These beats are called atrial escape beats. The characteristics of the late beat will be the same as the PAC. Escape beats require no treatment. It is important, however, to identify the cause of the pause so that appropriate intervention can be initiated, if necessary.

NONCONDUCTED PAC

A nonconducted PAC occurs when a premature discharge of an ectopic atrial focus occurs so early it finds the AV node refractory, and the impulse is not conducted to the ventricles. The nonconducted PAC is characterized by a premature, abnormal P

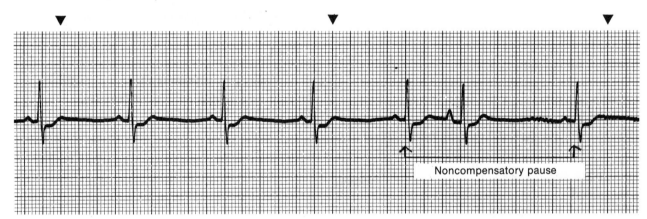

Noncompensatory pause

Figure 7-5. Normal Sinus Rhythm with Premature Atrial Contraction

Rhythm: Basic rhythm regular, irregular with PAC

Rate: Basic rhythm rate 60

P wave: Sinus P waves with basic rhythm, premature, abnormal P wave with PAC

PR: 0.12 to 0.16 seconds (basic rhythm)

QRS: 0.08 seconds

Comment: To determine the type of pause following premature beats, measure from the QRS preceding the premature beat to the QRS following the premature beat. If the measurement equals two RR intervals, the pause is compensatory. If the measurement is less than two RR intervals, the pause is noncompensatory. ST segment depression is present.

wave not accompanied by a QRS but followed by a pause.

Like the PAC, the P wave of the nonconducted PAC is often hidden in the preceding T wave, distorting the T wave contour, and the pause is noncompensatory. The nonconducted PAC also occurs in conjunction with the sinus rhythms (normal sinus rhythm, sinus bradycardia, and sinus tachycardia). It is the most common cause of pauses in regular sinus rhythms.

The nonconducted PAC can be confused with sinus arrest or sinus block. All produce a sudden pause in the rhythm. To distinguish these rhythms, one must examine and compare T wave contours.

The early P wave of the nonconducted PAC will distort the preceding T wave. In sinus arrest or sinus block there is no P wave, and the T wave contours remain unchanged.

Nonconducted PACs have the same significance as PACs and can be treated in the same manner (Box 7-3) (Figures 7-6 and 7-7).

PAT   *poroxysmal atrial tachy*

PAT is caused by a rapid discharge of an ectopic focus in the atrium, occurring at a regular rate of 150 to 250 per minute. The P waves associated with this rhythm are abnormal but seldom can be identified because they are hidden in the preceding T waves. The PR cannot be measured because the P waves are obscured. The QRS will be normal and, in most instances, the atrial and ventricular rates will be the same.

This rhythm begins suddenly and ends suddenly (paroxysmal), in contrast to sinus tachycardia, and is often preceded by frequent PACs. PAT can be considered as a series of three or more consecutive PACs occurring at a rapid rate.

PAT can occur in individuals with no evidence of heart disease. It often is precipitated by sympathetic nervous system stimulation, such as that seen in anxiety states, caffeine ingestion, fatigue, smoking, and excessive alcohol intake.

Box 7-3.	Nonconducted PACs—Identifying ECG Features
Rhythm:	Irregular owing to premature P wave and pause
Rate:	Usually normal but can occur with sinus bradycardia or sinus tachycardia
P wave:	P wave of nonconducted PAC is premature, abnormal, and often found hidden in preceding T wave distorting the T wave contour
PR:	Absent; impulse not conducted to ventricles
QRS:	Absent; impulse not conducted to ventricles

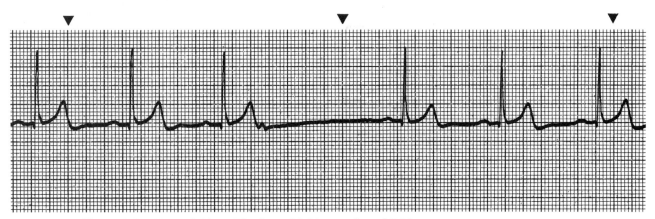

Figure 7-6. Normal Sinus Rhythm with Nonconducted PAC

Rhythm: Basic rhythm regular; irregular with nonconducted PAC

Rate: Basic rate 60; rate slows following nonconducted PAC; rate suppression can occur following a pause in the basic rhythm. After several cycles, the rate will return to the basic rhythm rate.

P wave: Sinus P waves with basic rhythm; premature, abnormal P wave with nonconducted PAC

PR: 0.20 seconds with basic rhythm

QRS: 0.06 to 0.08 seconds with basic rhythm

Comment: A U wave is present.

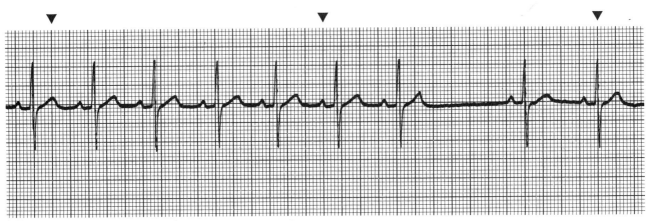

Figure 7-7. Normal Sinus Rhythm with Nonconducted PAC

Rhythm: Basic rhythm regular; irregular with nonconducted PACs

Rate: Basic rhythm rate 88

P wave: Sinus P waves with basic rhythm; p wave of nonconducted PAC is premature, abnormal, and hidden in the preceding T wave

PR: 0.16 to 0.18 seconds (basic rhythm); not present with nonconducted PAC

QRS: 0.06 to 0.08 seconds (basic rhythm); not present with nonconducted PAC

PAT is well tolerated by young people with healthy hearts but poorly tolerated by older people with unhealthy hearts. Rapid rate arrhythmias decrease cardiac output and increase myocardial oxygen demands. This impairment predisposes the person to left ventricular failure and myocardial ischemia.

Priorities of treatment depend on the person's tolerance of the rhythm. If the patient is stable, vagal maneuvers (valsalva, ice water facial immersion, carotid sinus massage) may be tried. If vagal maneuvers fail, adenosine (6 to 12 mg intravenously rapidly) is the drug of choice. Patients who fail to respond to adenosine can be treated with verapamil (5 to 10 mg intravenously slowly). Cardioversion is the initial treatment in patients who are hemodynamically unstable (Box 7-4) (Figures 7-8 and 7-9).

Box 7-4.	Paroxysmal Atrial Tachycardia—Identifying ECG Features
Rhythm:	Regular
Rate:	150 to 250
P waves:	Abnormal P waves precede each QRS; P waves are seldom identified because they are hidden in the preceding T wave
PR:	Not measurable
QRS:	Normal (less than 0.12 seconds)

ATRIAL FLUTTER

Atrial flutter, like PAT, is caused by rapid discharge of an ectopic focus in the atrium. The atrial rate is 250 to 400 per minute. The atrial muscles respond to this rapid stimulation by producing P wave deflections with a sawtooth appearance called flutter waves. These sawtooth waves affect the whole baseline to such a degree that there is no isoelectric line between flutter waves, and the T waves are usually masked or deformed. Atrial flutter is primarily recognized by this sawtooth baseline.

The AV node is bombarded with the rapid atrial impulses and usually conduct only some of them to the ventricles; the rest are blocked. The AV node conducts the impulses in various ratios. For example, the AV node might allow every second, fourth, or sixth atrial impulse to pass through the junction to the ventricles. The resulting disparity between the atrial and ventricular rates is described as atrial flutter with 2:1, 4:1, or 6:1 block. Even ratios (2:1, 4:1) are more common than odd ratios (3:1, 5:1). If the conduction ratio remains the same (eg, 4:1), the rhythm remains regular, and the rhythm is described as atrial flutter with 4:1 block. If the conduction ratio fluctuates (from 4:1 to 6:1 to 2:1), the rhythm is irregular, and the rhythm is described as atrial flutter with variable block.

Atrial flutter is less common than atrial fibrillation. Paroxysmal atrial flutter can occur in patients without structural heart disease, whereas chronic

Adenosine to slow the rate
push i dissipated in 30 sec.
may be given again

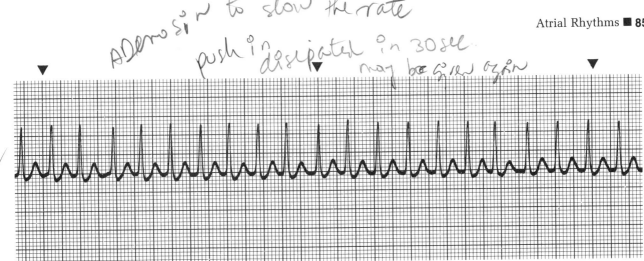

Figure 7-8. **Paroxysmal Atrial Tachycardia**

Lidocaine worser on ventricular tissue

Rhythm:	Regular
Rate:	188
P wave:	Hidden in preceding T wave
PR:	Not measurable
QRS:	0.06 to 0.08 seconds

atrial flutter is usually associated with underlying heart disease such as cardiomyopathy. It also may occur as a result of pulmonary emboli, mitral or tricuspid valve disease, or chronic heart failure. Cardioversion is the initial treatment of choice because cardioversion promptly and effectively restores sinus rhythm, often requiring relatively low energy levels (< 50 joules). Drug therapy is seldom successful in restoring normal sinus rhythm. However, diltiazem, verapamil, propranolol (or other beta-blockers), or digoxin can be used to slow the ventricular rate (Box 7-5) (Figures 7-10 and 7-11).

Box 7-5. **Atrial Flutter—Identifying ECG Features**

Rhythm:	Regular or irregular (depends on AV conduction ratios)
Rate:	Atrial: 250 to 400 Vent: Varies with number of impulses conducted to ventricles
P waves:	Sawtooth deflection called flutter waves
PR:	Not measurable
QRS:	Normal (less than 0.12 seconds)

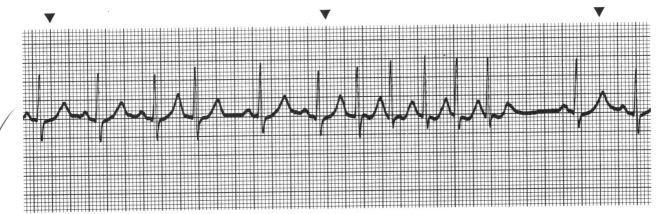

Figure 7-9. **Normal Sinus Rhythm with PAC and Burst of PAT**

Rhythm:	Basic rhythm regular; irregular with PAC and burst of PAT
Rate:	Basic rhythm rate 94; PAT rate (167)
P waves:	Sinus P waves with basic rhythm; premature, abnormal P waves with PAC and PAT
PR:	0.16 seconds (basic rhythm)
QRS:	0.08 seconds
Comment:	A run of three or more consecutive PACs is considered PAT.

QUINIDINE / PRONESTYL CHANNEL CA BLOCKERS

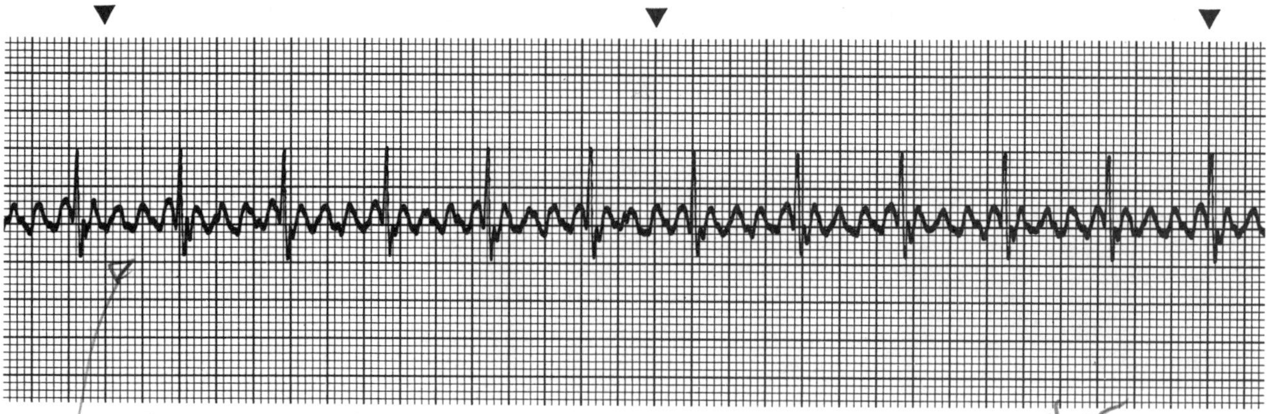

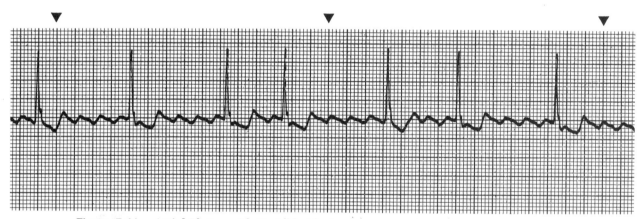

(handwritten note, left margin:) 4 to 1

(handwritten note, right of figure:) it can be very regular no atrial kicks

Figure 7-10. Atrial Flutter with 4:1 Block

Rhythm: Regular

Rate: Atrial: 428

Ventricular: 107

Note: If the ventricular rate is regular, multiply the number of flutter waves before each QRS × the ventricular rate to determine atrial rate.

P wave: Four flutter waves before each QRS

PR: Not measurable

QRS: 0.06 to 0.08 seconds

Figure 7-11. Atrial Flutter with Variable Block

Rhythm: Irregular

Rate: Atrial: 280

Ventricular: 60

Note: If the ventricular rate is irregular, count the number of flutter waves in a 6-second strip and multiply × 10 to obtain atrial rate.

P waves: Flutter waves before each QRS (varying ratios)

PR: Not measurable

QRS: 0.06 to 0.08 seconds

[handwritten annotations at top: "CONTROLLED ÷ 70-100 UNCONTROLLED ATRIAL FIB ē RVR = rapid vert. response >100 SVR = slow"]

ATRIAL FIBRILLATION

Atrial fibrillation, like PAT and atrial flutter, is caused by the rapid discharge of an ectopic focus in the atrium. The atrial rate is 400 or more per minute. The atria respond to this extremely rapid stimulation by merely twitching instead of contracting. The muscle twitching results in P wave deflections with a wavy appearance called fibrillatory waves. These wavy deflections affect the whole baseline.

The atrial impulses bombard the AV node, but the node can conduct only a small percentage of them to the ventricles; the rest are blocked. The impulses that pass through the AV node do so at irregular intervals, creating an irregular ventricular rhythm. When the ventricular rate is less than 100 per minute, the rhythm is called controlled atrial fibrillation. When the ventricular rate is greater than 100 per minute, the rhythm is called uncontrolled atrial fibrillation or atrial fibrllation with rapid ventricular response. Atrial fibrillation is primarily recognized by the wavy baseline and the grossly irregular ventricular rhythm. When the ventricular rate is very rapid or very slow, it may appear more regular.

Flutter waves often can be seen mixed in with the wavy fibrillatory waves of atrial fibrillation. Some authorities call this mixed rhythm fib-flutter.

Atrial fibrillation is common in older people with coronary artery disease, mitral or tricuspid valve disease, pulmonary embolism, cardiomyopathy, and heart failure. The main danger with this rhythm is a decrease in cardiac output not only from an increased ventricular rate but also from the loss of atrial contraction. Atrial contraction contributes as much as 20% to cardiac output. The noncontracting atria also tend to pool blood in the atrial chambers, increasing the potential for formation of atrial thrombi and subsequent embolization.

Priorities of treatment depend on the patient's tolerance of the rhythm. If the patient is stable, he or she can be treated with digitalis; beta-blockers, such as Inderal, or the calcium antagonists (diltiazem and verapamil). If drug therapy fails, atrial fibrillation can be treated with cardioversion. Cardioversion is the initial treatment in patients who are hemodynamically unstable (Box 7-6) (Figures 7-12 and 7-13).

Box 7-6.	Atrial Fibrillation—Identifying ECG Features
Rhythm:	Totally irregular
Rate:	Ventricular rate varies with number of impulses conducted to ventricles
P wave:	Wavy deflections called fibrillatory waves
PR:	Not measurable
QRS:	Normal (less than 0.12 seconds)

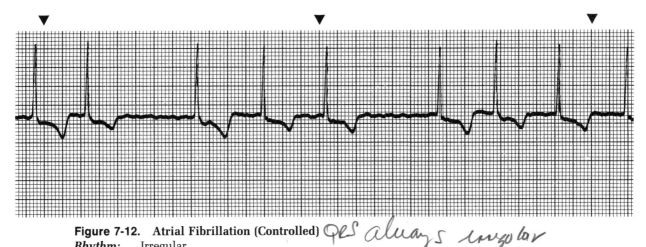

Figure 7-12. Atrial Fibrillation (Controlled) *[handwritten: QRS always irregular]*

Rhythm:	Irregular
Rate:	Ventricular rate 70
P waves:	Fibrillatory waves present
PR:	Not measurable
QRS:	0.04 to 0.06 seconds
Comment:	ST segment depression and T wave inversion are present

[handwritten notes: "Dig is a cardiotonic antiarrhythmic. Can be used ē quinidine. Cause PVC any arrhythmic. ē verapamil, inderal"]

[handwritten at bottom: "difference ÷ 3 HEART BLOCK B blockers"]

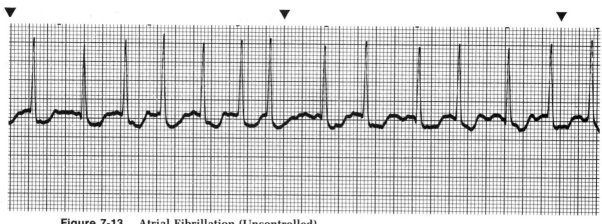

Figure 7-13. Atrial Fibrillation (Uncontrolled)

Rhythm: Irregular

Rate: Ventricular rate 130

P wave: Fibrillatory waves present

PR: Not measurable

QRS: 0.06 to 0.08 seconds

Comment: ST segment depression is present.

Cardioversion: elective
   synchronized to QRS
start at w/sec 25-50J lower
Dr → Premedication: Versed, valium, MS. O₂ Sat, suction, naloxin   reverses resp.

Defibrillation:
immediate
not synchronized
start 50-100, 200, 300-350 J

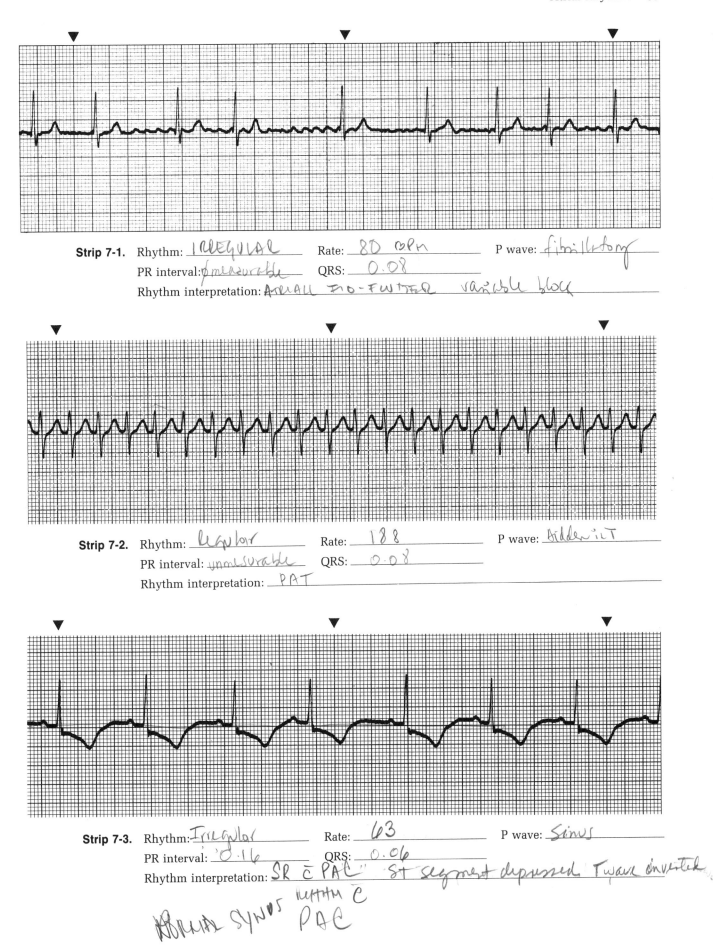

Strip 7-1. Rhythm: IRREGULAR   Rate: 80 bpm   P wave: fibrillatory

PR interval: unmeasurable   QRS: 0.08

Rhythm interpretation: ATRIAL FIB-FLUTTER variable block

Strip 7-2. Rhythm: Regular   Rate: 188   P wave: hidden in T

PR interval: unmeasurable   QRS: 0.08

Rhythm interpretation: PAT

Strip 7-3. Rhythm: Irregular   Rate: 63   P wave: Sinus

PR interval: 0.16   QRS: 0.06

Rhythm interpretation: SR c̄ PAC   ST segment depressed T wave inverted

NORMAL SINUS RHYTHM c̄ PAC

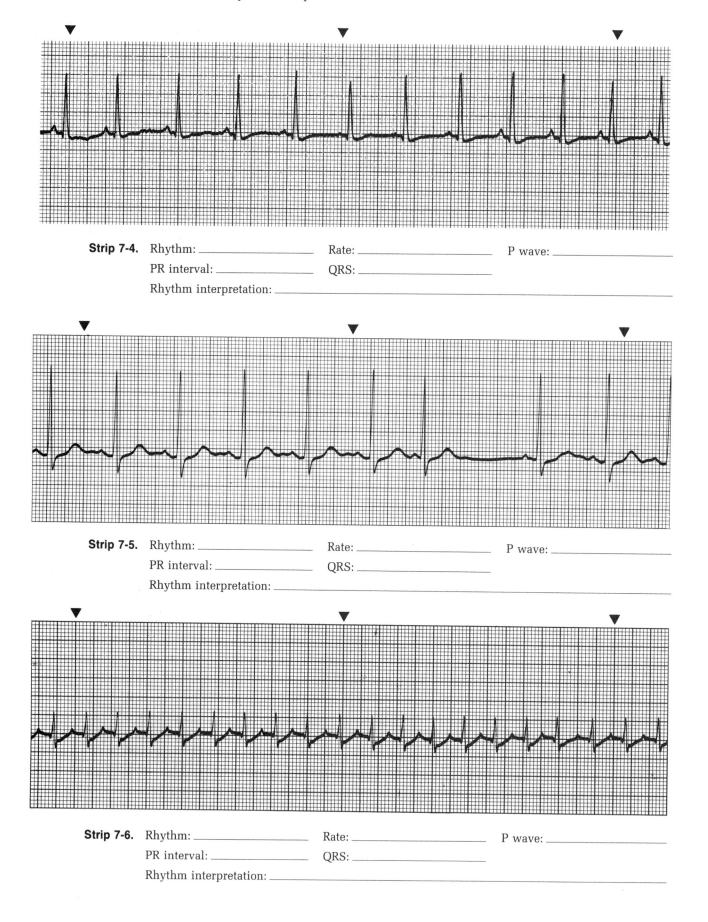

Strip 7-4. Rhythm: _____ Rate: _____ P wave: _____

PR interval: _____ QRS: _____

Rhythm interpretation: _____

Strip 7-5. Rhythm: _____ Rate: _____ P wave: _____

PR interval: _____ QRS: _____

Rhythm interpretation: _____

Strip 7-6. Rhythm: _____ Rate: _____ P wave: _____

PR interval: _____ QRS: _____

Rhythm interpretation: _____

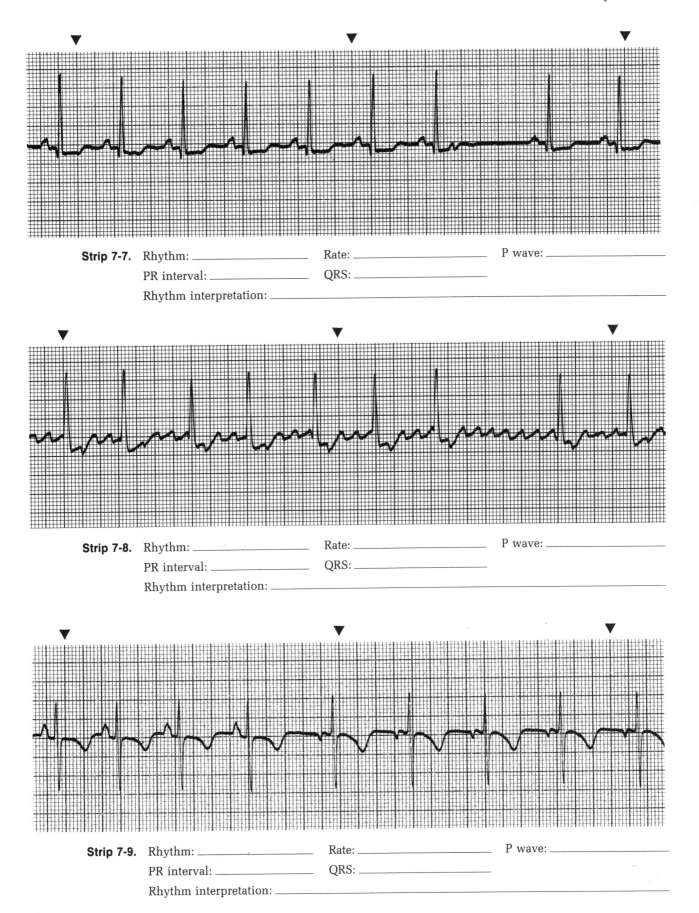

Strip 7-7. Rhythm: _____ Rate: _____ P wave: _____

PR interval: _____ QRS: _____

Rhythm interpretation: _____

Strip 7-8. Rhythm: _____ Rate: _____ P wave: _____

PR interval: _____ QRS: _____

Rhythm interpretation: _____

Strip 7-9. Rhythm: _____ Rate: _____ P wave: _____

PR interval: _____ QRS: _____

Rhythm interpretation: _____

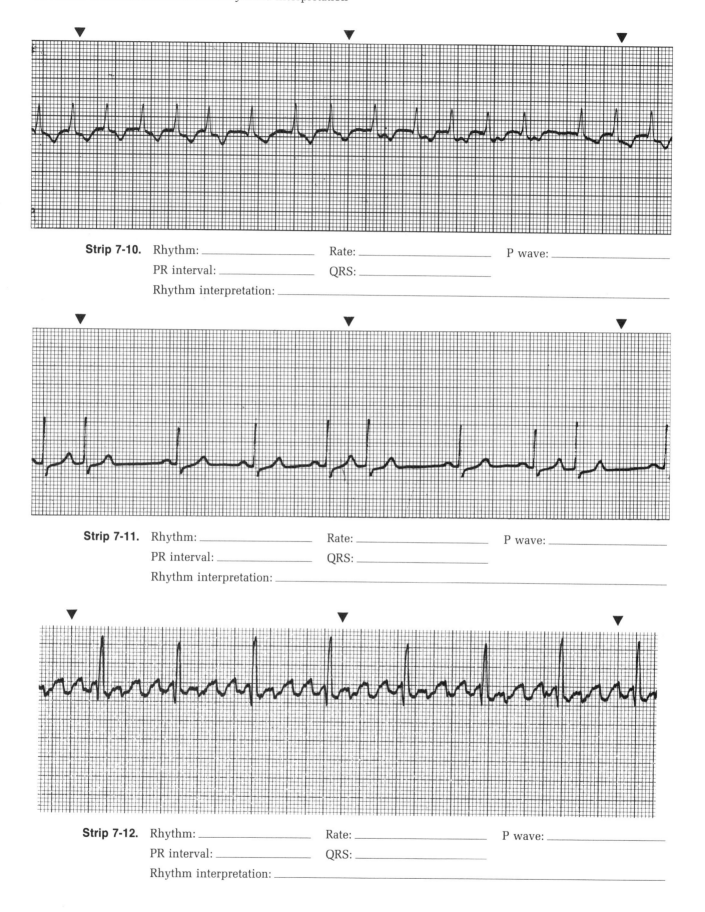

Strip 7-10. Rhythm: _____ Rate: _____ P wave: _____

PR interval: _____ QRS: _____

Rhythm interpretation: _____

Strip 7-11. Rhythm: _____ Rate: _____ P wave: _____

PR interval: _____ QRS: _____

Rhythm interpretation: _____

Strip 7-12. Rhythm: _____ Rate: _____ P wave: _____

PR interval: _____ QRS: _____

Rhythm interpretation: _____

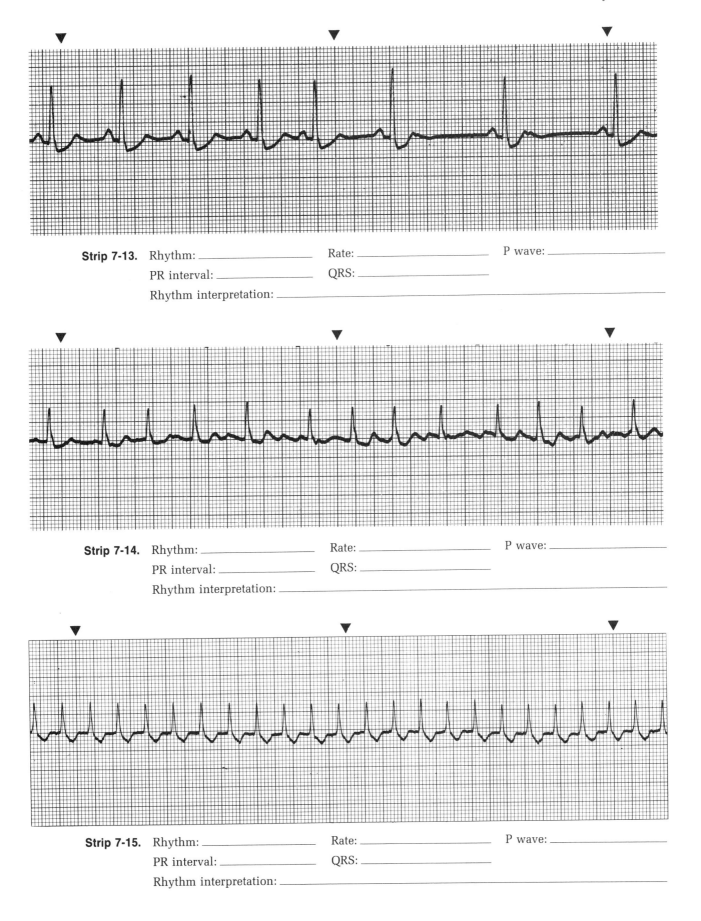

Strip 7-13. Rhythm: _____ Rate: _____ P wave: _____

PR interval: _____ QRS: _____

Rhythm interpretation: _____

Strip 7-14. Rhythm: _____ Rate: _____ P wave: _____

PR interval: _____ QRS: _____

Rhythm interpretation: _____

Strip 7-15. Rhythm: _____ Rate: _____ P wave: _____

PR interval: _____ QRS: _____

Rhythm interpretation: _____

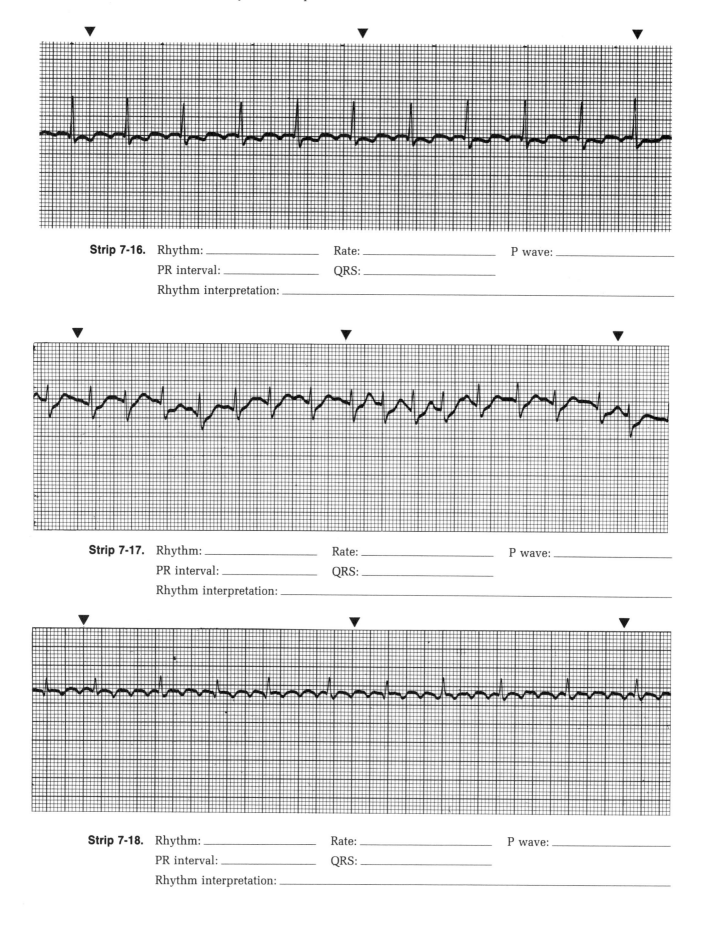

Strip 7-16. Rhythm: _____ Rate: _____ P wave: _____

PR interval: _____ QRS: _____

Rhythm interpretation: _____

Strip 7-17. Rhythm: _____ Rate: _____ P wave: _____

PR interval: _____ QRS: _____

Rhythm interpretation: _____

Strip 7-18. Rhythm: _____ Rate: _____ P wave: _____

PR interval: _____ QRS: _____

Rhythm interpretation: _____

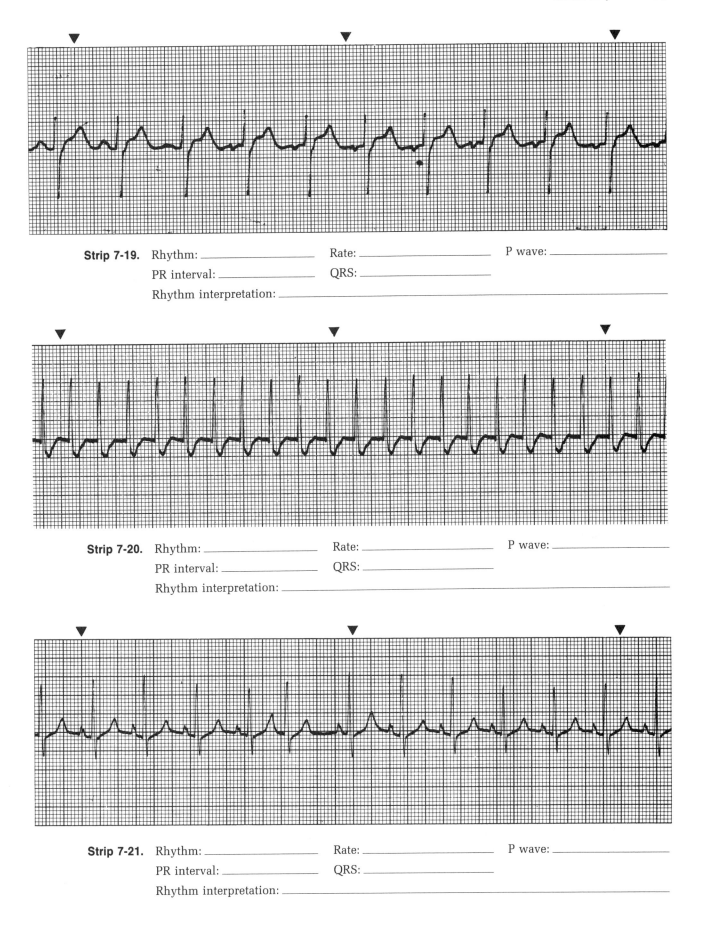

Strip 7-19. Rhythm: _____ Rate: _____ P wave: _____

PR interval: _____ QRS: _____

Rhythm interpretation: _____

Strip 7-20. Rhythm: _____ Rate: _____ P wave: _____

PR interval: _____ QRS: _____

Rhythm interpretation: _____

Strip 7-21. Rhythm: _____ Rate: _____ P wave: _____

PR interval: _____ QRS: _____

Rhythm interpretation: _____

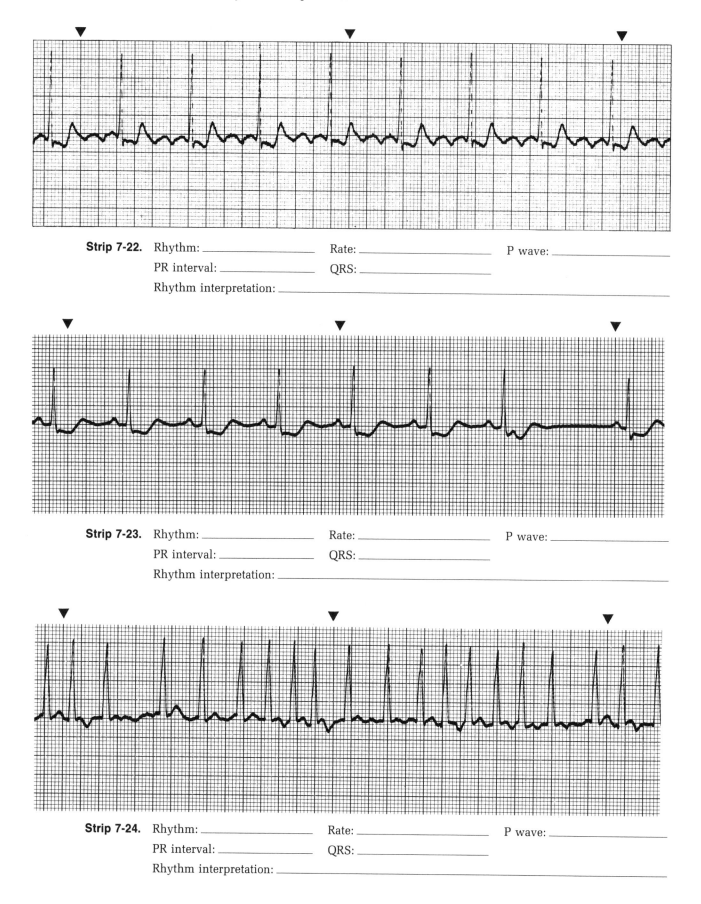

Strip 7-22. Rhythm: _____ Rate: _____ P wave: _____

PR interval: _____ QRS: _____

Rhythm interpretation: _____

Strip 7-23. Rhythm: _____ Rate: _____ P wave: _____

PR interval: _____ QRS: _____

Rhythm interpretation: _____

Strip 7-24. Rhythm: _____ Rate: _____ P wave: _____

PR interval: _____ QRS: _____

Rhythm interpretation: _____

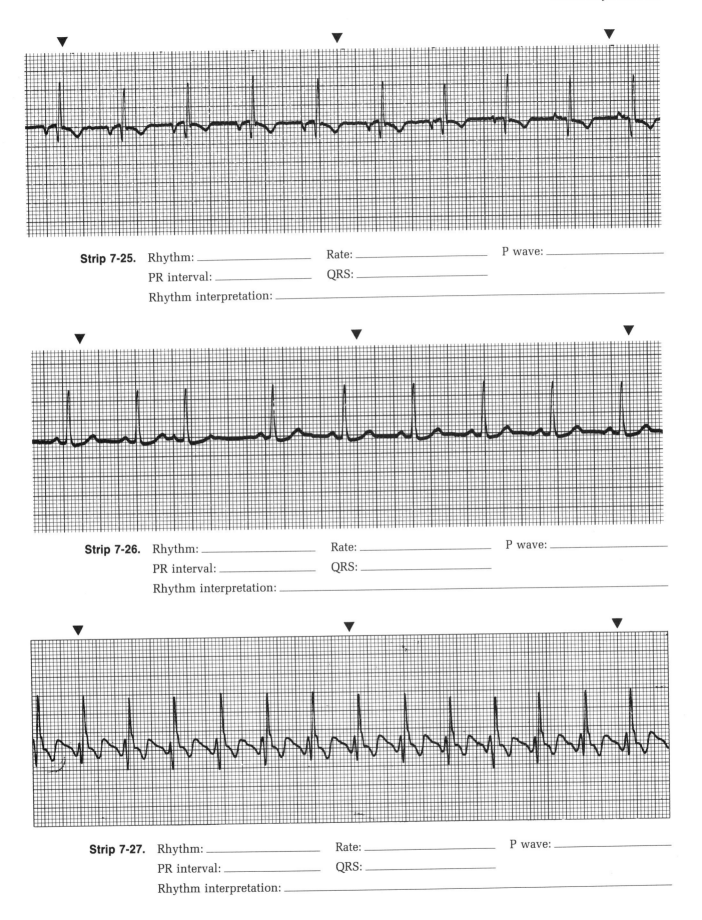

Strip 7-25. Rhythm: _____ Rate: _____ P wave: _____

PR interval: _____ QRS: _____

Rhythm interpretation: _____

Strip 7-26. Rhythm: _____ Rate: _____ P wave: _____

PR interval: _____ QRS: _____

Rhythm interpretation: _____

Strip 7-27. Rhythm: _____ Rate: _____ P wave: _____

PR interval: _____ QRS: _____

Rhythm interpretation: _____

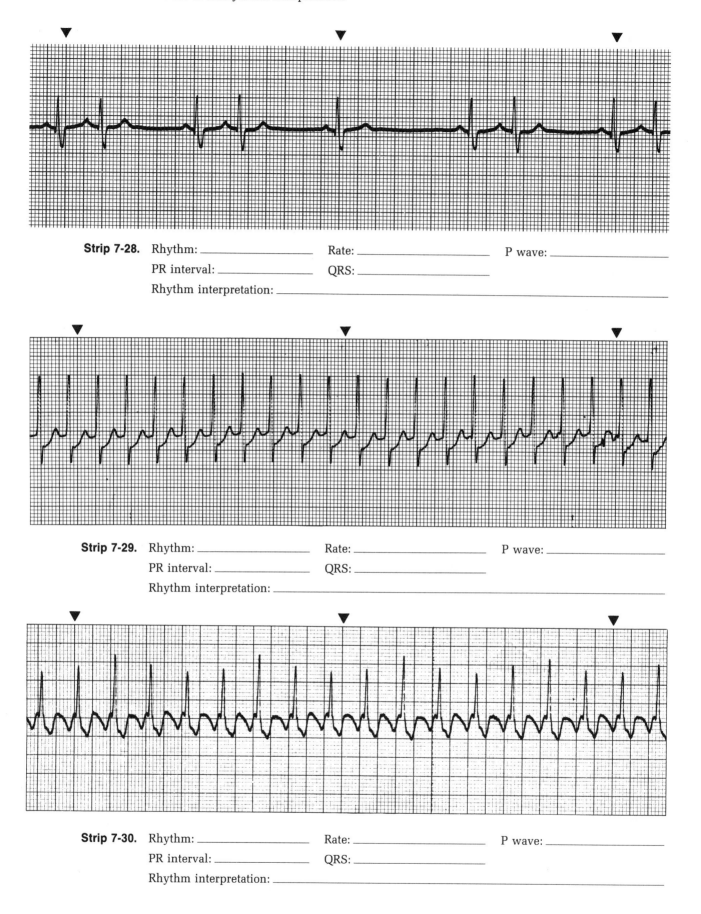

Strip 7-28.   Rhythm: _____   Rate: _____   P wave: _____

PR interval: _____   QRS: _____

Rhythm interpretation: _____

Strip 7-29.   Rhythm: _____   Rate: _____   P wave: _____

PR interval: _____   QRS: _____

Rhythm interpretation: _____

Strip 7-30.   Rhythm: _____   Rate: _____   P wave: _____

PR interval: _____   QRS: _____

Rhythm interpretation: _____

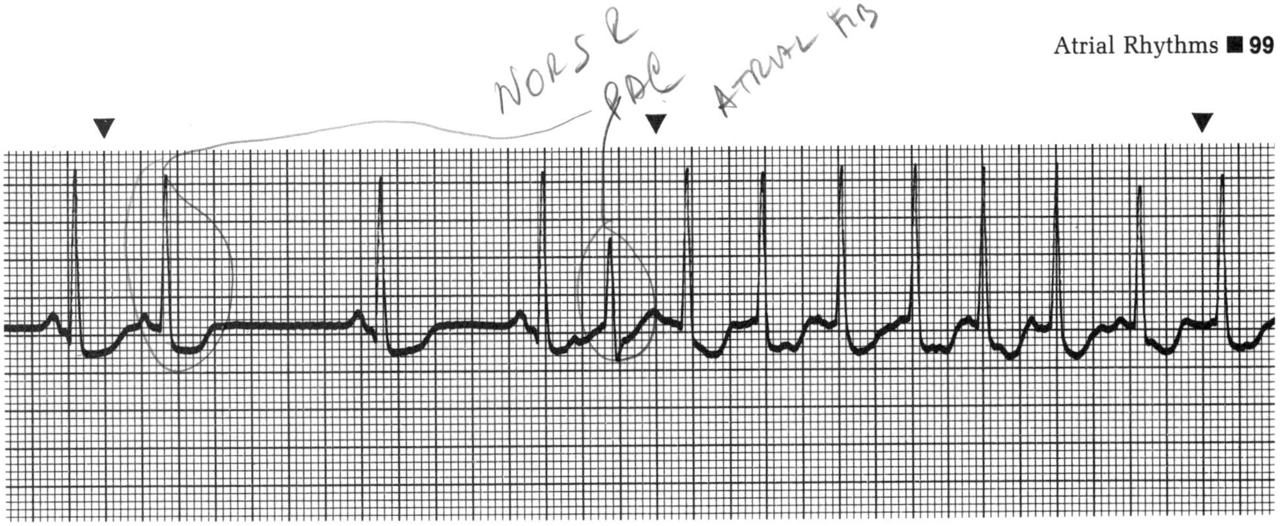

NORS R
PAC   ATRIAL FIB

Strip 7-31. Rhythm: _____ Rate: _____ P wave: _____

PR interval: _____ QRS: _____

Rhythm interpretation: _____

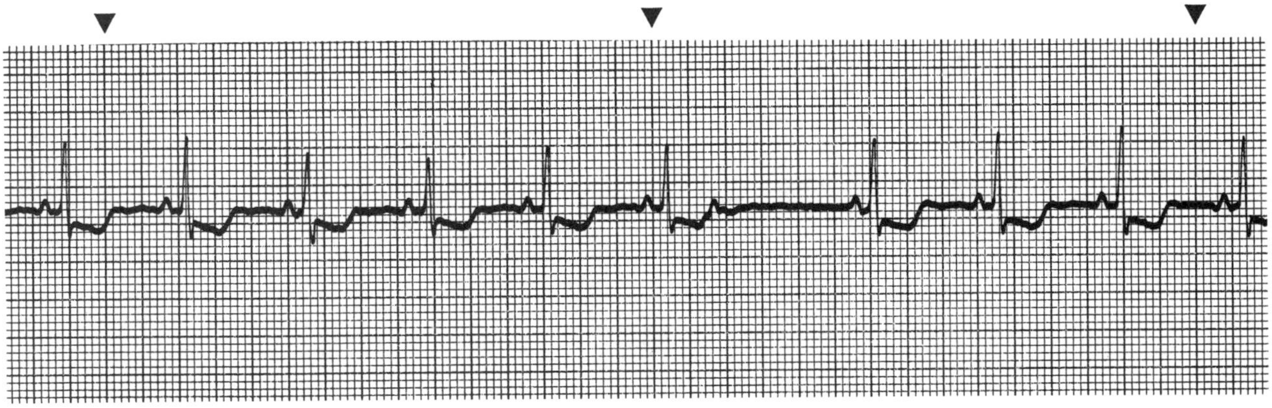

Strip 7-32. Rhythm: _____ Rate: _____ P wave: _____

PR interval: _____ QRS: _____

Rhythm interpretation: _____

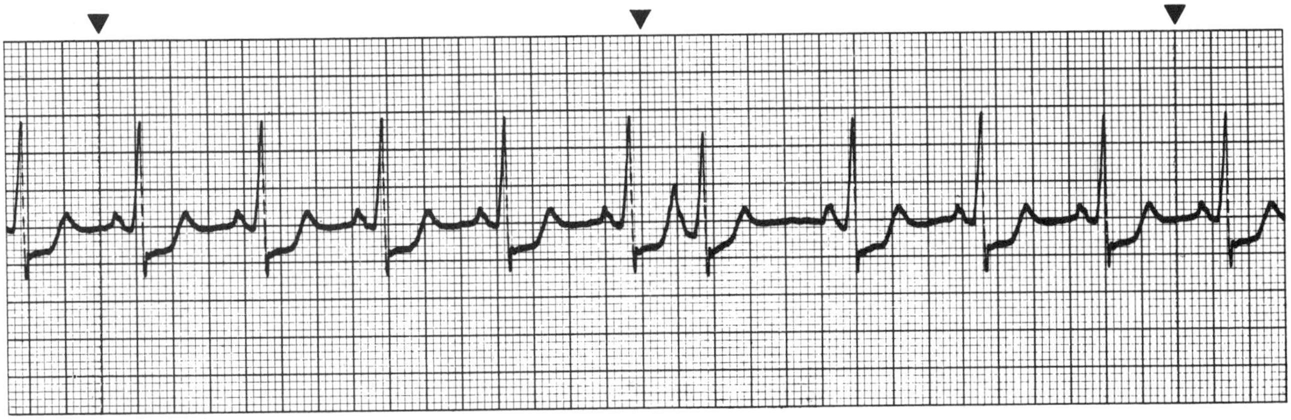

Strip 7-33. Rhythm: _____ Rate: _____ P wave: _____

PR interval: _____ QRS: _____

Rhythm interpretation: _____

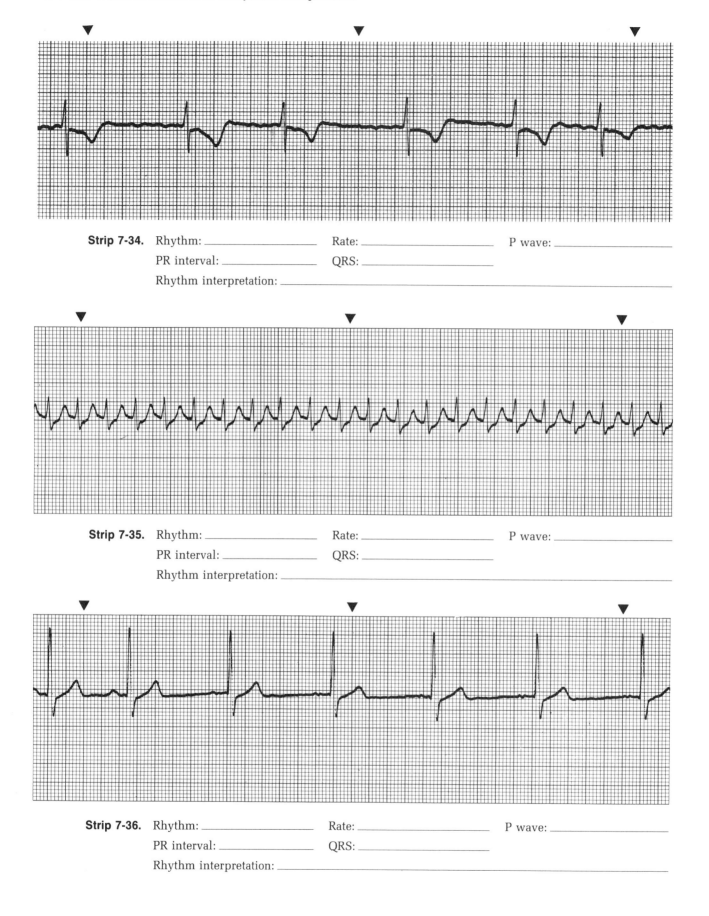

Strip 7-34. Rhythm: _____ Rate: _____ P wave: _____

PR interval: _____ QRS: _____

Rhythm interpretation: _____

Strip 7-35. Rhythm: _____ Rate: _____ P wave: _____

PR interval: _____ QRS: _____

Rhythm interpretation: _____

Strip 7-36. Rhythm: _____ Rate: _____ P wave: _____

PR interval: _____ QRS: _____

Rhythm interpretation: _____

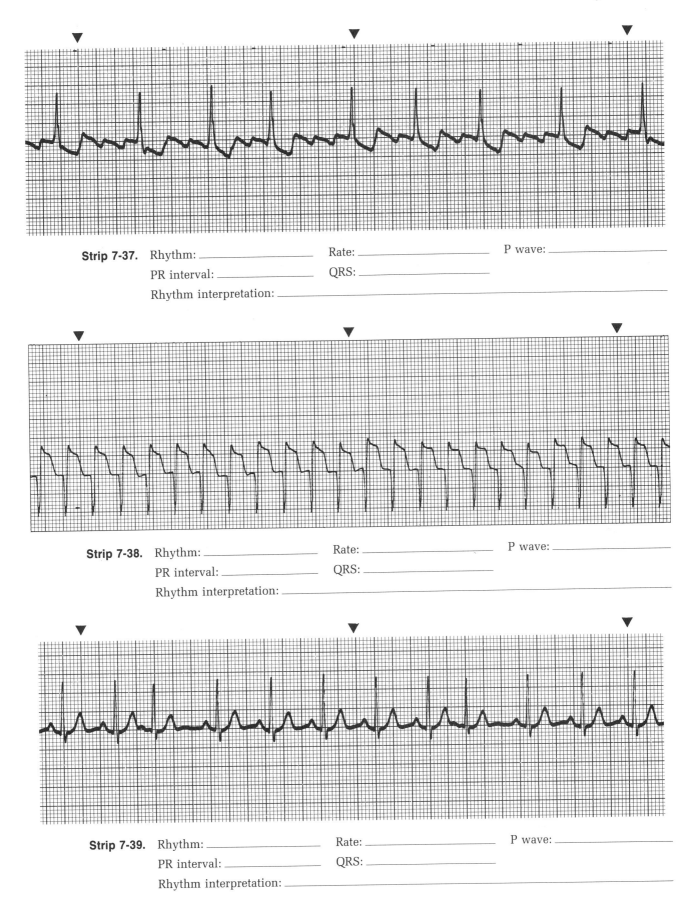

Strip 7-37. Rhythm: _____ Rate: _____ P wave: _____

PR interval: _____ QRS: _____

Rhythm interpretation: _____

Strip 7-38. Rhythm: _____ Rate: _____ P wave: _____

PR interval: _____ QRS: _____

Rhythm interpretation: _____

Strip 7-39. Rhythm: _____ Rate: _____ P wave: _____

PR interval: _____ QRS: _____

Rhythm interpretation: _____

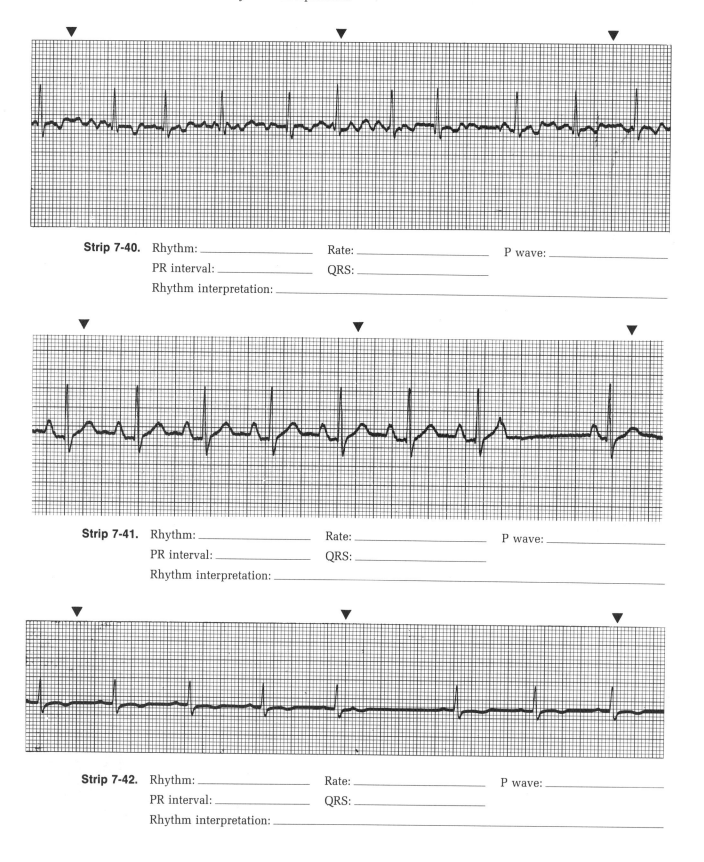

Strip 7-40. Rhythm: _____ Rate: _____ P wave: _____

PR interval: _____ QRS: _____

Rhythm interpretation: _____

Strip 7-41. Rhythm: _____ Rate: _____ P wave: _____

PR interval: _____ QRS: _____

Rhythm interpretation: _____

Strip 7-42. Rhythm: _____ Rate: _____ P wave: _____

PR interval: _____ QRS: _____

Rhythm interpretation: _____

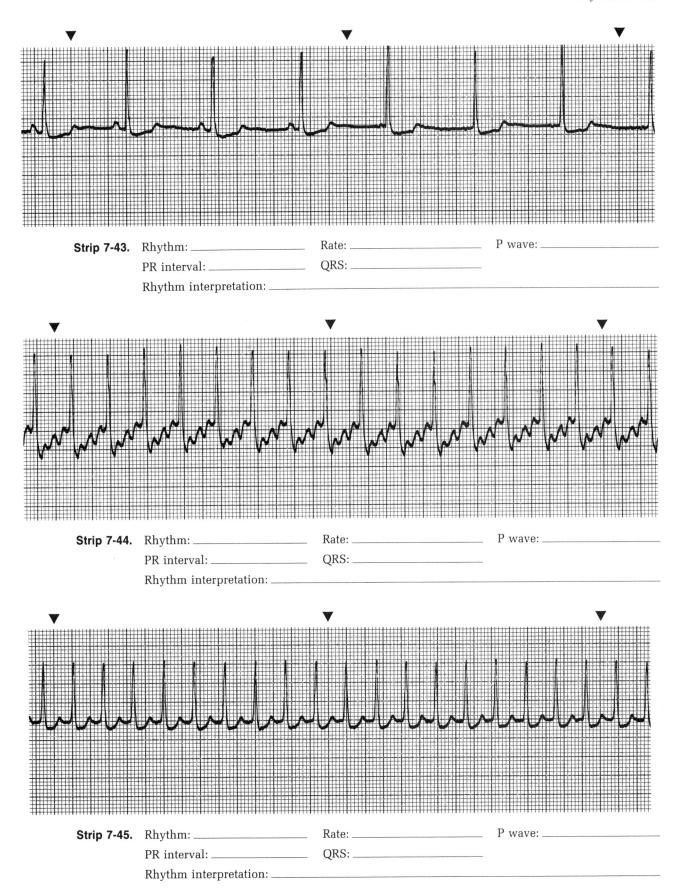

Strip 7-43. Rhythm: _____ Rate: _____ P wave: _____

PR interval: _____ QRS: _____

Rhythm interpretation: _____

Strip 7-44. Rhythm: _____ Rate: _____ P wave: _____

PR interval: _____ QRS: _____

Rhythm interpretation: _____

Strip 7-45. Rhythm: _____ Rate: _____ P wave: _____

PR interval: _____ QRS: _____

Rhythm interpretation: _____

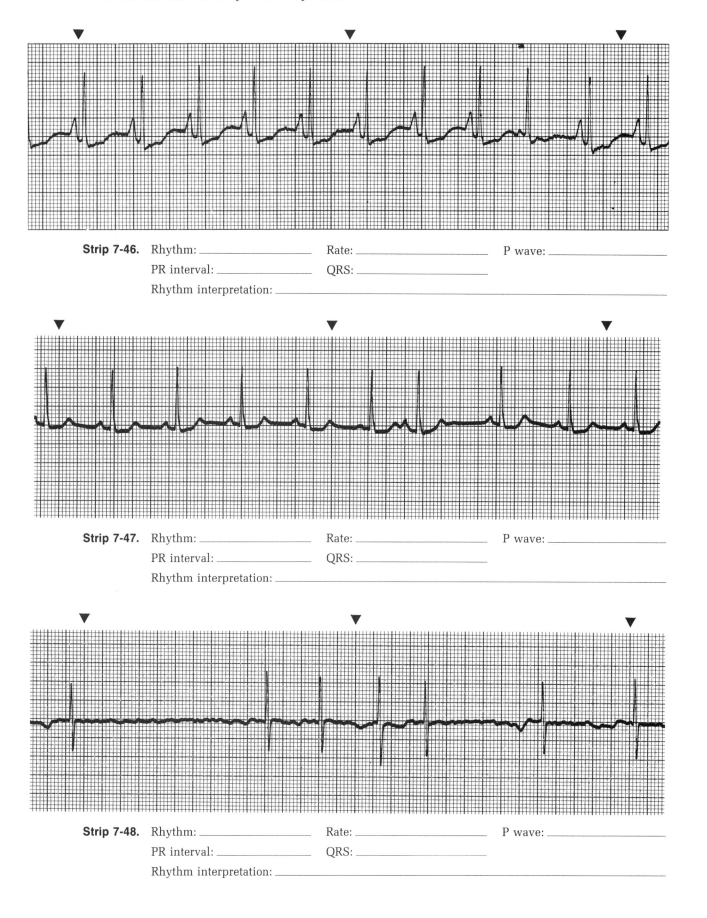

Strip 7-46. Rhythm: _____ Rate: _____ P wave: _____

PR interval: _____ QRS: _____

Rhythm interpretation: _____

Strip 7-47. Rhythm: _____ Rate: _____ P wave: _____

PR interval: _____ QRS: _____

Rhythm interpretation: _____

Strip 7-48. Rhythm: _____ Rate: _____ P wave: _____

PR interval: _____ QRS: _____

Rhythm interpretation: _____

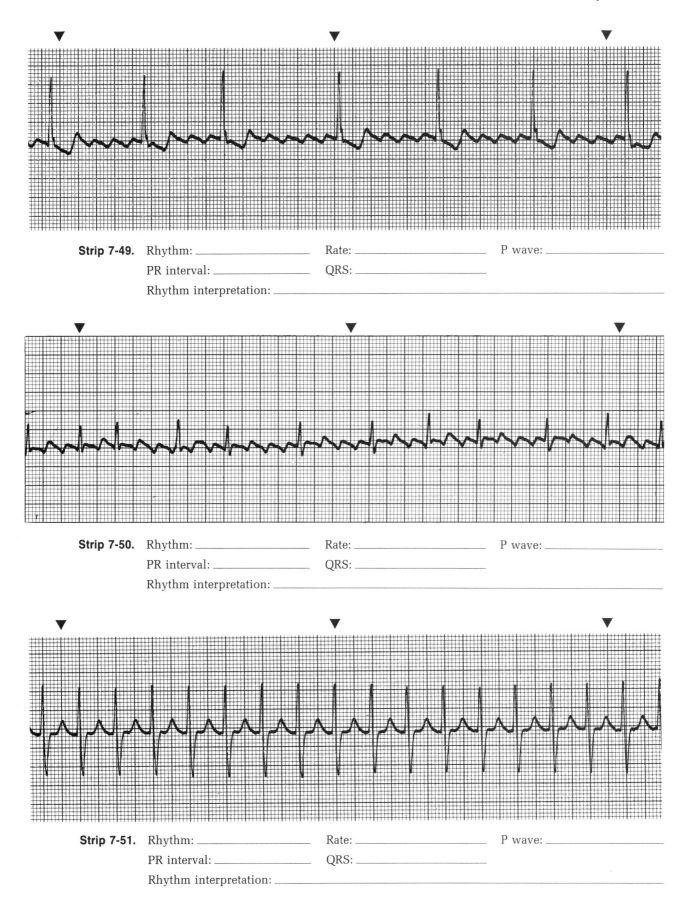

Strip 7-49. Rhythm: _____ Rate: _____ P wave: _____

PR interval: _____ QRS: _____

Rhythm interpretation: _____

Strip 7-50. Rhythm: _____ Rate: _____ P wave: _____

PR interval: _____ QRS: _____

Rhythm interpretation: _____

Strip 7-51. Rhythm: _____ Rate: _____ P wave: _____

PR interval: _____ QRS: _____

Rhythm interpretation: _____

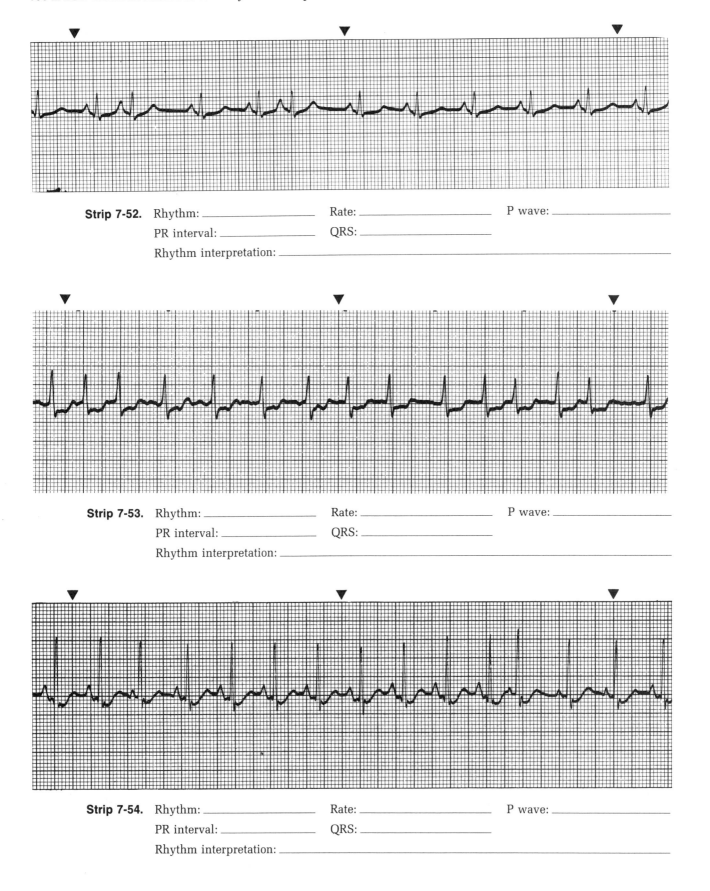

Strip 7-52. Rhythm: _____ Rate: _____ P wave: _____

PR interval: _____ QRS: _____

Rhythm interpretation: _____

Strip 7-53. Rhythm: _____ Rate: _____ P wave: _____

PR interval: _____ QRS: _____

Rhythm interpretation: _____

Strip 7-54. Rhythm: _____ Rate: _____ P wave: _____

PR interval: _____ QRS: _____

Rhythm interpretation: _____

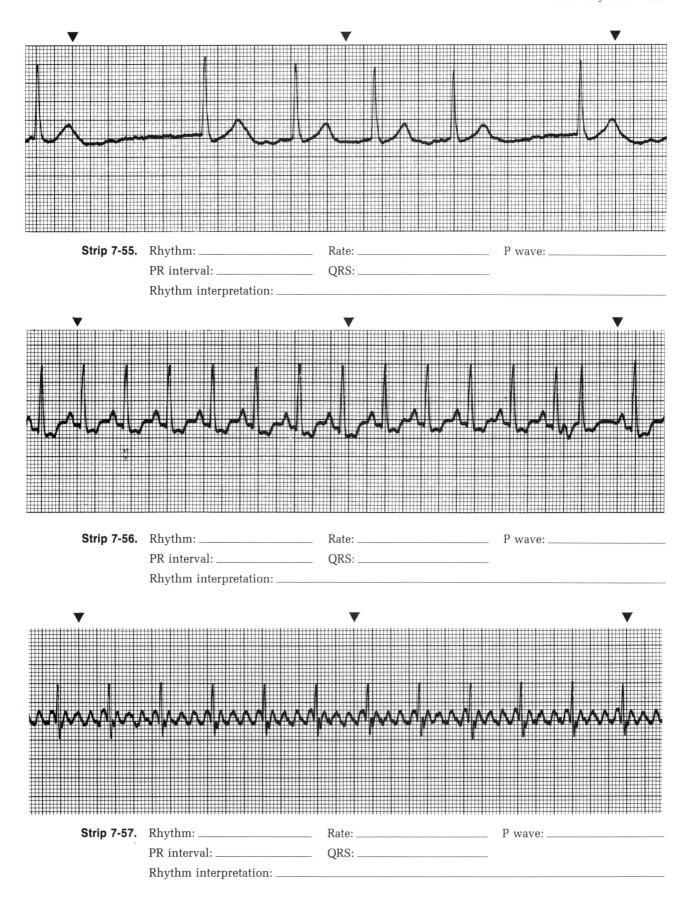

Strip 7-55. Rhythm: _____ Rate: _____ P wave: _____

PR interval: _____ QRS: _____

Rhythm interpretation: _____

Strip 7-56. Rhythm: _____ Rate: _____ P wave: _____

PR interval: _____ QRS: _____

Rhythm interpretation: _____

Strip 7-57. Rhythm: _____ Rate: _____ P wave: _____

PR interval: _____ QRS: _____

Rhythm interpretation: _____

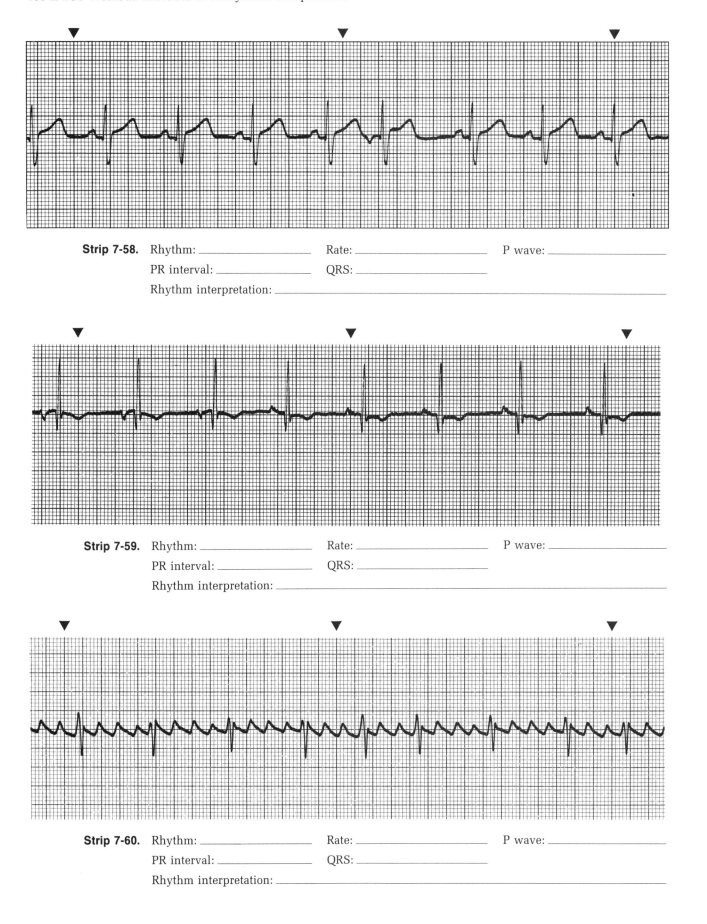

Strip 7-58. Rhythm: _____ Rate: _____ P wave: _____

PR interval: _____ QRS: _____

Rhythm interpretation: _____

Strip 7-59. Rhythm: _____ Rate: _____ P wave: _____

PR interval: _____ QRS: _____

Rhythm interpretation: _____

Strip 7-60. Rhythm: _____ Rate: _____ P wave: _____

PR interval: _____ QRS: _____

Rhythm interpretation: _____

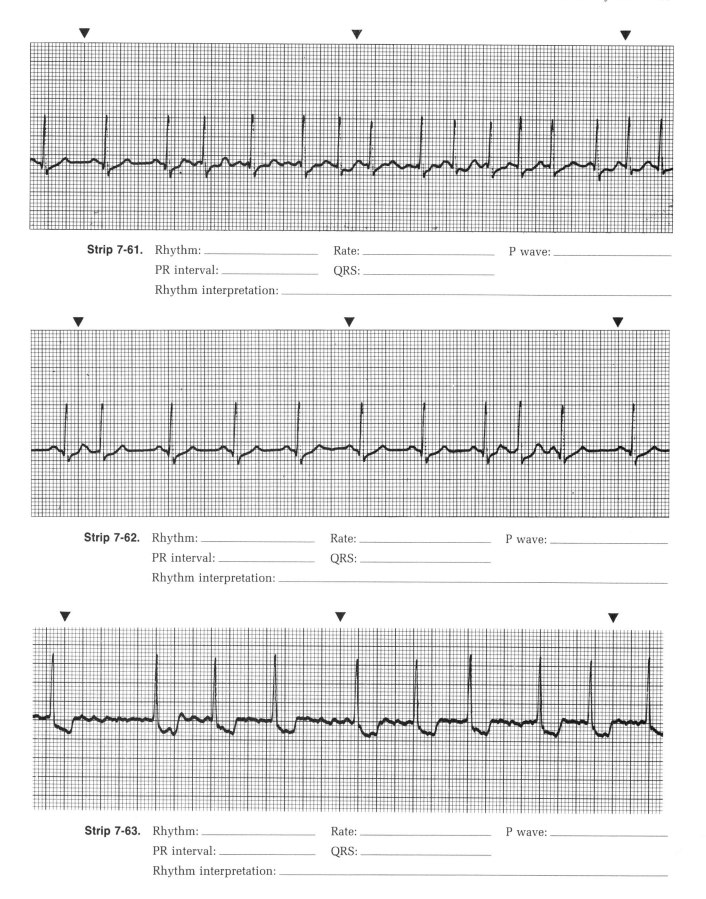

Strip 7-61. Rhythm: _____ Rate: _____ P wave: _____

PR interval: _____ QRS: _____

Rhythm interpretation: _____

Strip 7-62. Rhythm: _____ Rate: _____ P wave: _____

PR interval: _____ QRS: _____

Rhythm interpretation: _____

Strip 7-63. Rhythm: _____ Rate: _____ P wave: _____

PR interval: _____ QRS: _____

Rhythm interpretation: _____

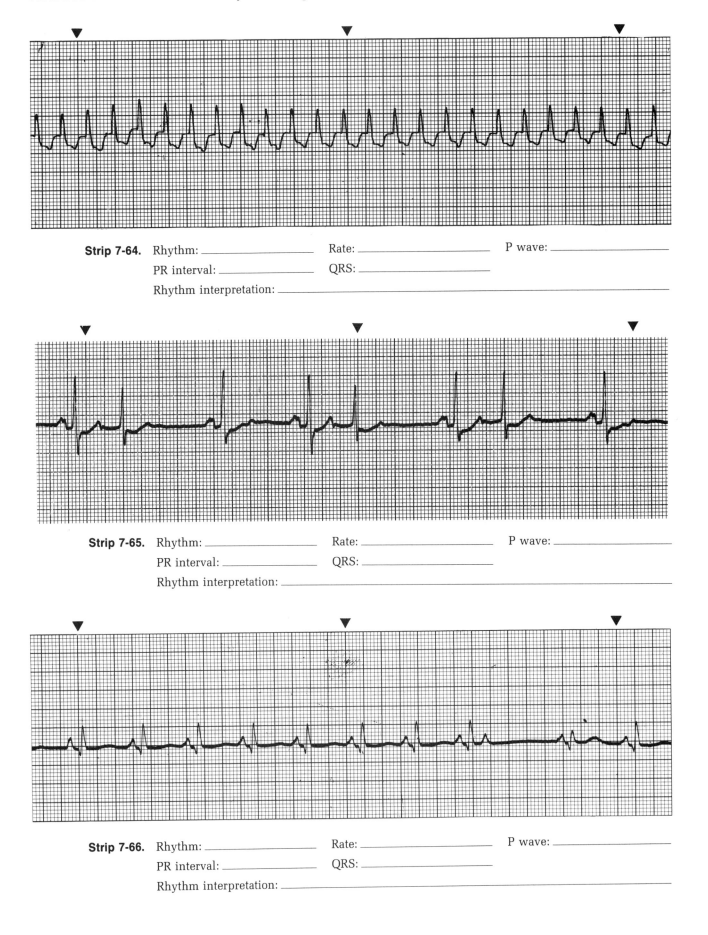

Strip 7-64. Rhythm: _____ Rate: _____ P wave: _____

PR interval: _____ QRS: _____

Rhythm interpretation: _____

Strip 7-65. Rhythm: _____ Rate: _____ P wave: _____

PR interval: _____ QRS: _____

Rhythm interpretation: _____

Strip 7-66. Rhythm: _____ Rate: _____ P wave: _____

PR interval: _____ QRS: _____

Rhythm interpretation: _____

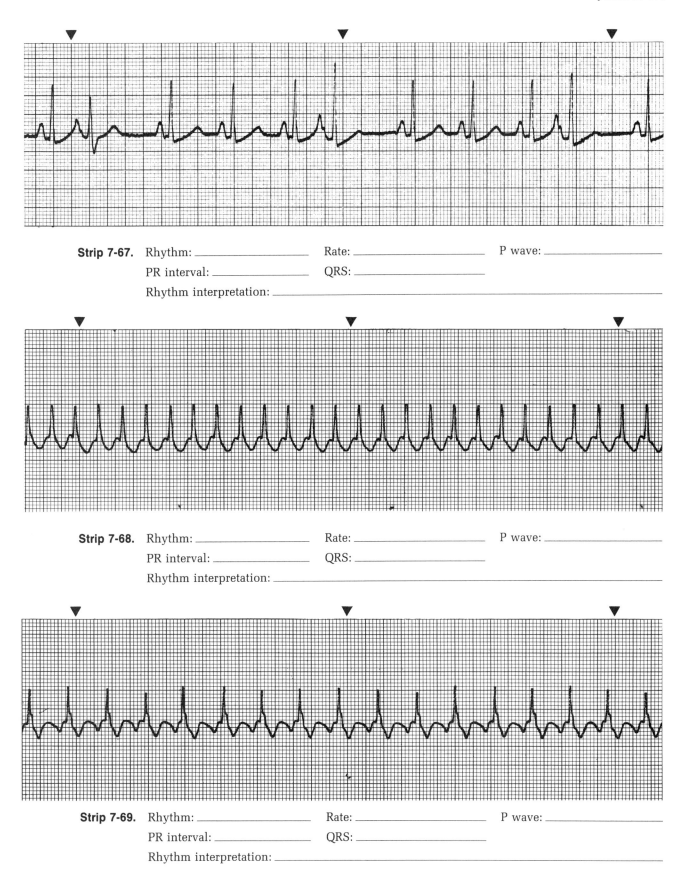

Strip 7-67. Rhythm: _____ Rate: _____ P wave: _____

PR interval: _____ QRS: _____

Rhythm interpretation: _____

Strip 7-68. Rhythm: _____ Rate: _____ P wave: _____

PR interval: _____ QRS: _____

Rhythm interpretation: _____

Strip 7-69. Rhythm: _____ Rate: _____ P wave: _____

PR interval: _____ QRS: _____

Rhythm interpretation: _____

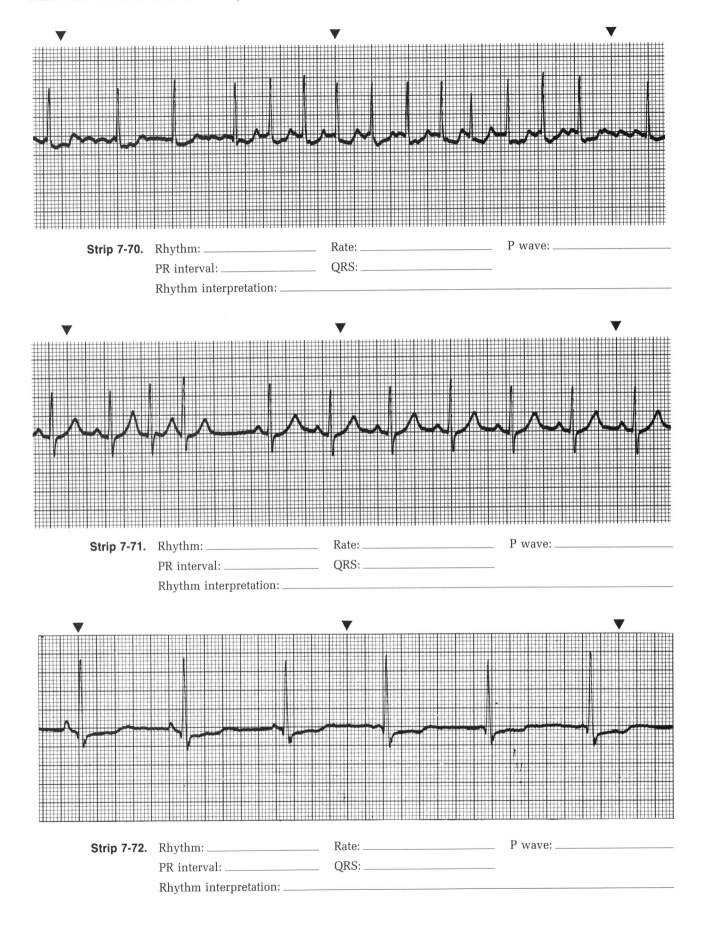

Strip 7-70. Rhythm: _____ Rate: _____ P wave: _____

PR interval: _____ QRS: _____

Rhythm interpretation: _____

Strip 7-71. Rhythm: _____ Rate: _____ P wave: _____

PR interval: _____ QRS: _____

Rhythm interpretation: _____

Strip 7-72. Rhythm: _____ Rate: _____ P wave: _____

PR interval: _____ QRS: _____

Rhythm interpretation: _____

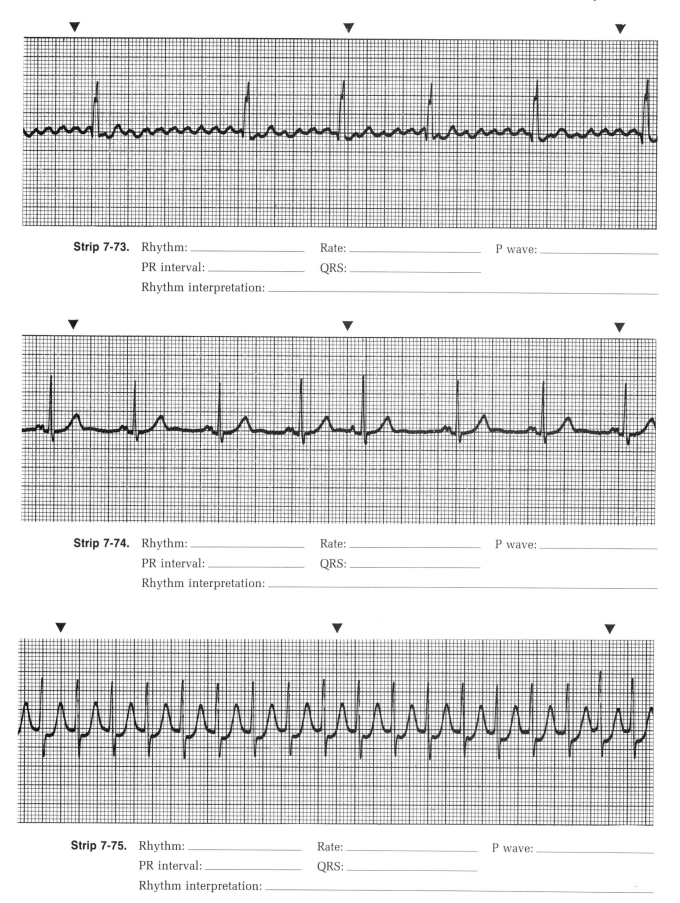

Strip 7-73. Rhythm: _____ Rate: _____ P wave: _____

PR interval: _____ QRS: _____

Rhythm interpretation: _____

Strip 7-74. Rhythm: _____ Rate: _____ P wave: _____

PR interval: _____ QRS: _____

Rhythm interpretation: _____

Strip 7-75. Rhythm: _____ Rate: _____ P wave: _____

PR interval: _____ QRS: _____

Rhythm interpretation: _____

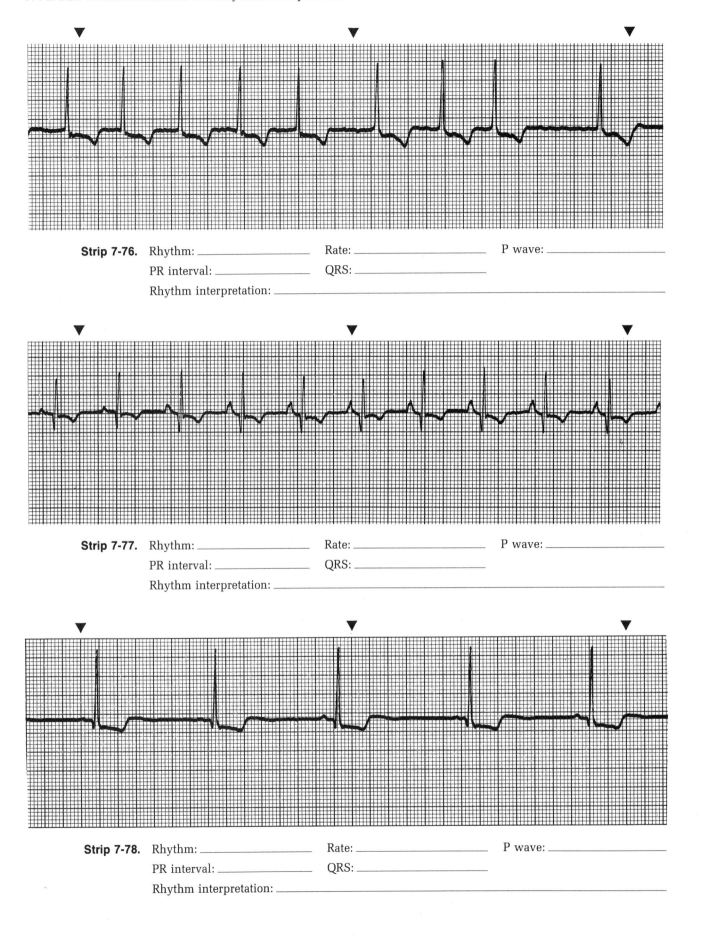

Strip 7-76. Rhythm: _____ Rate: _____ P wave: _____

PR interval: _____ QRS: _____

Rhythm interpretation: _____

Strip 7-77. Rhythm: _____ Rate: _____ P wave: _____

PR interval: _____ QRS: _____

Rhythm interpretation: _____

Strip 7-78. Rhythm: _____ Rate: _____ P wave: _____

PR interval: _____ QRS: _____

Rhythm interpretation: _____

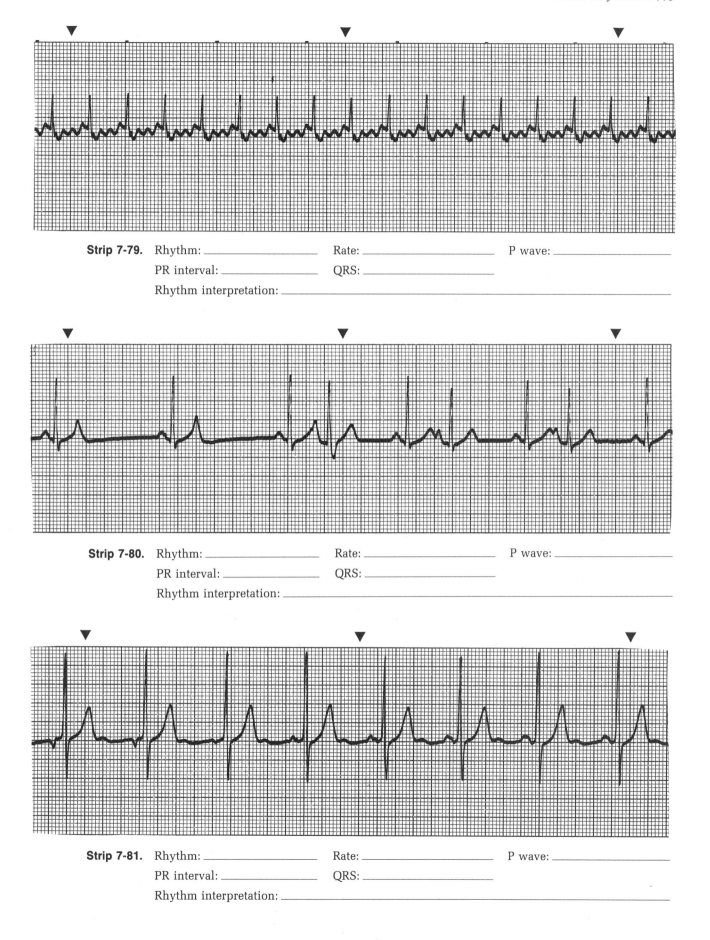

Strip 7-79. Rhythm: _____ Rate: _____ P wave: _____

PR interval: _____ QRS: _____

Rhythm interpretation: _____

Strip 7-80. Rhythm: _____ Rate: _____ P wave: _____

PR interval: _____ QRS: _____

Rhythm interpretation: _____

Strip 7-81. Rhythm: _____ Rate: _____ P wave: _____

PR interval: _____ QRS: _____

Rhythm interpretation: _____

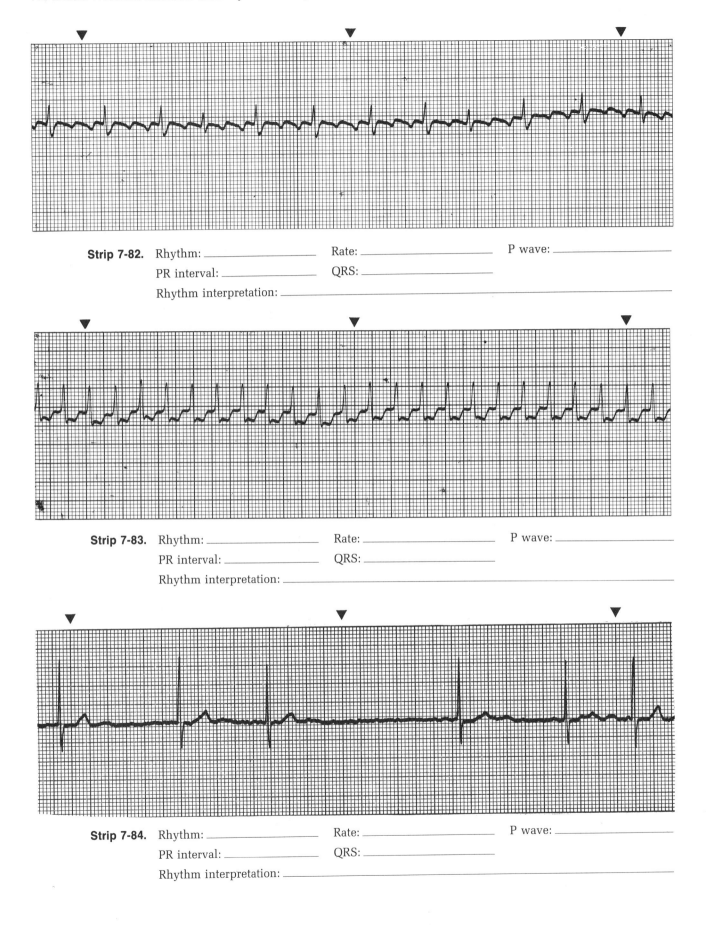

Strip 7-82. Rhythm: _____ Rate: _____ P wave: _____

PR interval: _____ QRS: _____

Rhythm interpretation: _____

Strip 7-83. Rhythm: _____ Rate: _____ P wave: _____

PR interval: _____ QRS: _____

Rhythm interpretation: _____

Strip 7-84. Rhythm: _____ Rate: _____ P wave: _____

PR interval: _____ QRS: _____

Rhythm interpretation: _____

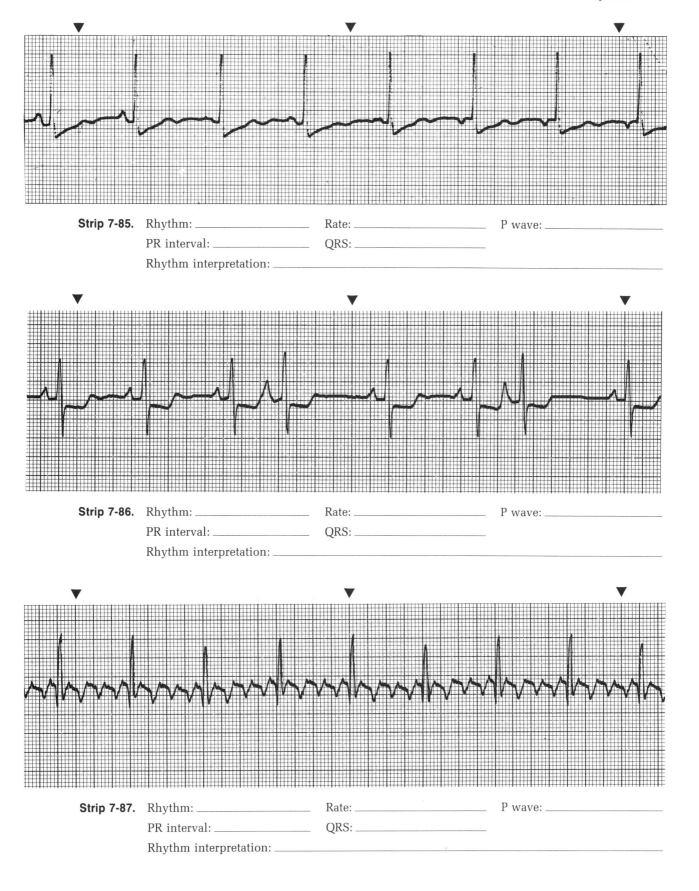

Strip 7-85. Rhythm: _____ Rate: _____ P wave: _____

PR interval: _____ QRS: _____

Rhythm interpretation: _____

Strip 7-86. Rhythm: _____ Rate: _____ P wave: _____

PR interval: _____ QRS: _____

Rhythm interpretation: _____

Strip 7-87. Rhythm: _____ Rate: _____ P wave: _____

PR interval: _____ QRS: _____

Rhythm interpretation: _____

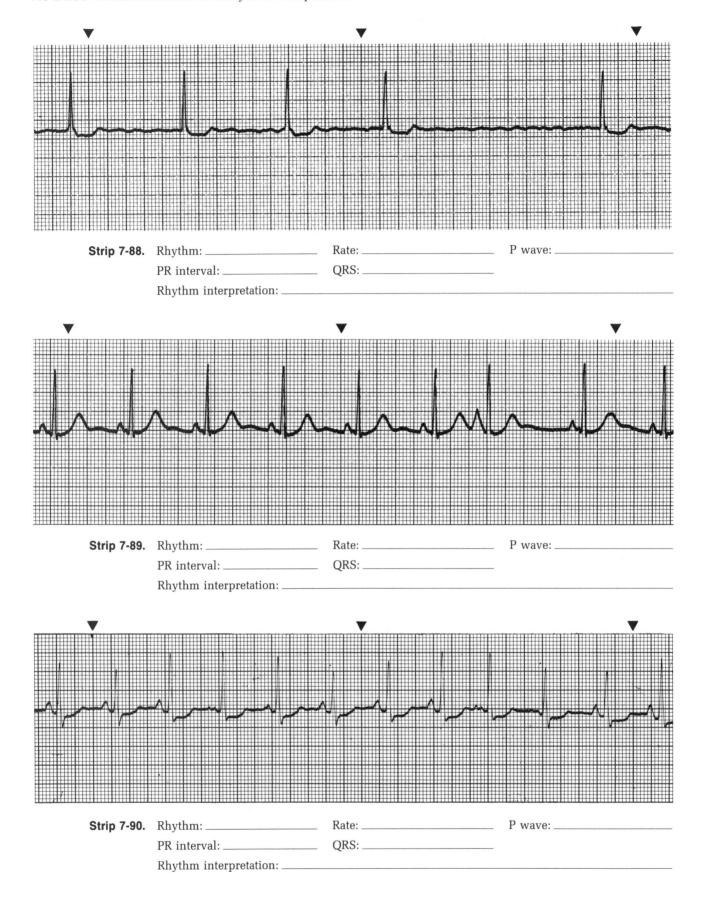

Strip 7-88. Rhythm: _____ Rate: _____ P wave: _____

PR interval: _____ QRS: _____

Rhythm interpretation: _____

Strip 7-89. Rhythm: _____ Rate: _____ P wave: _____

PR interval: _____ QRS: _____

Rhythm interpretation: _____

Strip 7-90. Rhythm: _____ Rate: _____ P wave: _____

PR interval: _____ QRS: _____

Rhythm interpretation: _____

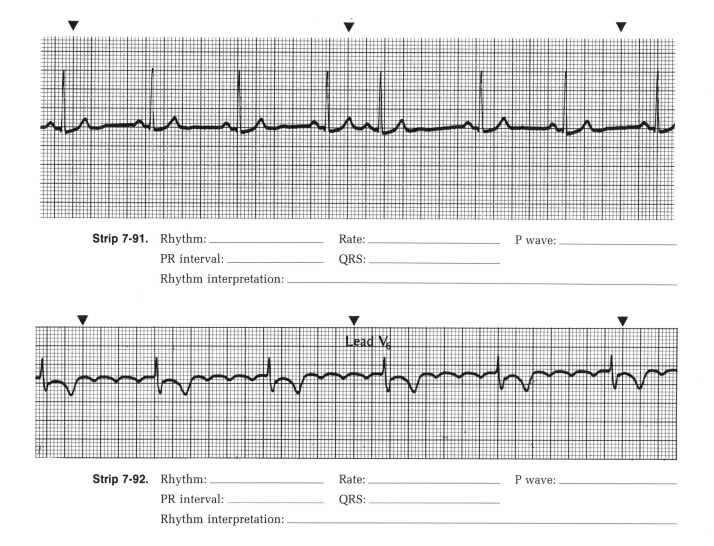

Strip 7-91. Rhythm: _____ Rate: _____ P wave: _____

PR interval: _____ QRS: _____

Rhythm interpretation: _____

Strip 7-92. Rhythm: _____ Rate: _____ P wave: _____

PR interval: _____ QRS: _____

Rhythm interpretation: _____

8

Atrioventricular Junctional Rhythms and Atrioventricular Blocks

Huff J, Doernbach DP, White RD: *ECG WORKOUT: EXERCISES IN ARRHYTHMIA INTERPRETATION, 2nd ed.* © 1993 J.B. Lippincott Company.

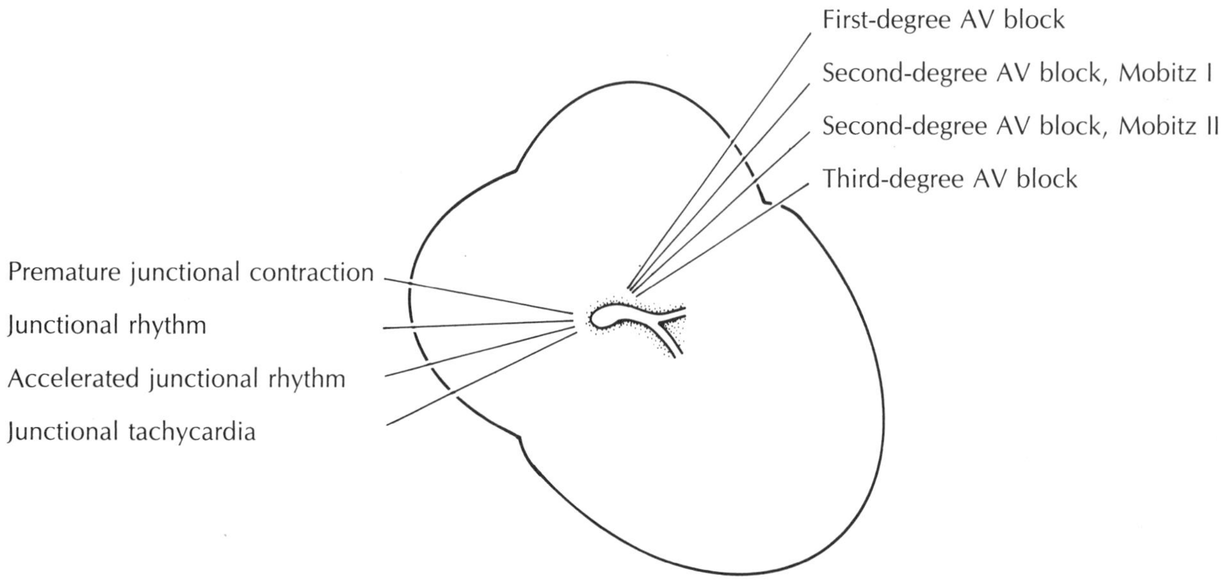

Figure 8-1. AV Junctional Rhythms and AV Blocks

There are two types of dysrhythmias that center in or around the atrioventricular (AV) node: those that are caused by an ectopic focus (AV junctional rhythms) and those caused by a blockage in the AV node area (AV blocks) (Figure 8-1).

AV JUNCTIONAL RHYTHMS

AV junctional rhythms originate in the junctional tissue surrounding the AV node. The junction contains a small cluster of pacemaker cells (p-cells) and can serve as a secondary pacemaker site. The inherent firing rate of these cells is 40 to 60 per minute. A rhythm occurring at this rate is called a junctional rhythm. On some occasions, the rate is accelerated beyond the basic firing rate. Two dysrhythmias may result from this increased activity in the AV junction: accelerated junctional rhythm and junctional tachycardia. The AV junction also can produce premature beats. Junctional rhythms usually occur owing to suppression of the sinoatrial (SA) node as a result of increased parasympathetic activity.

There is a particular conduction sequence that distinguishes these rhythms from others. As the electrical impulse leaves the junctional tissue, it is conducted backward (retrograde) to the atria and forward (antegrade) to the ventricles. Three conduction sequences are possible:

1. If the impulse from the junction depolarizes the atria first and then depolarizes the ventricles, the P wave is in front of the QRS.

2. If the impulse from the junction depolarizes the ventricles first and then depolarizes the atria, the P wave is after the QRS.

3. If the electrical impulse from the junction depolarizes the atria and the ventricles simultaneously, the P wave is hidden within the QRS complex.

In all these conduction sequences, the atria are depolarized in a retrograde fashion. Retrograde conduction produces an inverted P wave in positive electrocardiogram (ECG) leads and an upright P wave in negative ECG leads. Because the junctional impulse does not follow the normal AV conduction pathway, the PR interval will be less than 0.12 seconds. Antegrade conduction of the impulse to the ventricles is usually normal, resulting in a normal QRS complex (Box 8-1).

Box 8-1. AV Junctional Rhythms—Identifying Features

1. P waves can be
   a. before the QRS
   b. after the QRS
   c. hidden in the QRS.
2. P waves will be inverted in positive leads and upright in negative leads.
3. PR interval will be less than 0.12 seconds.
4. QRS width will be normal.

AV BLOCKS

AV blocks originate in the sinus node. Because the SA node is the impulse origin, sinus P waves will be present. The electrical impulse is conducted normally to the AV node, where it is delayed or blocked.

AV blocks are categorized into first-degree AV block, second-degree AV block, and third-degree AV block. These classifications are based on the extent of the conduction defect between the atria and the ventricles. In first-degree AV block, the sinus impulse is delayed in the AV node, but each impulse is conducted to the ventricles. In second-degree AV block, some of the sinus impulses fail to be conducted to the ventricles. In third-degree AV block, no impulses are conducted to the ventricles. AV blocks usually develop because of ischemic injury to the AV node or the junctional tissue.

PREMATURE JUNCTIONAL CONTRACTION

A premature junctional contraction (PJC) results from the premature discharge of an ectopic junctional focus. Like the premature atrial contraction (PAC), the premature junctional beat will be accompanied by a normal QRS and followed by a pause that is usually noncompensatory. Owing to retrograde conduction to the atria, several features distinguish this premature beat from the atrial premature beat. The P wave of the PJC will be inverted in positive ECG leads and upright in negative ECG leads with a PR interval of less than 0.12 seconds. The P wave can occur in three different patterns: before the QRS, after the QRS, or hidden in the QRS complex.

PJCs do not constitute a basic rhythm but occur in conjunction with the sinus rhythms. They may occur as a single beat, every other beat (bigeminal PJCs), every third beat (trigeminal PJCs), in pairs, or

in runs. When PJCs occur in runs of three or more, the rhythm is called paroxysmal junctional tachycardia.

Treatment of PJCs generally is not necessary. PJCs usually reflect irritability of the junctional tissues secondary to ischemic injury to the AV node.

On some occasions, a junctional beat may occur late instead of early. These beats are called junctional escape beats. The characteristics of the late beat will be the same as the PJC. Junctional escape beats are common following any pause in the sinus rhythm (eg, sinus arrest or block, nonconducted PAC). Escape beats require no treatment. It is important, however, to identify the cause of the pause so that appropriate intervention can be initiated, if necessary (Box 8-2) (Figures 8-2 and 8-3).

Box 8-2. Premature Junctional Contraction— Identifying Features

Rhythm:	Irregular owing to premature beat and pause
Rate:	Usually normal but can occur with sinus bradycardia or sinus tachycardia
P wave:	Premature, abnormal; will be inverted in positive leads and upright in negative leads; can occur before, after, or be hidden in the QRS complex
PR:	Less than 0.12 seconds
QRS:	Normal

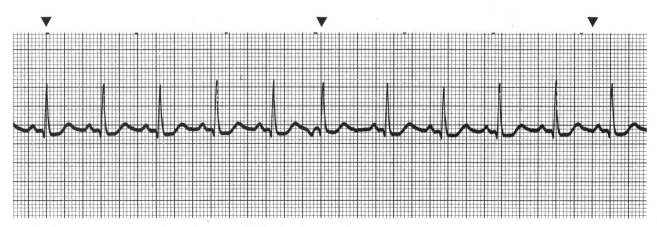

Figure 8-2. Normal Sinus Rhythm with One PJC

Rhythm:	Basic rhythm regular; irregular with PJC
Rate:	Basic rhythm rate 94
P waves:	Sinus P waves with basic rhythm; inverted P wave with PJC
PR:	0.14 to 0.16 seconds (basic rhythm) 0.08 seconds (PJC)
QRS:	0.08 seconds
Comment:	ST segment depression is present.

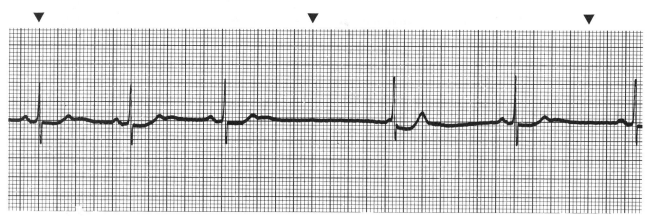

Figure 8-3. Normal Sinus Rhythm with a Junctional Escape Beat

Rhythm: Basic rhythm regular; irregular with escape beat

Rate: Basic rhythm 60; rate slows to 45 after escape beat. Rate suppression can occur following a premature or escape beat. After several cycles the rate will return to the basic rate.

P waves: Sinus P waves with basic rhythm; hidden P wave with escape beat

PR: 0.16 seconds

QRS: 0.06 seconds

Comment: ST segment depression and a U wave are present.

JUNCTIONAL RHYTHM

A junctional rhythm occurs when the impulse originates in the junctional tissue surrounding the AV node and impulses are discharged at a rate of 40 to 60 per minute. The junctional impulse is conducted backward to the atria and forward to the ventricles. Depending on the speed of retrograde and antegrade conduction, the P waves may precede, follow, or be hidden within the QRS complex. The P waves will be inverted in positive leads and upright in negative leads. The PR interval is short (less than 0.12 seconds), and the QRS is normal.

A junctional rhythm (often called junctional escape rhytnm) is basically a slow, passive rhythm that takes over when the SA node discharges impulses too slowly (as in sinus bradycardia) or during pauses in the basic sinus rhythm (sinus arrest or block, nonconducted PAC, or Mobitz I). The suppression of the SA node, which permits a junctional rhythm to develop, is often the result of excessive vagal activity.

Although some individuals tolerate a junctional rhythm without difficulty, the rhythm is potentially dangerous because the AV node is a less dependable pacemaker. The slow rate may decrease cardiac output and lead to myocardial ischemia or heart failure. The slow rate may also allow PVCs to occur.

Atropine can be used to increase the discharge rate of the SA node, allowing it to regain control. If the slow heart rate compromises circulation, a transvenous pacemaker should be used to increase

cardiac output. If PVCs develop in the presence of a junctional rhythm, they are best controlled by rate acceleration (atropine or cardiac pacing). Lidocaine is less effective in controlling PVCs that develop during slow heart rates (Box 8-3) (Figures 8-4 and 8-5).

Box 8-3.	Junctional Rhythm—Identifying Features
Rhythm:	Regular
Rate:	40 to 60
P waves:	Inverted in positive leads and upright in negative leads; can occur before, after, or be hidden in the QRS complex
PR:	Short (less than 0.12 seconds)
QRS:	Normal

ACCELERATED JUNCTIONAL RHYTHM

An accelerated junctional rhythm occurs when the impulse originates in the junctional tissue surrounding the AV node and impulses are discharged at a rate between 60 and 100 per minute. The term "accelerated" denotes a rate faster than the inherent AV nodal rate (40 to 60) but less than 100 per minute.

Like junctional rhythm, the impulse is conducted retrograde to the atria and antegrade to the

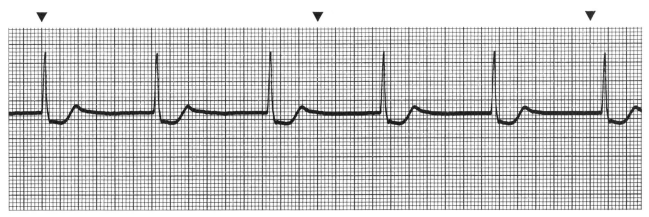

Figure 8-4. Junctional Rhythm

Rhythm: Regular

Rate: 50

P waves: Hidden in QRS complexes

PR: Not measurable

QRS: 0.06 to 0.08 seconds

Comment: ST segment depression is present.

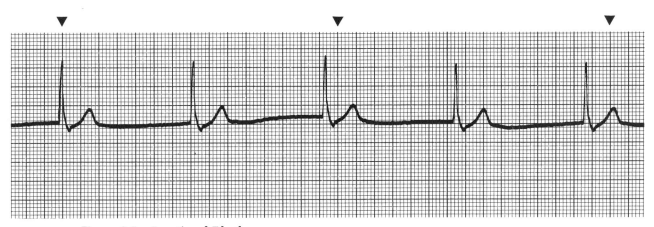

Figure 8-5. Junctional Rhythm

Rhythm: Regular

Rate: 42

P waves: Inverted after QRS

PR: 0.04 seconds

QRS: 0.08 seconds

ventricles. The ECG features are identical to those of junctional rhythm except for the ventricular rate.

The most common cause of the rhythm is digitalis excess, although it can occur following open heart surgery and myocardial infarction. If the patient tolerates the dysrhythmia well, careful monitoring and attention to the underlying heart disease is usually all that is required. If digitalis toxicity is the cause, the drug must be stopped (Box 8-4) (Figure 8-6).

Box 8-4. Accelerated Junctional Rhythm—Identifying Features

Rhythm: Regular

Rate: 60 to 100

P waves: Inverted in positive leads and upright in negative leads; can occur before, after, or be hidden in the QRS complex

PR: Short (less than 0.12 seconds)

QRS: Normal

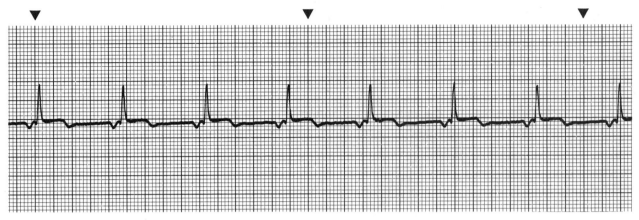

Figure 8-6. Accelerated Junctional Rhythm

Rhythm: Regular

Rate: 65

P waves: Inverted before each QRS

PR: 0.08 to 0.10 seconds

QRS: 0.08 seconds

Comment: ST segment elevation and T wave inversion are present.

PAROXYSMAL JUNCTIONAL TACHYCARDIA

Paroxysmal junctional tachycardia occurs when the impulse originates in the junctional tissue surrounding the AV node and impulses are discharged at a rate greater than 100 per minute. Paroxysmal junctional tachycardia will begin and end suddenly in a manner similar to paroxysmal atrial tachycardia. Paroxysmal junctional tachycardia can be considered as a series of three or more consecutive PJCs occurring at a rapid rate.

The conduction sequence and associated ECG features are identical to those of the other junctional rhythms. The only feature that differs is the ventricular rate.

It is often impossible to distinguish paroxysmal junctional tachycardia from paroxysmal atrial tachycardia electrocardiographically. The P waves are frequently obscured in both these rhythms. In this situation, the two dysrhythmias can be called paroxysmal supraventricular tachycardia, indicating that the location of the ectopic focus may be atrial or junctional.

Paroxysmal junctional tachycardia can occur in patients who have no structural heart disease. It also can occur from metabolic disturbances or develop secondary to ischemia in the AV junction. Paroxysmal junctional tachycardia may decrease cardiac output and increase myocardial oxygen demands, predisposing the individual to left ventricular failure and myocardial ischemia.

Priorities of treatment depend on the person's tolerance of the rhythm. If the patient is stable, vagal maneuvers (valsalva, ice water facial immersion, carotid sinus massage) serve as the first line of therapy. If vagal maneuvers fail, adenosine, verapamil, diltiazem, or propranolol intravenously may be used. Patients who fail to respond to drug therapy can be treated with synchronized electrical shock. Cardioversion is the initial treatment in patients who are hemodynamically unstable (Box 8-5) (Figure 8-7).

Box 8-5.	Paroxysmal Junctional Tachycardia—Identifying Features
Rhythm:	Regular
Rate:	Over 100
P waves:	Inverted in positive leads and upright in negative leads; can occur before, after, or be hidden in the QRS complex
PR:	Short (less than 0.12 seconds)
QRS:	Normal

FIRST-DEGREE AV BLOCK

In first-degree AV block, the sinus impulses are delayed in the AV node, but all are conducted to the ventricles. The sinus impulse is conducted normally to the AV node. On arrival at the AV junction, the impulse is temporarily delayed before being con-

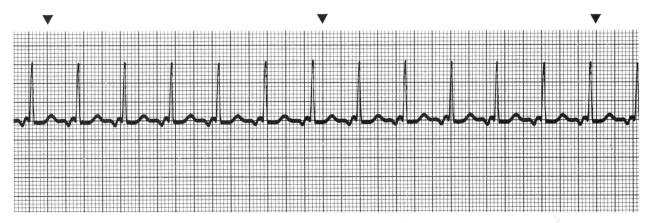

Figure 8-7. Paroxysmal Junctional Tachycardia

Rhythm: Regular

Rate: 115

P waves: Inverted before each QRS

PR: 0.08 seconds

QRS: 0.06 to 0.08 seconds

ducted to the ventricles. The delay results in a prolonged PR interval. This rhythm is reflected on the ECG as a regular rhythm with one P wave to each QRS complex and a PR interval greater than 0.20 seconds.

First-degree AV block may be caused by ischemic injury to the AV node or surrounding tissue secondary to acute myocardial infarction. Drugs such as digitalis, the beta-blockers, and the calcium antagonists (other than nifedipine) prolong AV conduction time and may be responsible for the development of first-degree AV block. This rhythm does not reduce hemodynamic efficiency and requires no specific

treatment. One should observe the rhythm to detect progression to a more severe degree of AV block (Box 8-6) (Figure 8-8).

Box 8-6.	First-degree AV Block—Identifying Features
Rhythm:	Regular
Rate:	Usually normal
P waves:	Sinus P waves present; one P wave to each QRS
PR:	Prolonged (greater than 0.20 seconds)
QRS:	Normal

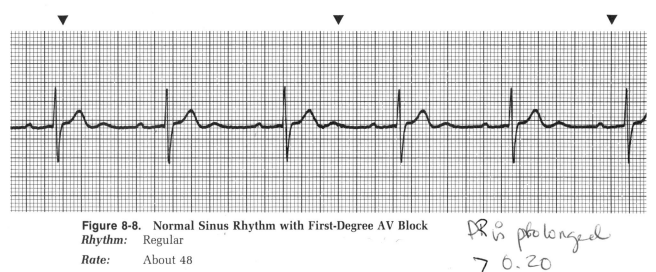

Figure 8-8. Normal Sinus Rhythm with First-Degree AV Block

Rhythm: Regular

Rate: About 48

P waves: Sinus P waves present; One P wave to each QRS

PR: 0.28 to 0.32 seconds

QRS: 0.08 to 0.10 seconds.

Note: A U wave is present.

PR is prolonged 7 0.20

usually not treated

SECOND-DEGREE AV BLOCK, MOBITZ I

In second-degree AV block, Mobitz I, some of the sinus impulses are not conducted to the ventricles. The sinus impulse is transmitted normally to the AV node. Transmission through the AV node takes longer with each successive impulse until an impulse fails to be conducted to the ventricles. This intermittent failure of impulse conduction through the AV node is reflected on the ECG by progressively lengthening PR intervals followed by a dropped QRS complex and a pause. This sequence is then repeated in cyclic fashion.

Mobitz I can be confused with the nonconducted PAC. Both rhythms have P waves not accompanied by a QRS but followed by a pause. To distinguish between these two rhythms, one must examine the configuration of the P waves and the PP regularity. The nonconducted PAC will have an abnormal P wave and occur prematurely. In Mobitz I, the P wave configuration remains the same, and the P wave will occur on schedule.

Common causes of Mobitz I include ischemia to the AV node usually secondary to inferior myocardial infarction. It is usually a temporary disorder and subsides spontaneously within 72 to 96 hours. This type of second-degree AV block usually does not require therapy (Box 8-7) (Figure 8-9).

Box 8-7.	Second-degree AV Block, Mobitz I—Identifying Features
Rhythm:	Irregular
Rate:	Usually slow but can be normal
P waves:	Sinus P waves present; some not followed by QRS complexes
PR:	Progressively lengthens
QRS:	Normal

SECOND-DEGREE AV BLOCK, MOBITZ II

Like Mobitz I, second-degree AV block Mobitz II is characterized by failure of some of the sinus impulses to conduct to the ventricles. The sinus impulse is conducted normally to the AV node. The conduction defect is located below the level of the AV node in the bundle of His or the bundle branch area. The sinus impulses usually are blocked at regular intervals, allowing only every second, third, or fourth impulse to be conducted to the ventricles. If the conduction defect is in the bundle of His, the QRS will be normal. The QRS is wide if the conduction defect involves the bundle branches.

This rhythm is reflected on the ECG paper as a regular rhythm with two, three, or four P waves before each QRS and a constant PR interval. The rhythm can be irregular if the conduction ratio varies.

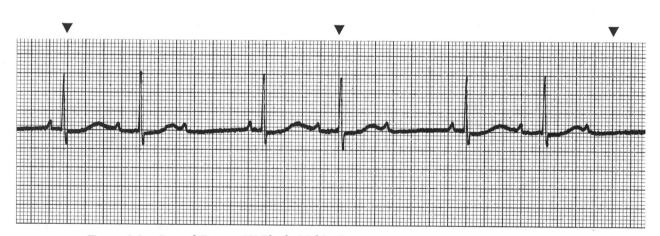

Figure 8-9. Second-Degree AV Block, Mobitz I

Rhythm: Irregular ventricular rhythm

Rate: Atria: 79

Ventricular: 50

P waves: Sinus P waves are present; some P waves not followed by QRS complexes

PR: Progresses from 0.16 to 0.28 seconds

QRS: 0.06 to 0.08 seconds

Mobitz II is much less common than Mobitz I but is far more serious. It is associated with anterior or anteroseptal myocardial infarction and involves ischemic injury to the bundle of His or the bundle branch area. Mobitz II may progress abruptly to third-degree AV block or ventricular standstill.

Because of the unpredictable course of Mobitz II and the threat of sudden third-degree AV block or ventricular standstill, a temporary transvenous pacemaker should be inserted when this rhythm is identified. While preparations are being made for pacemaker insertion, an external pacemaker can be applied. If hypotension is associated with the rhythm, dopamine at a rate of 5 to 20 μg/kg/min or epinephrine at a rate of 2 to 10 μg/kg/min may be infused. Acceleration of the sinus rate in Mobitz II block with vagolytic (atropine) or sympathomimetic (isoproterenol) drugs can worsen the degree of AV

block or produce complete heart block (third-degree AV block). Transcutaneous or transvenous pacing is the intervention of choice (Box 8-8) (Figure 8-10).

THIRD-DEGREE AV BLOCK

In third-degree AV block, all sinus impulses are blocked and none reach the ventricles. The conduction defect is located below the level of the AV node in the bundle of His or the bundle branch area.

Regardless of the site of the block, the atria and ventricles beat independently of each other. The atria are activated by one pacemaker (usually the SA node), and the ventricles are activated by another (either junctional or ventricular). If the block is in the bundle of His, the ventricles will be paced at a rate of 40 to 60 per minute by the junctional tissue and the QRS will be normal. If the block is below the bundle of His in a bundle branch area, the ventricles will be paced at a rate of 30 to 40 per minute by the ventricular tissue, and the QRS will be wide.

This rhythm is reflected on the ECG by a regular rhythm (both atria and ventricles), a PR that varies, and P waves found hidden in QRS complexes and T waves. Third-degree AV block with a junctional pacemaker usually is associated with an inferior myocardial infarction. The rhythm is usually transient and has favorable prognosis. Third-degree AV block with a ventricular pacemaker usually is associated with an anterior myocardial infarction. This rhythm has a less favorable prognosis.

Box 8-8.	Second-degree AV Block, Mobitz II—Identifying Features
Rhythm:	Regular usually; can be irregular if conduction ratios vary
Rate:	Usually slow
P waves:	Two, three, or four P waves before each QRS
PR:	PR interval of beats with QRS is constant; PR interval may be normal or prolonged
QRS:	Normal if block in His bundle; wide if block involves bundle branches

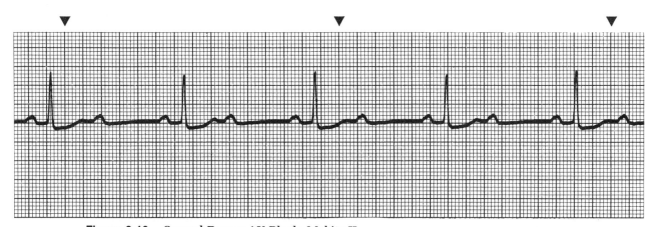

Figure 8-10. Second-Degree AV Block, Mobitz II

Rhythm: Regular

Rate: Atrial: 84

Ventricular: 42

P waves: Two P waves before each QRS

PR: 0.24 seconds

QRS: 0.04 to 0.06 seconds

Because of the unpredictable course of third-degree AV block and the threat of ventricular standstill, a temporary transvenous pacemaker should be inserted when this rhythm is identified. While preparations are being made for pacemaker insertion, an external pacemaker may be applied. Atropine can be used to increase the heart rate in narrow-complex third-degree heart block but is contraindicated in wide-complex third-degree heart block. If hypotension is associated with the rhythm, dopamine at a rate of 5 to 20 μg/kg/min or epinephrine at a rate of 2 to 10 μg/kg/min may be infused (Box 8-9) (Figure 8-11) (Table 8-1).

Box 8-9. Third-degree AV Block—Identifying Features

Rhythm:	Regular
Rate:	40 to 60 if block in His bundle; 30 to 40 if block involves bundle branches
P waves:	Sinus P waves present; bear no relationship to QRS; can be found hidden in QRS complexes and T waves
PR:	Varies greatly
QRS:	Normal if block in His bundle; wide if block involves bundle branches

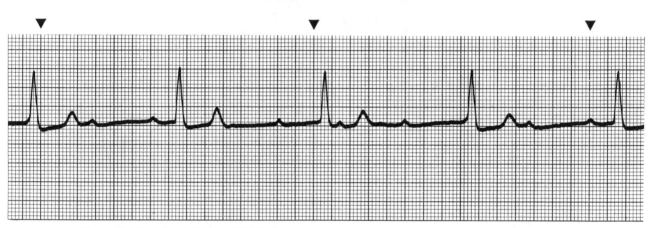

Figure 8-11. Third-degree AV block

Rhythm: Regular

Rate: Atrial: 84

Ventricular: 38

P waves: Sinus P waves present; bear no relationship to QRS; found hidden in QRS and T waves

PR: Varies greatly

QRS: 0.08 to 0.10 seconds.

Table 8-1. AV Block Comparisons

PR Constant	PR Varies
(First-degree)	(Mobitz I)
1. PR constant	1. PR varies
2. PR is long	2. PR progressively gets longer until QRS is dropped
3. One P wave to each QRS	3. Irregular ventricular rhythm in cyclic pattern
4. Regular ventricular rhythm	
(Mobitz II)	(Third-degree)
1. PR constant	1. PR varies
2. PR normal or long	2. P waves bear no relationship to QRS—found hidden in QRS and T waves
3. Two, three, or four P waves to each QRS	3. Regular ventricular rhythm
4. Regular ventricular rhythm (unless conduction ratios vary)	

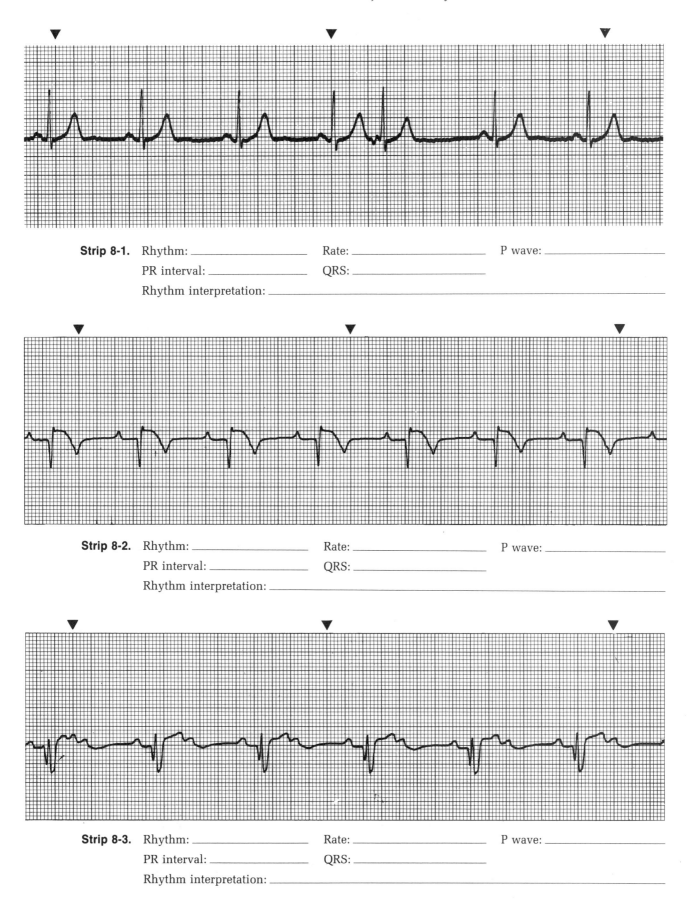

Strip 8-1. Rhythm: _____ Rate: _____ P wave: _____

PR interval: _____ QRS: _____

Rhythm interpretation: _____

Strip 8-2. Rhythm: _____ Rate: _____ P wave: _____

PR interval: _____ QRS: _____

Rhythm interpretation: _____

Strip 8-3. Rhythm: _____ Rate: _____ P wave: _____

PR interval: _____ QRS: _____

Rhythm interpretation: _____

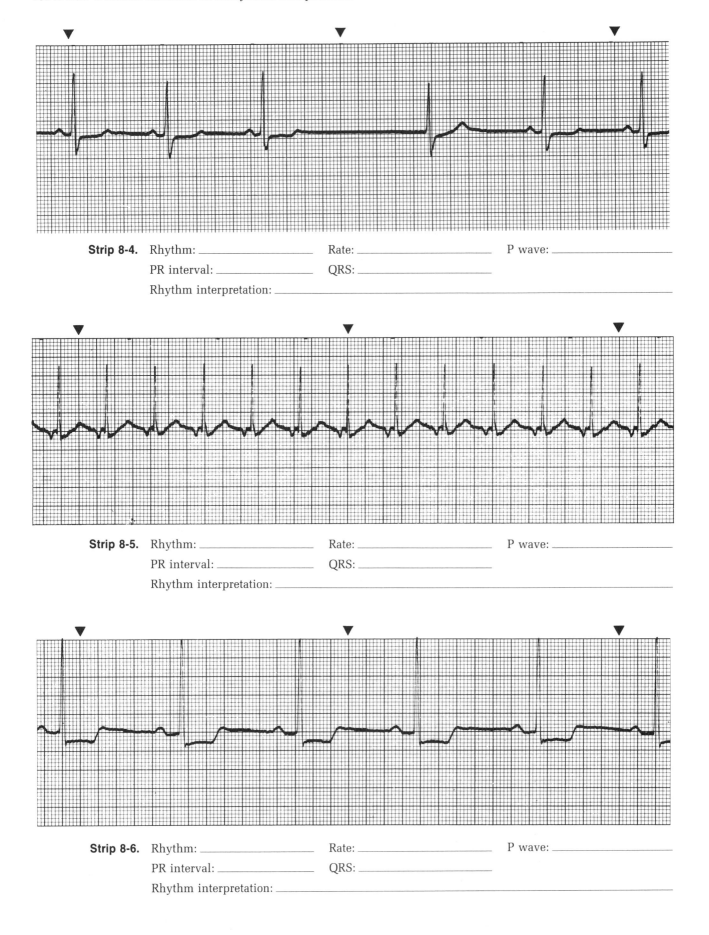

Strip 8-4. Rhythm: _____ Rate: _____ P wave: _____

PR interval: _____ QRS: _____

Rhythm interpretation: _____

Strip 8-5. Rhythm: _____ Rate: _____ P wave: _____

PR interval: _____ QRS: _____

Rhythm interpretation: _____

Strip 8-6. Rhythm: _____ Rate: _____ P wave: _____

PR interval: _____ QRS: _____

Rhythm interpretation: _____

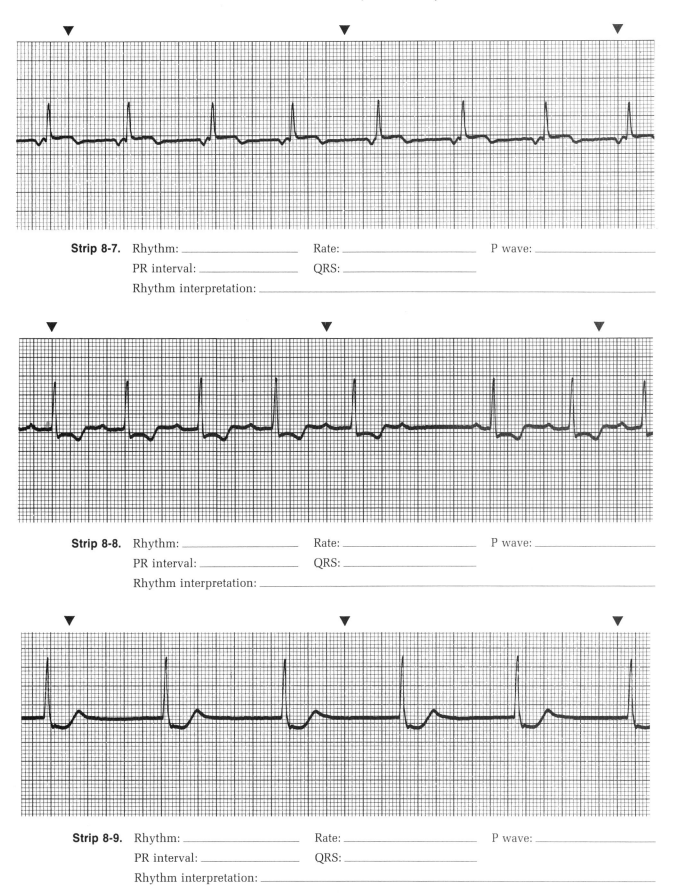

Strip 8-7. Rhythm: _____ Rate: _____ P wave: _____

PR interval: _____ QRS: _____

Rhythm interpretation: _____

Strip 8-8. Rhythm: _____ Rate: _____ P wave: _____

PR interval: _____ QRS: _____

Rhythm interpretation: _____

Strip 8-9. Rhythm: _____ Rate: _____ P wave: _____

PR interval: _____ QRS: _____

Rhythm interpretation: _____

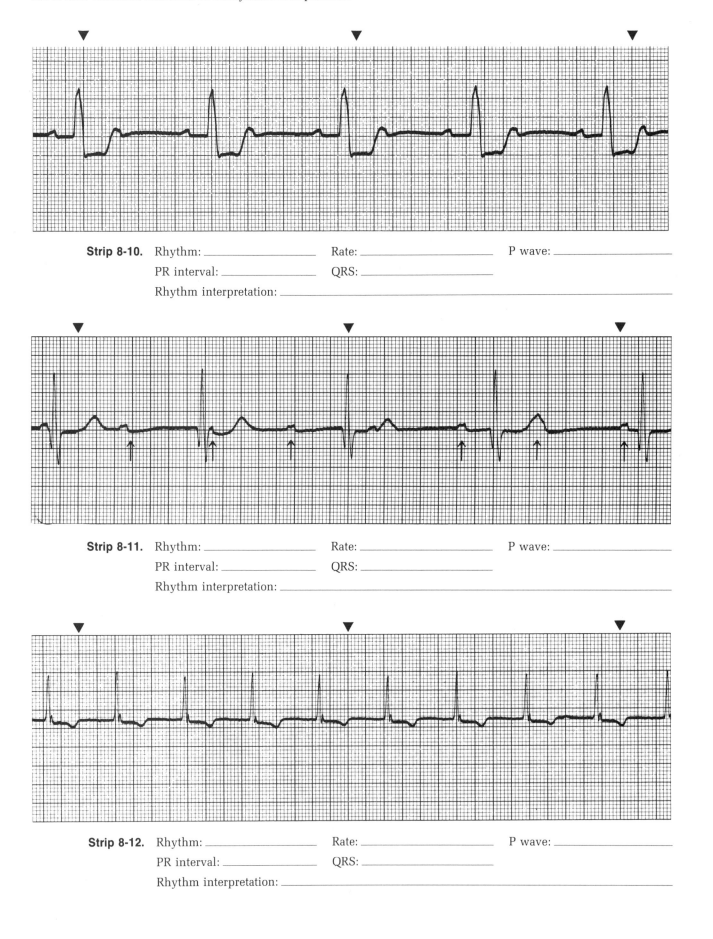

Strip 8-10. Rhythm: _____ Rate: _____ P wave: _____

PR interval: _____ QRS: _____

Rhythm interpretation: _____

Strip 8-11. Rhythm: _____ Rate: _____ P wave: _____

PR interval: _____ QRS: _____

Rhythm interpretation: _____

Strip 8-12. Rhythm: _____ Rate: _____ P wave: _____

PR interval: _____ QRS: _____

Rhythm interpretation: _____

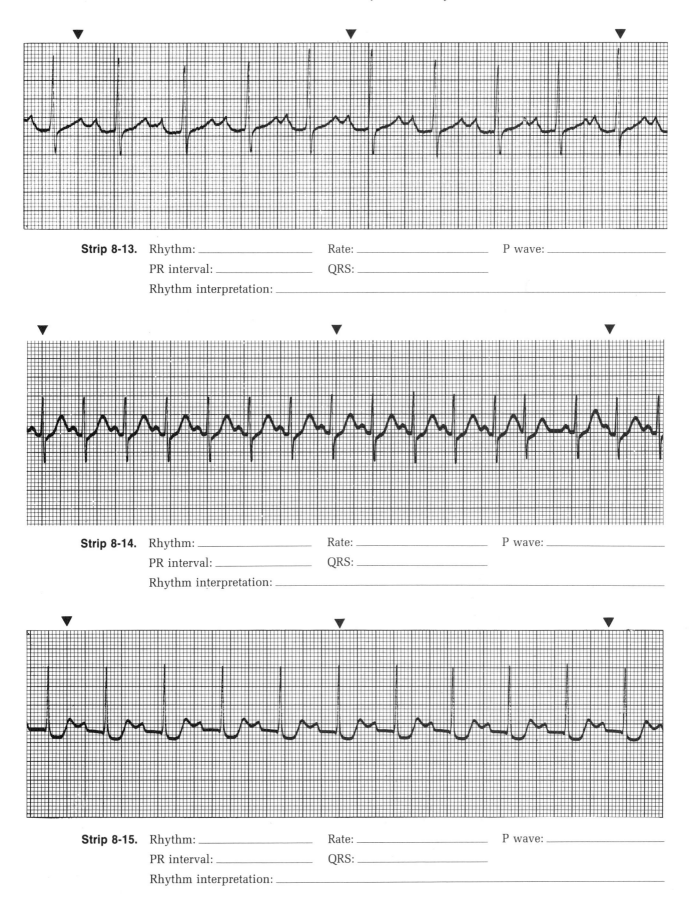

Strip 8-13. Rhythm: _____ Rate: _____ P wave: _____

PR interval: _____ QRS: _____

Rhythm interpretation: _____

Strip 8-14. Rhythm: _____ Rate: _____ P wave: _____

PR interval: _____ QRS: _____

Rhythm interpretation: _____

Strip 8-15. Rhythm: _____ Rate: _____ P wave: _____

PR interval: _____ QRS: _____

Rhythm interpretation: _____

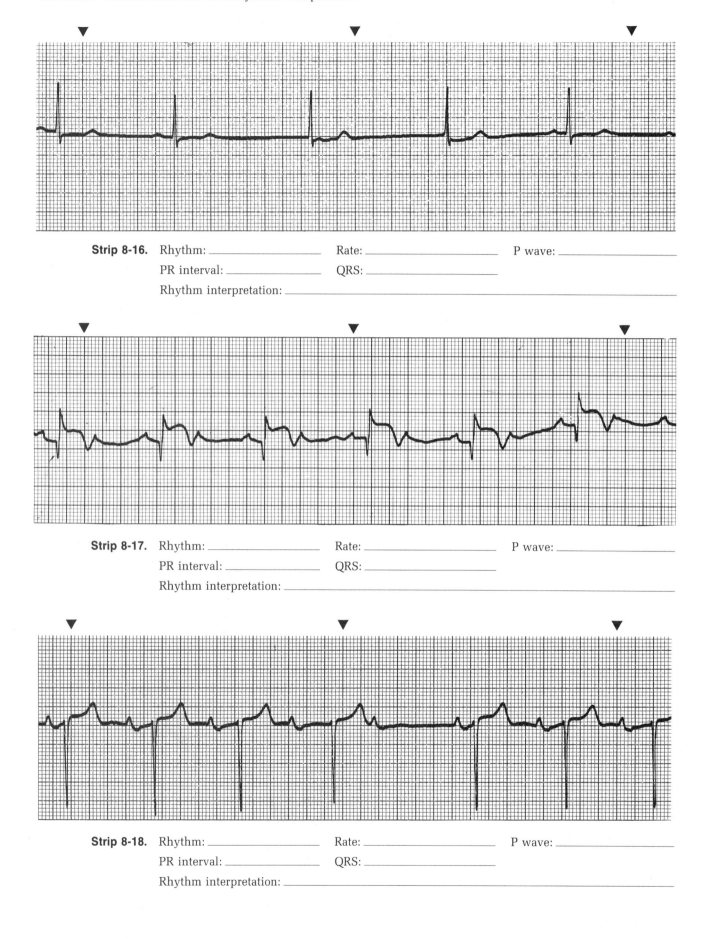

Strip 8-16. Rhythm: _____ Rate: _____ P wave: _____

PR interval: _____ QRS: _____

Rhythm interpretation: _____

Strip 8-17. Rhythm: _____ Rate: _____ P wave: _____

PR interval: _____ QRS: _____

Rhythm interpretation: _____

Strip 8-18. Rhythm: _____ Rate: _____ P wave: _____

PR interval: _____ QRS: _____

Rhythm interpretation: _____

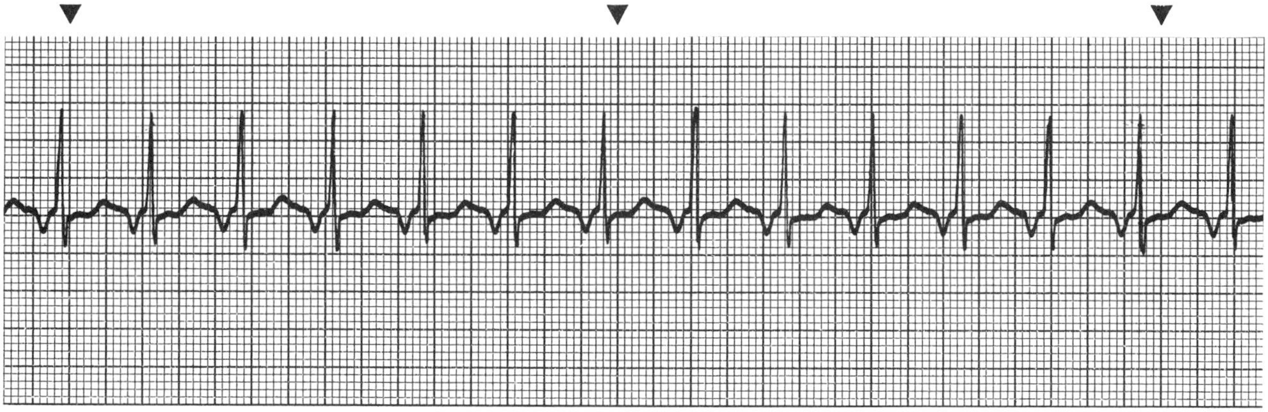

Strip 8-19. Rhythm: _____ Rate: _____ P wave: _____

PR interval: _____ QRS: _____

Rhythm interpretation: _____

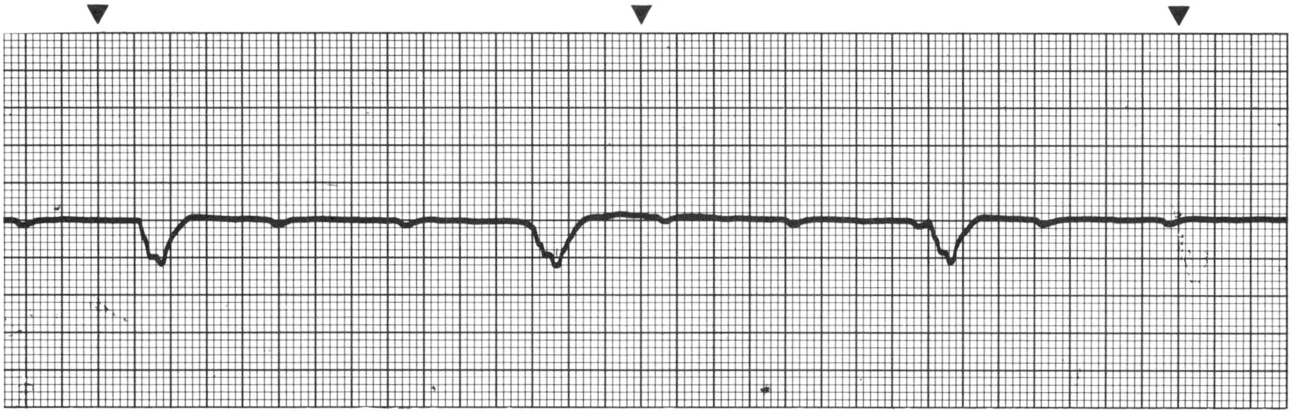

Strip 8-20. Rhythm: _____ Rate: _____ P wave: _____

PR interval: _____ QRS: _____

Rhythm interpretation: _____

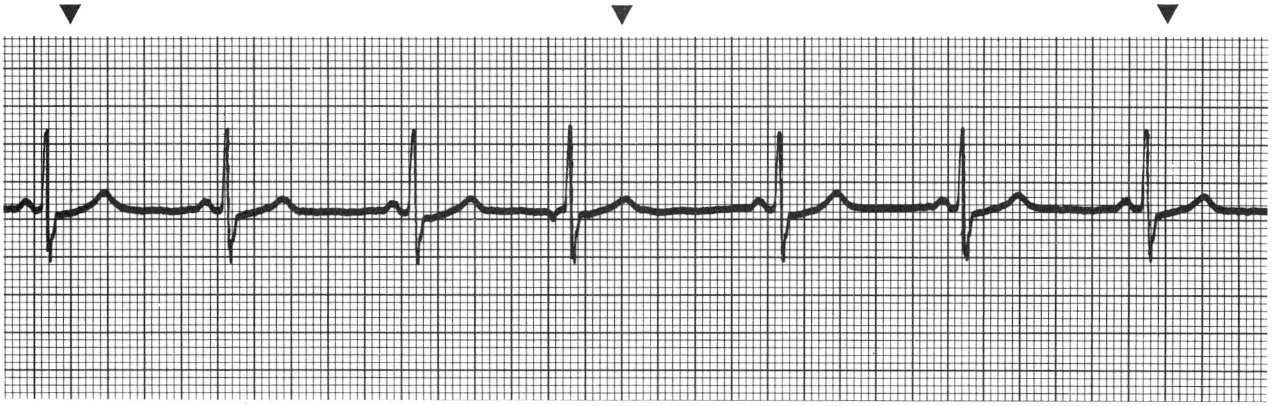

Strip 8-21. Rhythm: _____ Rate: _____ P wave: _____

PR interval: _____ QRS: _____

Rhythm interpretation: _____

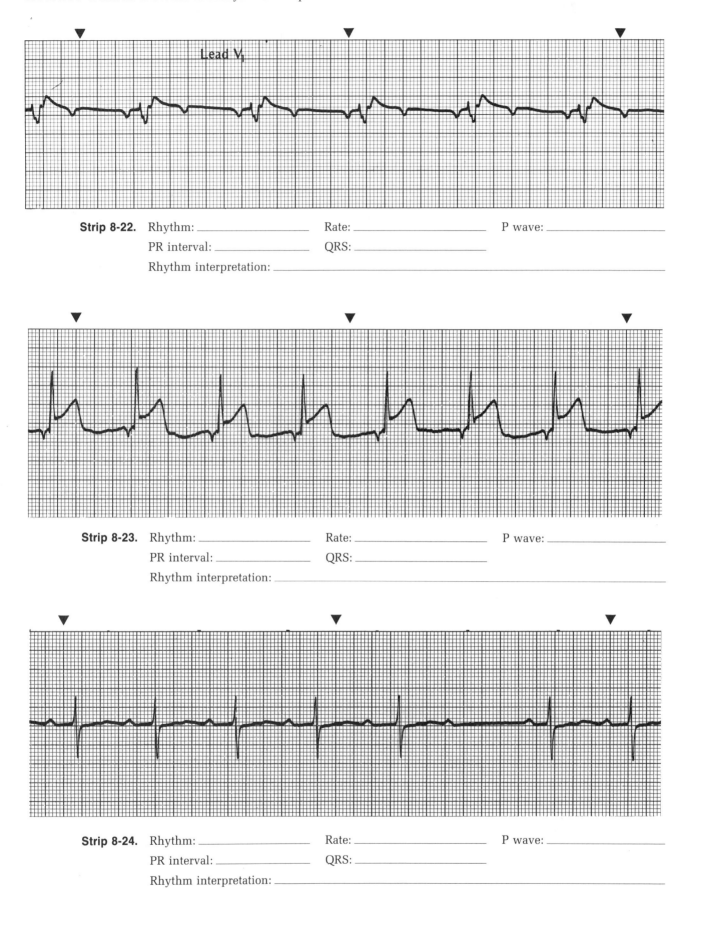

Lead V₁

Strip 8-22. Rhythm: _____ Rate: _____ P wave: _____

PR interval: _____ QRS: _____

Rhythm interpretation: _____

Strip 8-23. Rhythm: _____ Rate: _____ P wave: _____

PR interval: _____ QRS: _____

Rhythm interpretation: _____

Strip 8-24. Rhythm: _____ Rate: _____ P wave: _____

PR interval: _____ QRS: _____

Rhythm interpretation: _____

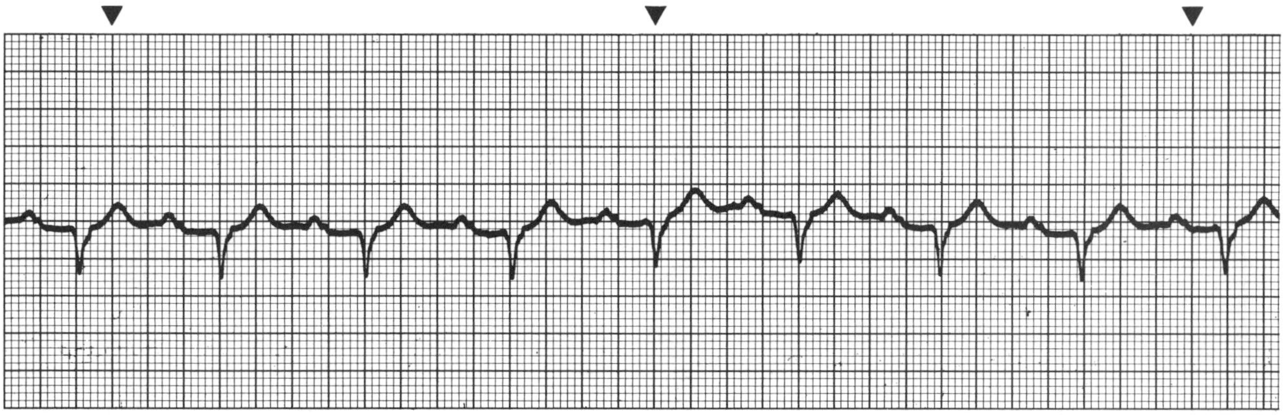

Strip 8-25. Rhythm: _____ Rate: _____ P wave: _____

PR interval: _____ QRS: _____

Rhythm interpretation: _____

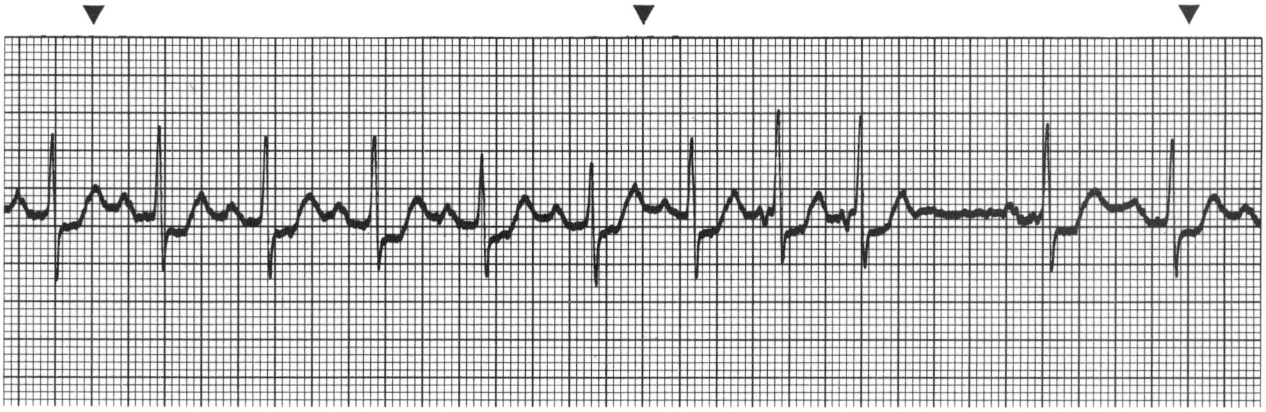

Strip 8-26. Rhythm: _____ Rate: _____ P wave: _____

PR interval: _____ QRS: _____

Rhythm interpretation: _____

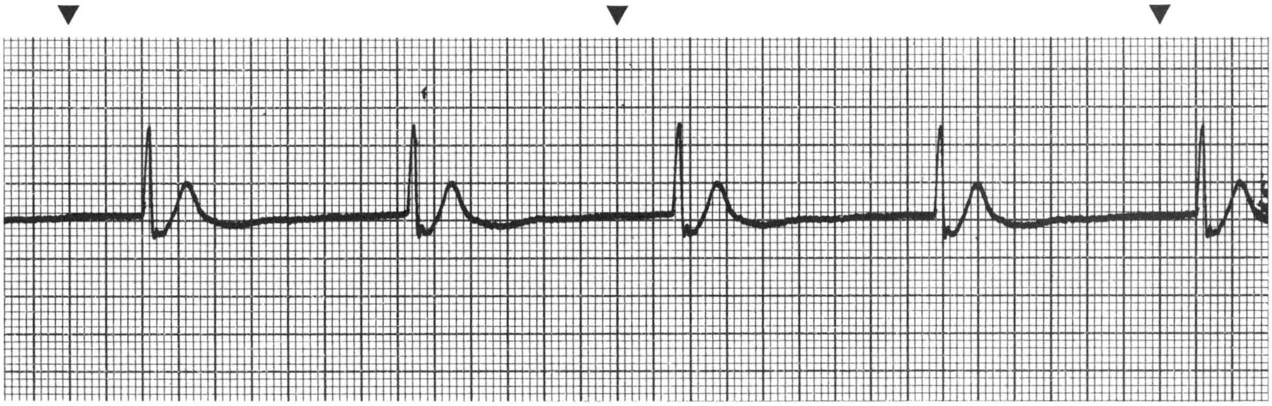

Strip 8-27. Rhythm: _____ Rate: _____ P wave: _____

PR interval: _____ QRS: _____

Rhythm interpretation: _____

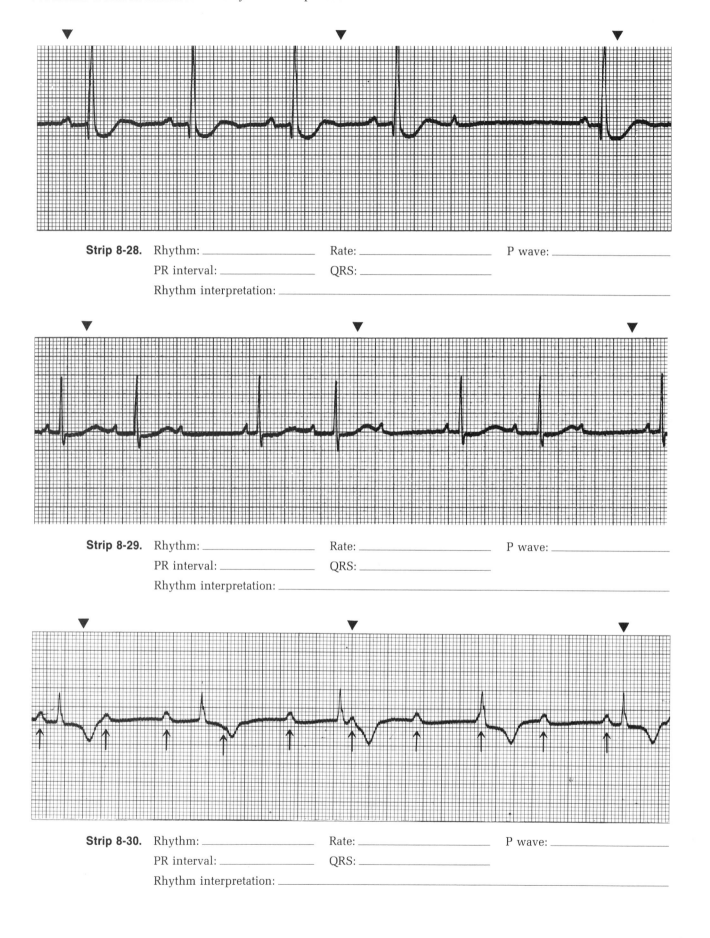

Strip 8-28. Rhythm: _____ Rate: _____ P wave: _____

PR interval: _____ QRS: _____

Rhythm interpretation: _____

Strip 8-29. Rhythm: _____ Rate: _____ P wave: _____

PR interval: _____ QRS: _____

Rhythm interpretation: _____

Strip 8-30. Rhythm: _____ Rate: _____ P wave: _____

PR interval: _____ QRS: _____

Rhythm interpretation: _____

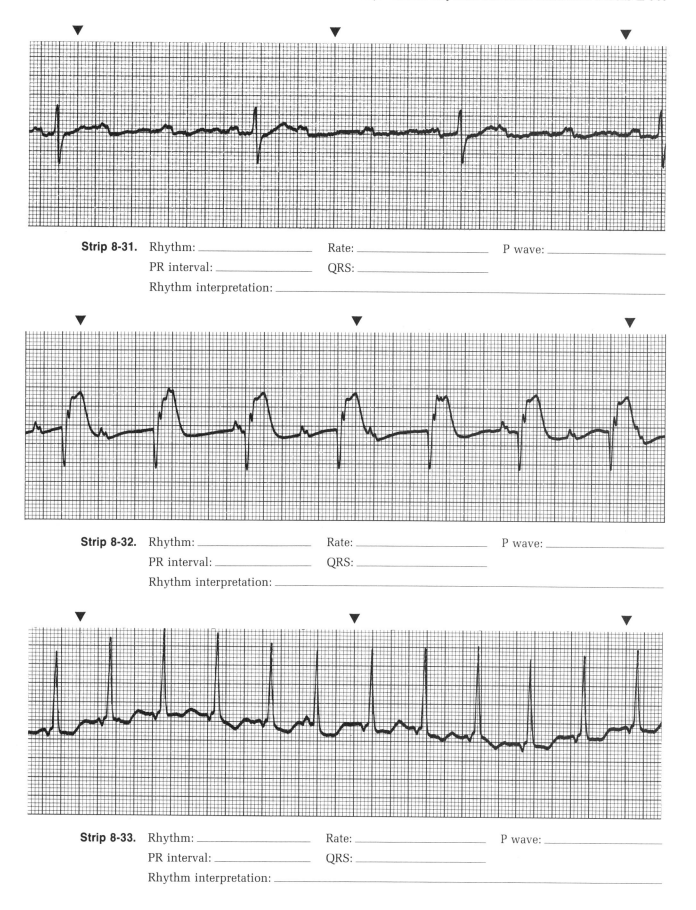

Strip 8-31. Rhythm: _____ Rate: _____ P wave: _____

PR interval: _____ QRS: _____

Rhythm interpretation: _____

Strip 8-32. Rhythm: _____ Rate: _____ P wave: _____

PR interval: _____ QRS: _____

Rhythm interpretation: _____

Strip 8-33. Rhythm: _____ Rate: _____ P wave: _____

PR interval: _____ QRS: _____

Rhythm interpretation: _____

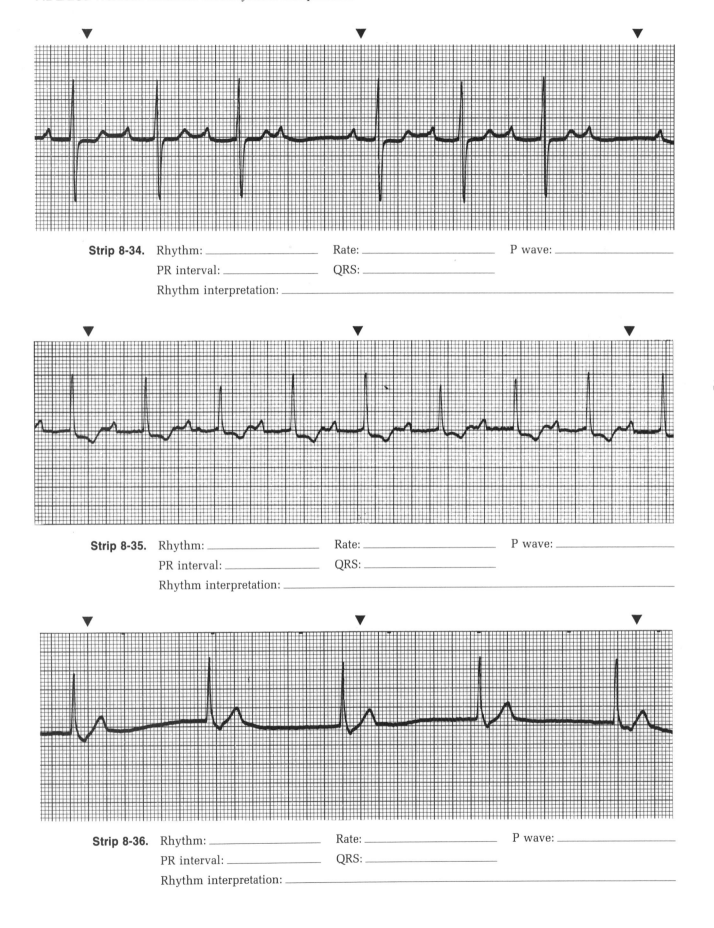

Strip 8-34. Rhythm: _____ Rate: _____ P wave: _____

PR interval: _____ QRS: _____

Rhythm interpretation: _____

Strip 8-35. Rhythm: _____ Rate: _____ P wave: _____

PR interval: _____ QRS: _____

Rhythm interpretation: _____

Strip 8-36. Rhythm: _____ Rate: _____ P wave: _____

PR interval: _____ QRS: _____

Rhythm interpretation: _____

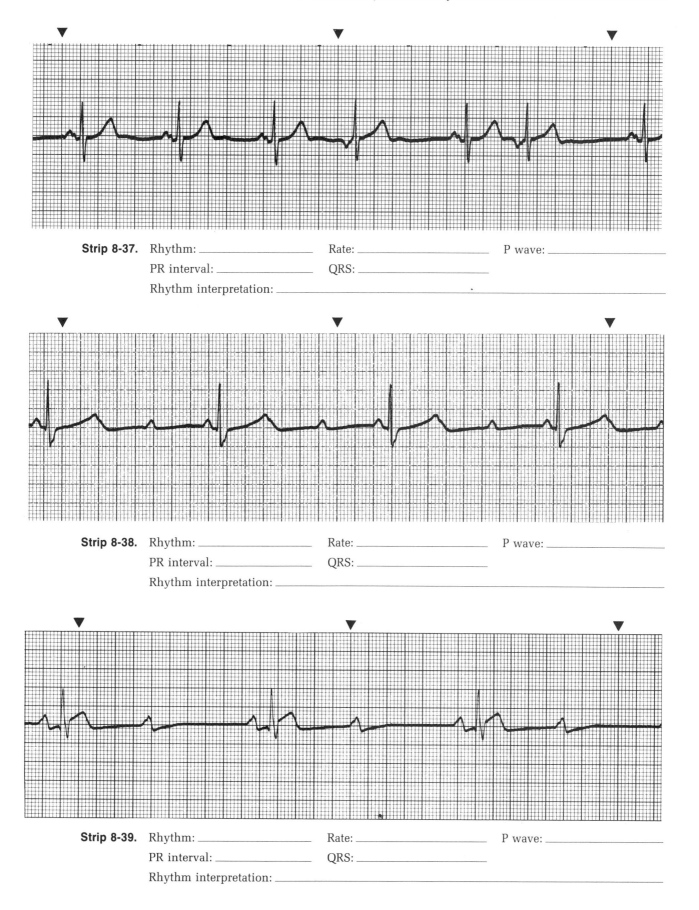

Strip 8-37. Rhythm: _____ Rate: _____ P wave: _____

PR interval: _____ QRS: _____

Rhythm interpretation: _____

Strip 8-38. Rhythm: _____ Rate: _____ P wave: _____

PR interval: _____ QRS: _____

Rhythm interpretation: _____

Strip 8-39. Rhythm: _____ Rate: _____ P wave: _____

PR interval: _____ QRS: _____

Rhythm interpretation: _____

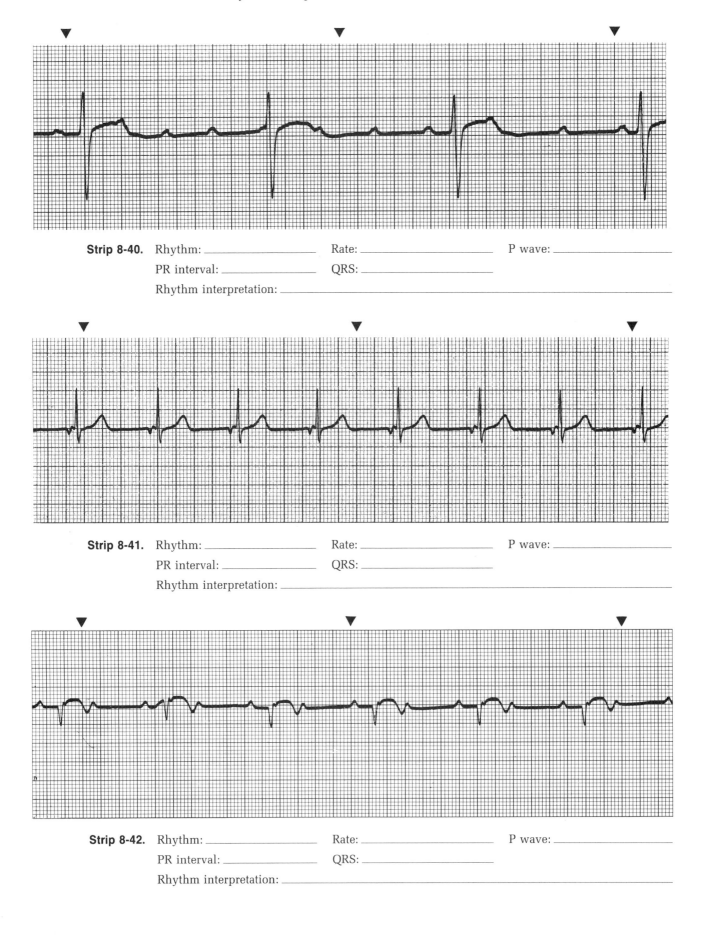

Strip 8-40. Rhythm: _____ Rate: _____ P wave: _____

PR interval: _____ QRS: _____

Rhythm interpretation: _____

Strip 8-41. Rhythm: _____ Rate: _____ P wave: _____

PR interval: _____ QRS: _____

Rhythm interpretation: _____

Strip 8-42. Rhythm: _____ Rate: _____ P wave: _____

PR interval: _____ QRS: _____

Rhythm interpretation: _____

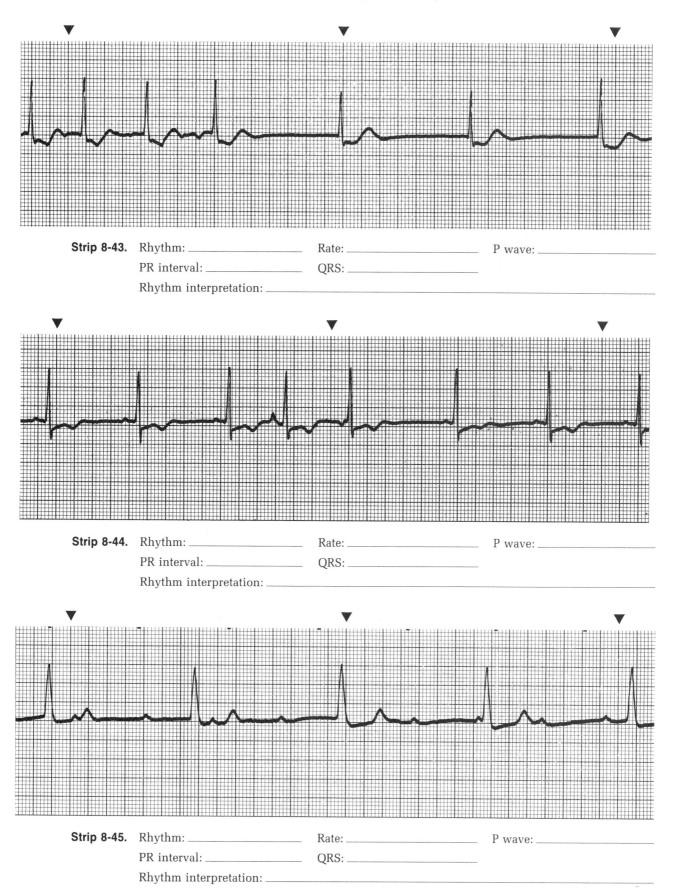

Strip 8-43. Rhythm: _____ Rate: _____ P wave: _____

PR interval: _____ QRS: _____

Rhythm interpretation: _____

Strip 8-44. Rhythm: _____ Rate: _____ P wave: _____

PR interval: _____ QRS: _____

Rhythm interpretation: _____

Strip 8-45. Rhythm: _____ Rate: _____ P wave: _____

PR interval: _____ QRS: _____

Rhythm interpretation: _____

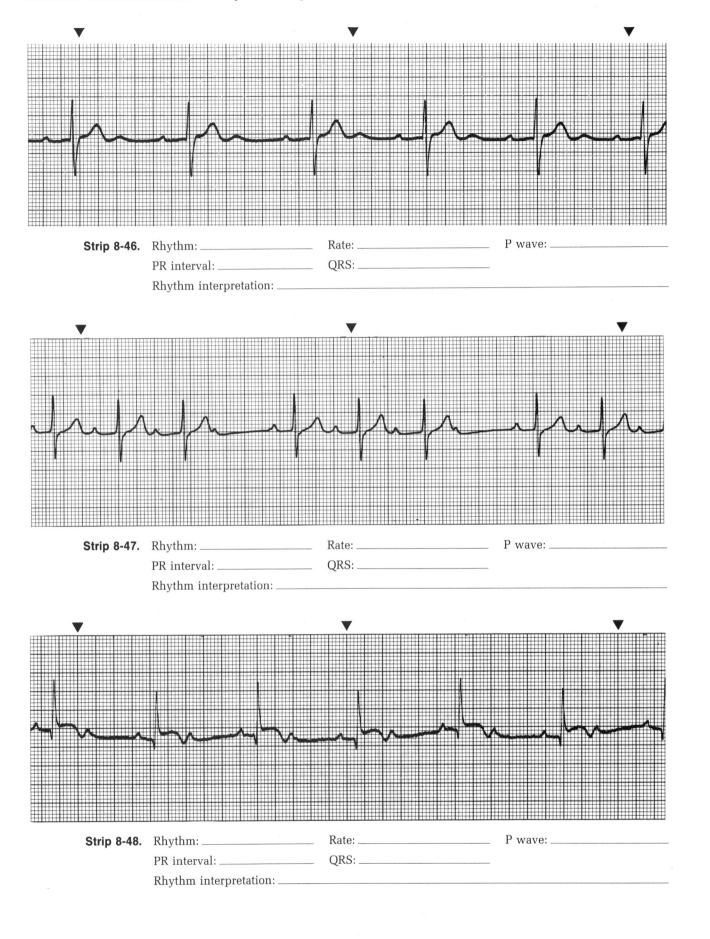

Strip 8-46. Rhythm: _____ Rate: _____ P wave: _____

PR interval: _____ QRS: _____

Rhythm interpretation: _____

Strip 8-47. Rhythm: _____ Rate: _____ P wave: _____

PR interval: _____ QRS: _____

Rhythm interpretation: _____

Strip 8-48. Rhythm: _____ Rate: _____ P wave: _____

PR interval: _____ QRS: _____

Rhythm interpretation: _____

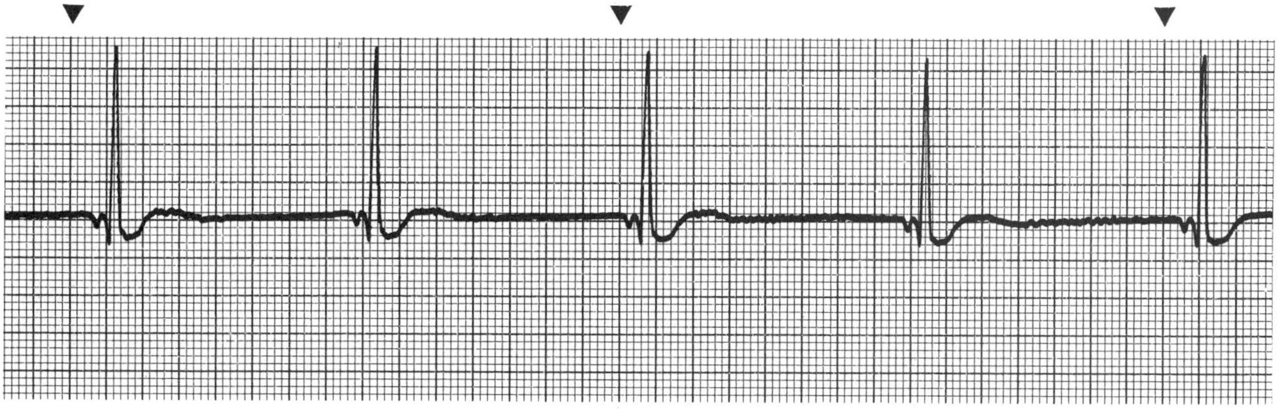

Strip 8-49. Rhythm: _____ Rate: _____ P wave: _____

PR interval: _____ QRS: _____

Rhythm interpretation: _____

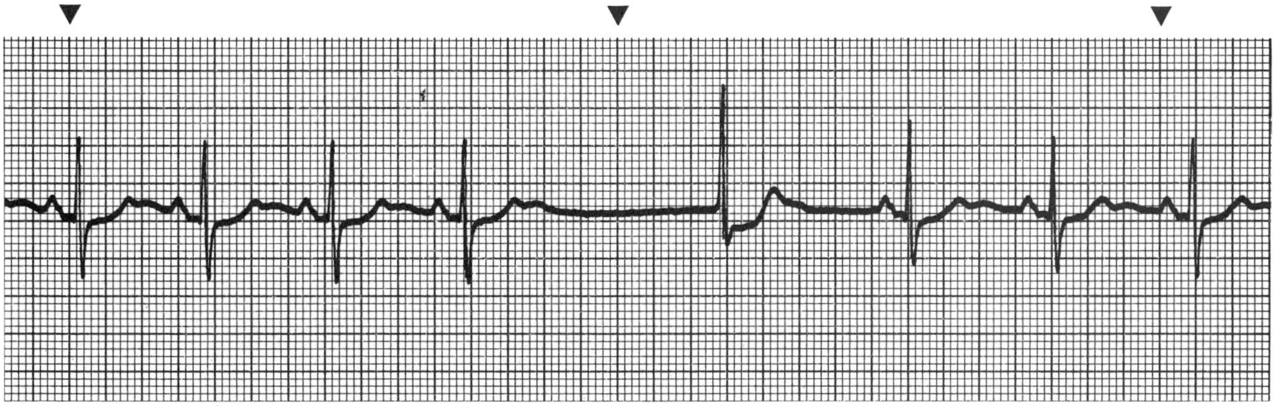

Strip 8-50. Rhythm: _____ Rate: _____ P wave: _____

PR interval: _____ QRS: _____

Rhythm interpretation: _____

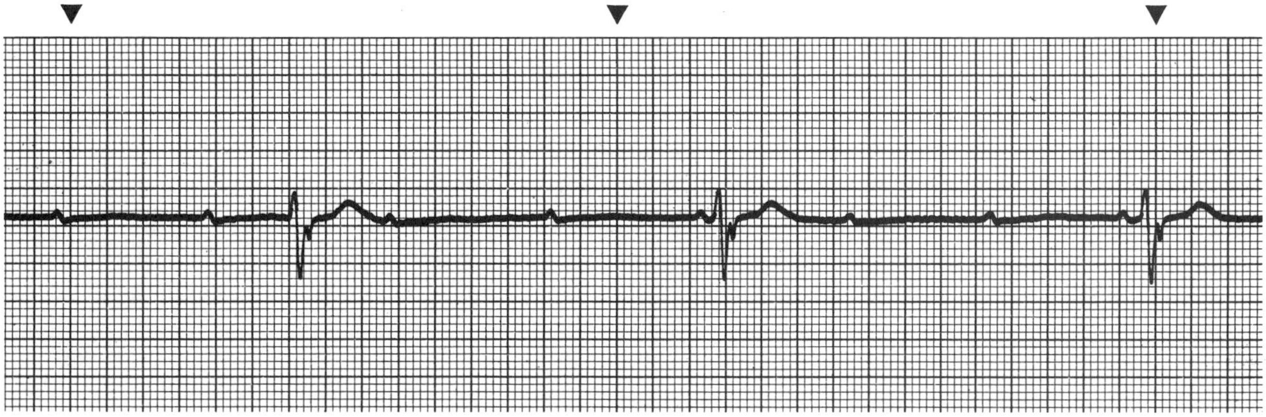

Strip 8-51. Rhythm: _____ Rate: _____ P wave: _____

PR interval: _____ QRS: _____

Rhythm interpretation: _____

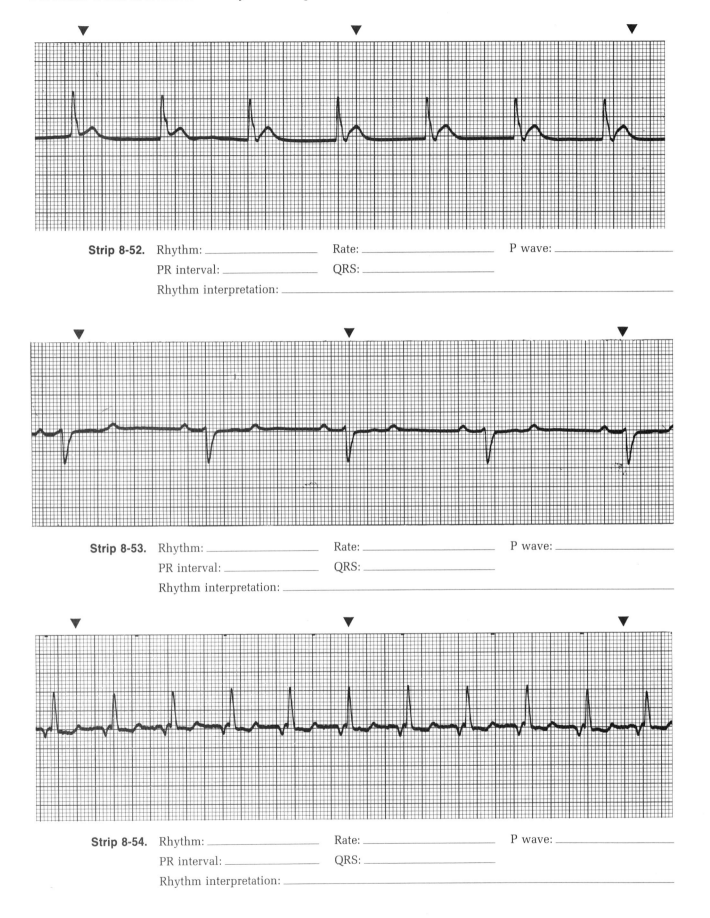

Strip 8-52. Rhythm: _____ Rate: _____ P wave: _____

PR interval: _____ QRS: _____

Rhythm interpretation: _____

Strip 8-53. Rhythm: _____ Rate: _____ P wave: _____

PR interval: _____ QRS: _____

Rhythm interpretation: _____

Strip 8-54. Rhythm: _____ Rate: _____ P wave: _____

PR interval: _____ QRS: _____

Rhythm interpretation: _____

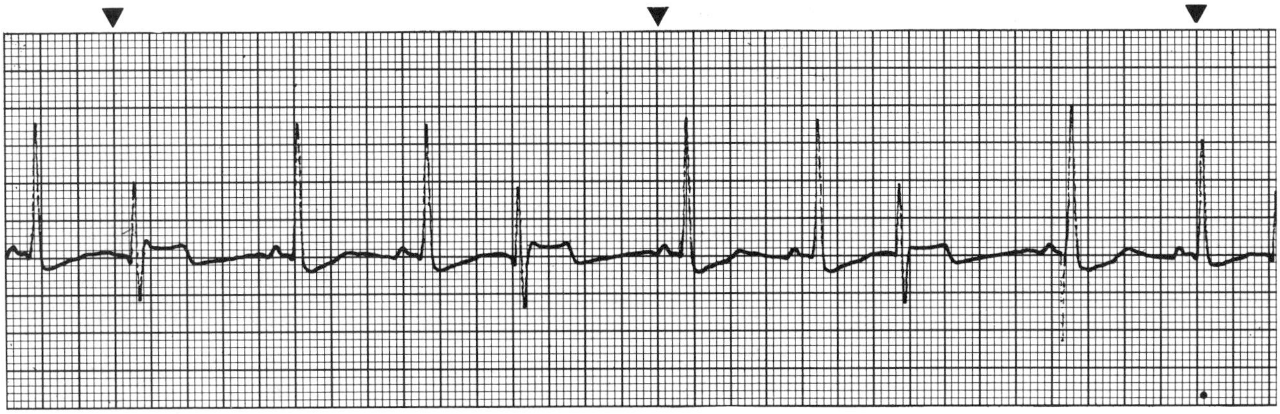

Strip 8-55. Rhythm: _____ Rate: _____ P wave: _____

PR interval: _____ QRS: _____

Rhythm interpretation: _____

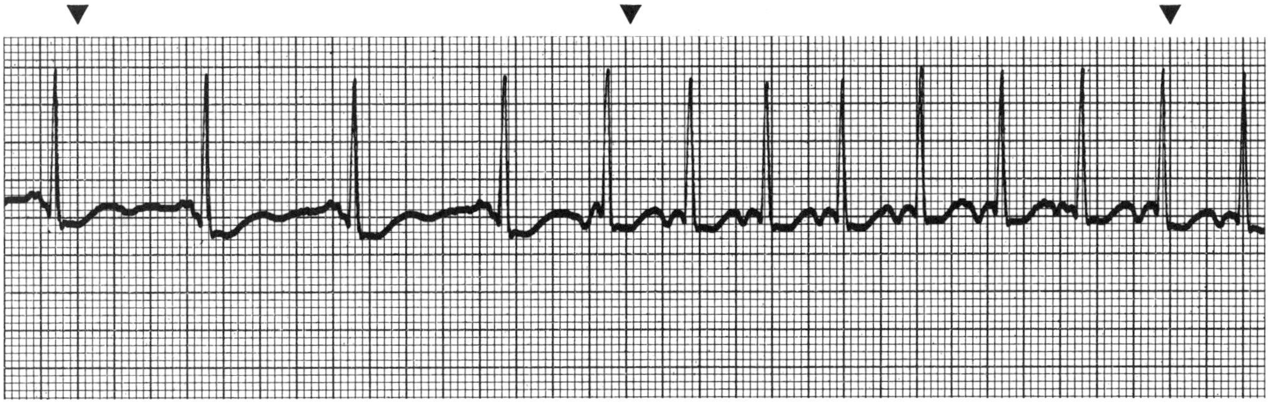

Strip 8-56. Rhythm: _____ Rate: _____ P wave: _____

PR interval: _____ QRS: _____

Rhythm interpretation: _____

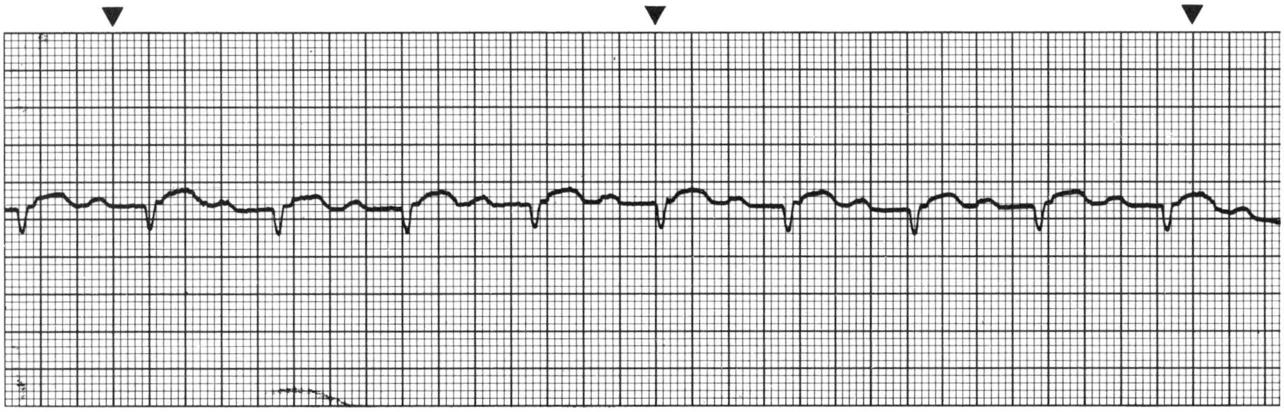

Strip 8-57. Rhythm: _____ Rate: _____ P wave: _____

PR interval: _____ QRS: _____

Rhythm interpretation: _____

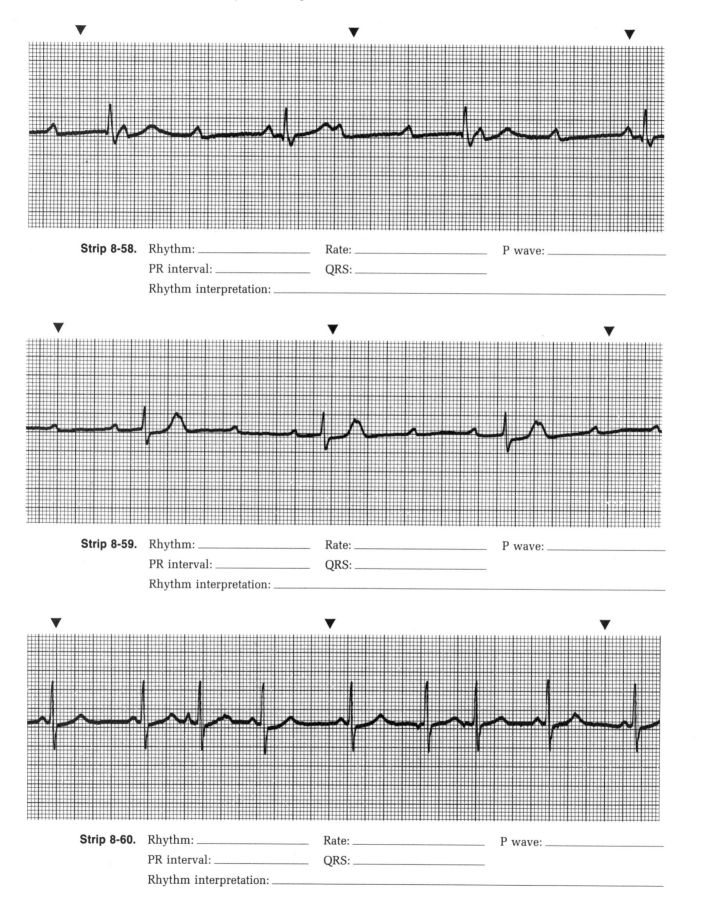

Strip 8-58. Rhythm: _____ Rate: _____ P wave: _____

PR interval: _____ QRS: _____

Rhythm interpretation: _____

Strip 8-59. Rhythm: _____ Rate: _____ P wave: _____

PR interval: _____ QRS: _____

Rhythm interpretation: _____

Strip 8-60. Rhythm: _____ Rate: _____ P wave: _____

PR interval: _____ QRS: _____

Rhythm interpretation: _____

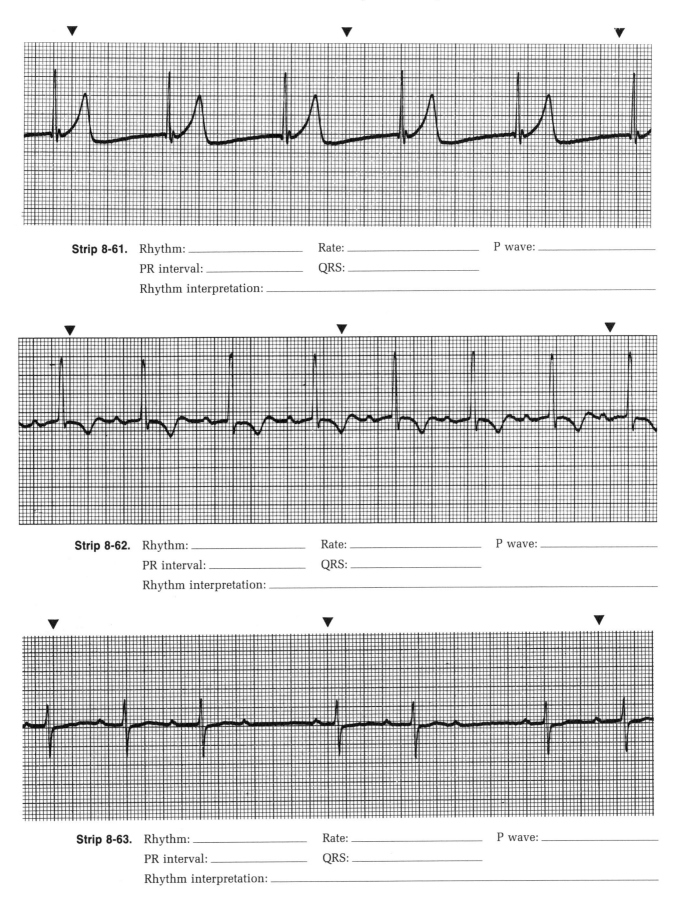

Strip 8-61. Rhythm: _____ Rate: _____ P wave: _____

PR interval: _____ QRS: _____

Rhythm interpretation: _____

Strip 8-62. Rhythm: _____ Rate: _____ P wave: _____

PR interval: _____ QRS: _____

Rhythm interpretation: _____

Strip 8-63. Rhythm: _____ Rate: _____ P wave: _____

PR interval: _____ QRS: _____

Rhythm interpretation: _____

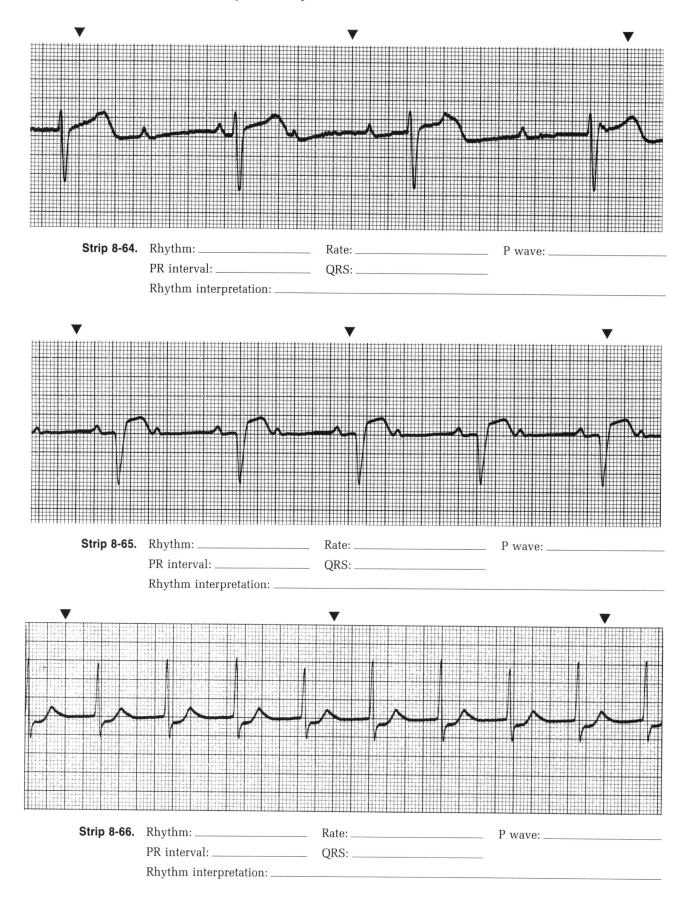

Strip 8-64. Rhythm: _____ Rate: _____ P wave: _____

PR interval: _____ QRS: _____

Rhythm interpretation: _____

Strip 8-65. Rhythm: _____ Rate: _____ P wave: _____

PR interval: _____ QRS: _____

Rhythm interpretation: _____

Strip 8-66. Rhythm: _____ Rate: _____ P wave: _____

PR interval: _____ QRS: _____

Rhythm interpretation: _____

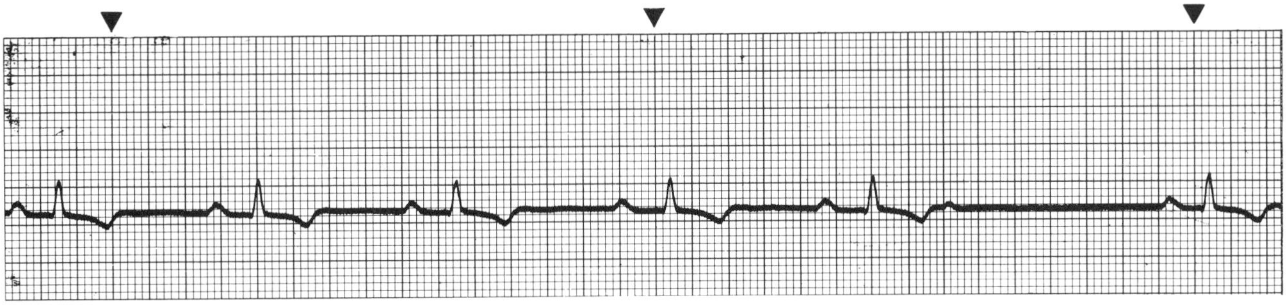

Strip 8-67. Rhythm: _____ Rate: _____ P wave: _____

PR interval: _____ QRS: _____

Rhythm interpretation: _____

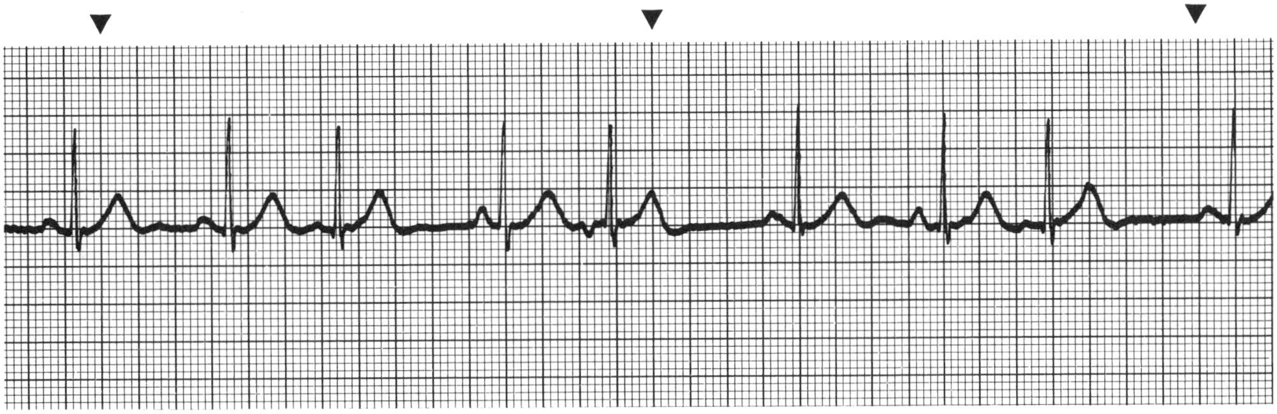

Strip 8-68. Rhythm: _____ Rate: _____ P wave: _____

PR interval: _____ QRS: _____

Rhythm interpretation: _____

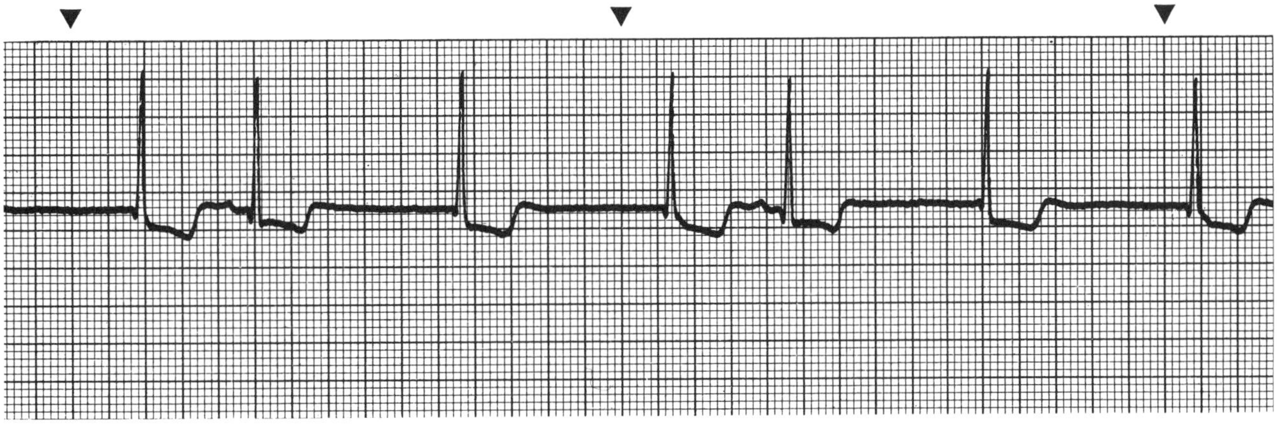

Strip 8-69. Rhythm: _____ Rate: _____ P wave: _____

PR interval: _____ QRS: _____

Rhythm interpretation: _____

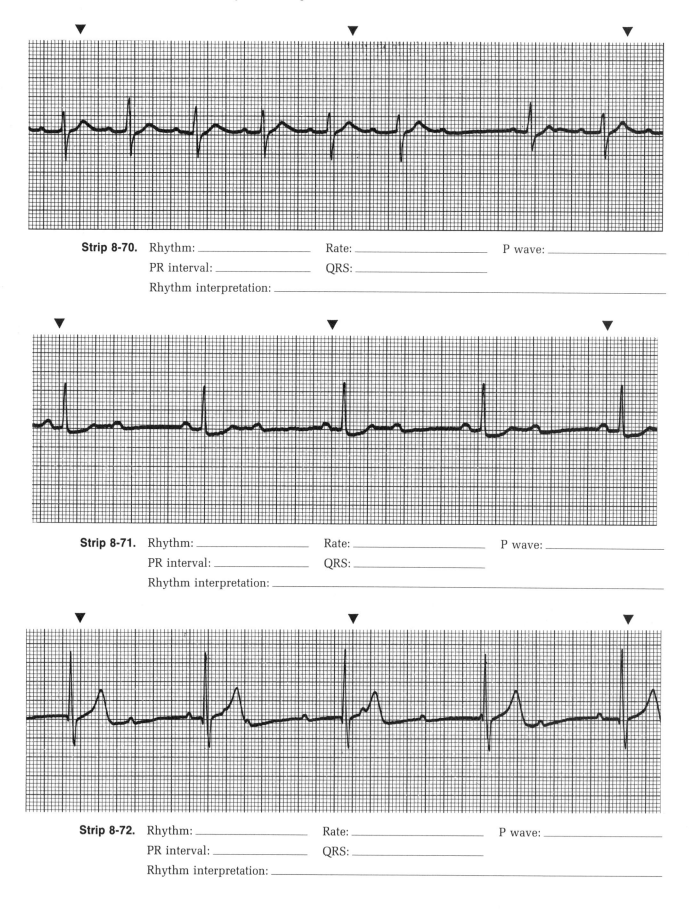

Strip 8-70. Rhythm: _____ Rate: _____ P wave: _____

PR interval: _____ QRS: _____

Rhythm interpretation: _____

Strip 8-71. Rhythm: _____ Rate: _____ P wave: _____

PR interval: _____ QRS: _____

Rhythm interpretation: _____

Strip 8-72. Rhythm: _____ Rate: _____ P wave: _____

PR interval: _____ QRS: _____

Rhythm interpretation: _____

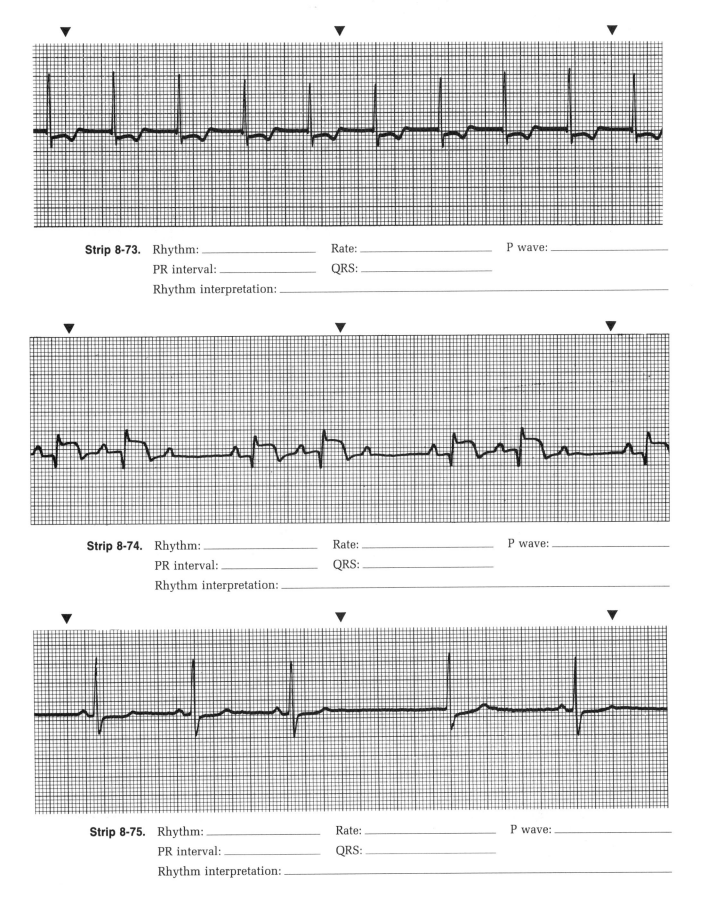

Strip 8-73. Rhythm: _____ Rate: _____ P wave: _____

PR interval: _____ QRS: _____

Rhythm interpretation: _____

Strip 8-74. Rhythm: _____ Rate: _____ P wave: _____

PR interval: _____ QRS: _____

Rhythm interpretation: _____

Strip 8-75. Rhythm: _____ Rate: _____ P wave: _____

PR interval: _____ QRS: _____

Rhythm interpretation: _____

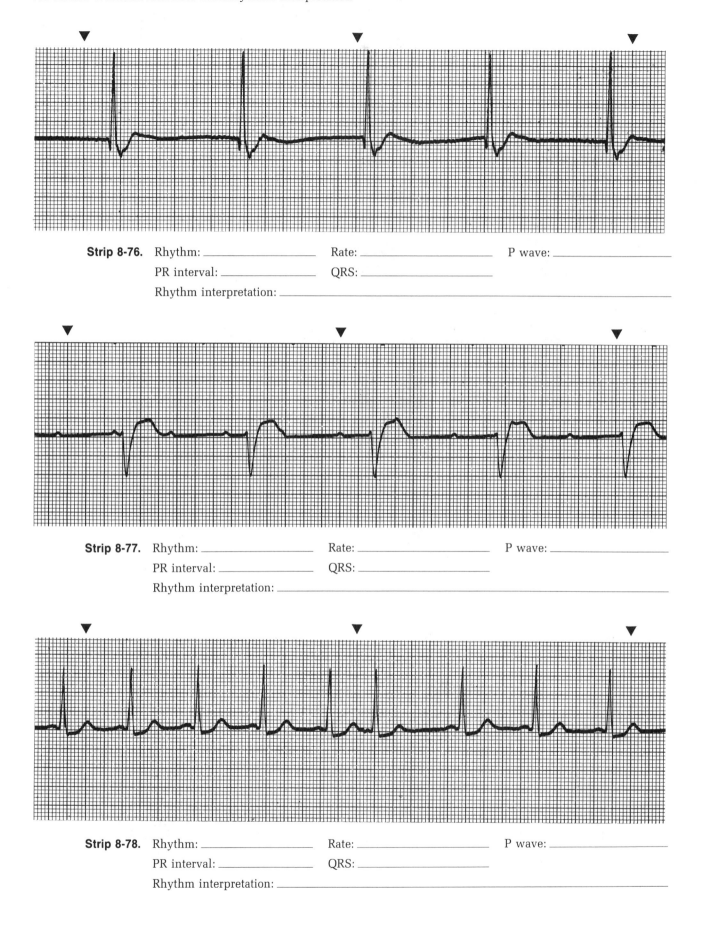

Strip 8-76. Rhythm: _____ Rate: _____ P wave: _____

PR interval: _____ QRS: _____

Rhythm interpretation: _____

Strip 8-77. Rhythm: _____ Rate: _____ P wave: _____

PR interval: _____ QRS: _____

Rhythm interpretation: _____

Strip 8-78. Rhythm: _____ Rate: _____ P wave: _____

PR interval: _____ QRS: _____

Rhythm interpretation: _____

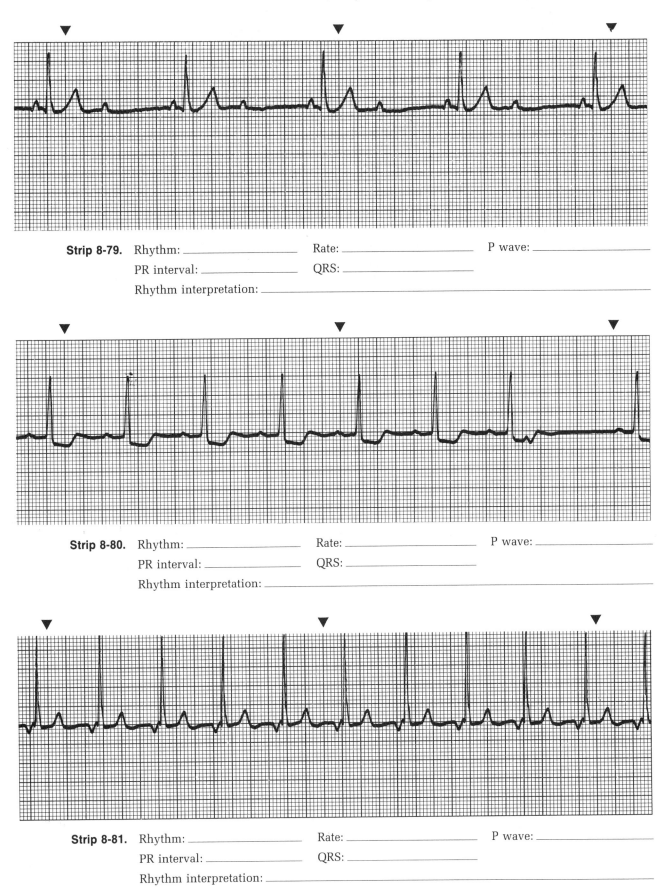

Strip 8-79. Rhythm: _____ Rate: _____ P wave: _____

PR interval: _____ QRS: _____

Rhythm interpretation: _____

Strip 8-80. Rhythm: _____ Rate: _____ P wave: _____

PR interval: _____ QRS: _____

Rhythm interpretation: _____

Strip 8-81. Rhythm: _____ Rate: _____ P wave: _____

PR interval: _____ QRS: _____

Rhythm interpretation: _____

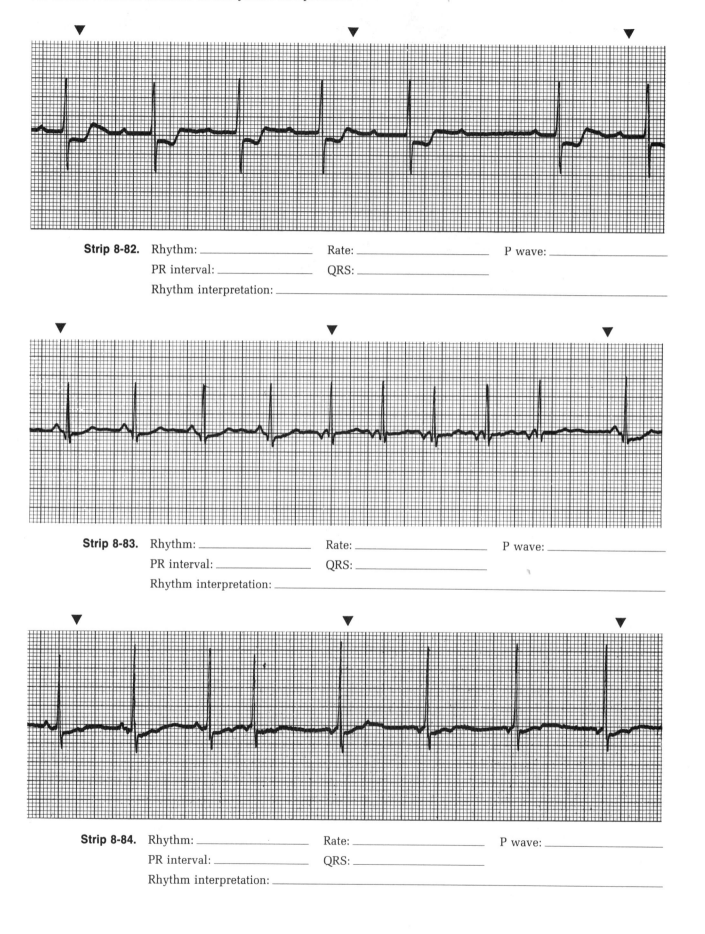

Strip 8-82. Rhythm: _____ Rate: _____ P wave: _____

PR interval: _____ QRS: _____

Rhythm interpretation: _____

Strip 8-83. Rhythm: _____ Rate: _____ P wave: _____

PR interval: _____ QRS: _____

Rhythm interpretation: _____

Strip 8-84. Rhythm: _____ Rate: _____ P wave: _____

PR interval: _____ QRS: _____

Rhythm interpretation: _____

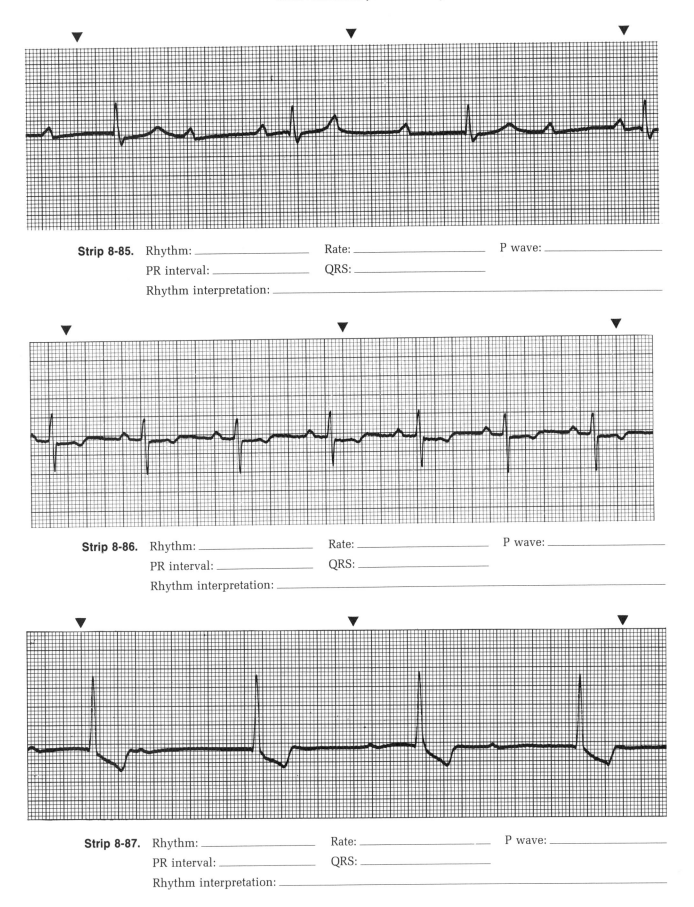

Strip 8-85. Rhythm: _____ Rate: _____ P wave: _____

PR interval: _____ QRS: _____

Rhythm interpretation: _____

Strip 8-86. Rhythm: _____ Rate: _____ P wave: _____

PR interval: _____ QRS: _____

Rhythm interpretation: _____

Strip 8-87. Rhythm: _____ Rate: _____ P wave: _____

PR interval: _____ QRS: _____

Rhythm interpretation: _____

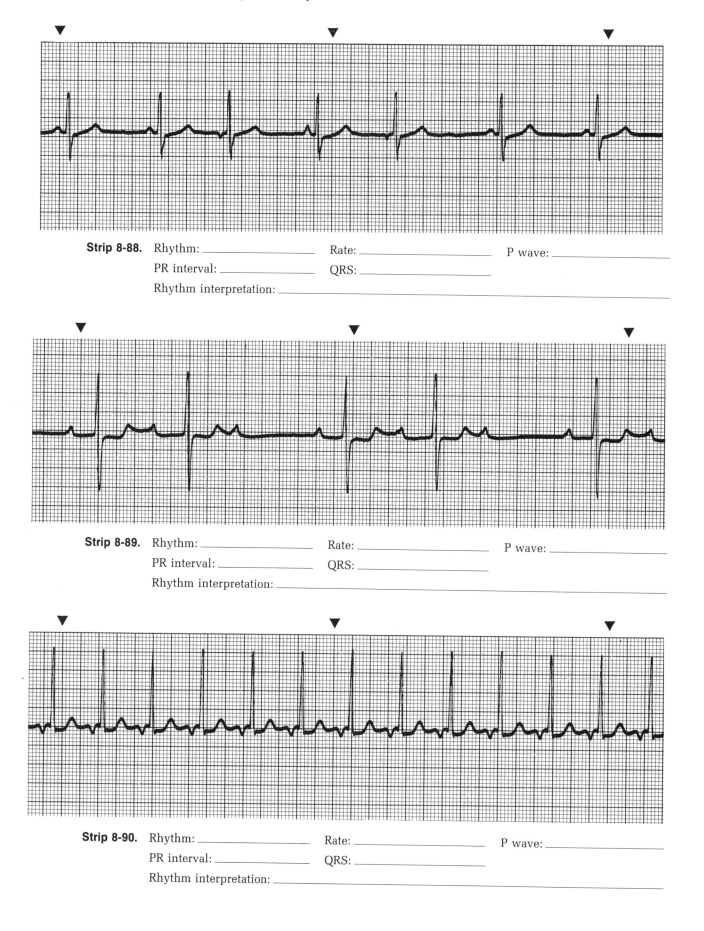

Strip 8-88. Rhythm: _____ Rate: _____ P wave: _____

PR interval: _____ QRS: _____

Rhythm interpretation: _____

Strip 8-89. Rhythm: _____ Rate: _____ P wave: _____

PR interval: _____ QRS: _____

Rhythm interpretation: _____

Strip 8-90. Rhythm: _____ Rate: _____ P wave: _____

PR interval: _____ QRS: _____

Rhythm interpretation: _____

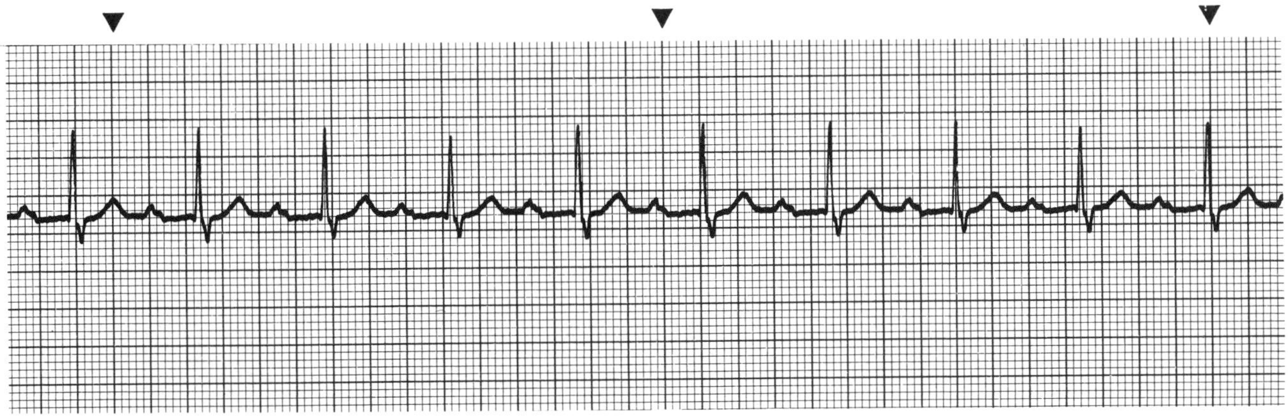

Strip 8-91. Rhythm: _____ Rate: _____ P wave: _____

PR interval: _____ QRS: _____

Rhythm interpretation: _____

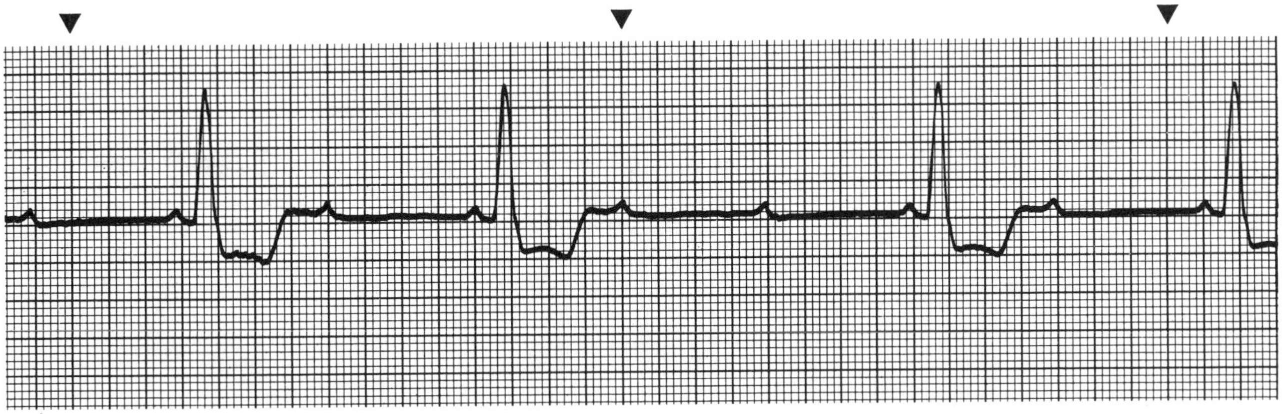

Strip 8-92. Rhythm: _____ Rate: _____ P wave: _____

PR interval: _____ QRS: _____

Rhythm interpretation: _____

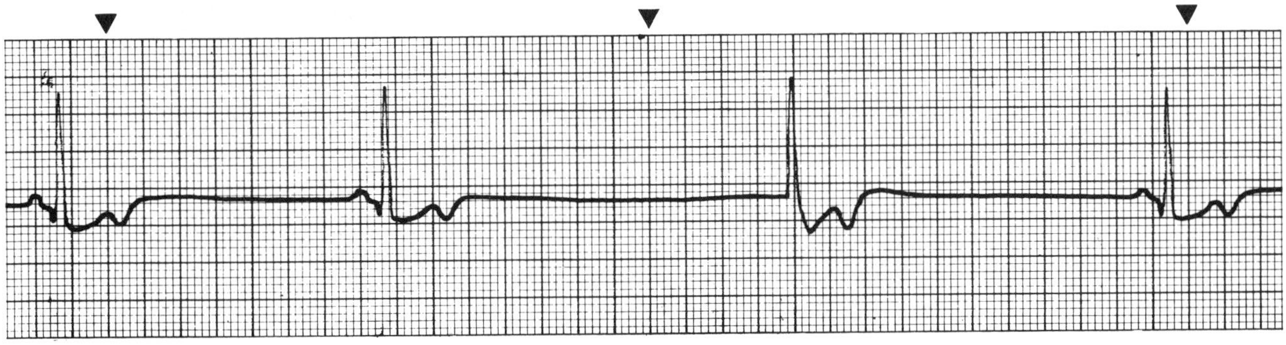

Strip 8-93. Rhythm: _____ Rate: _____ P wave: _____

PR interval: _____ QRS: _____

Rhythm interpretation: _____

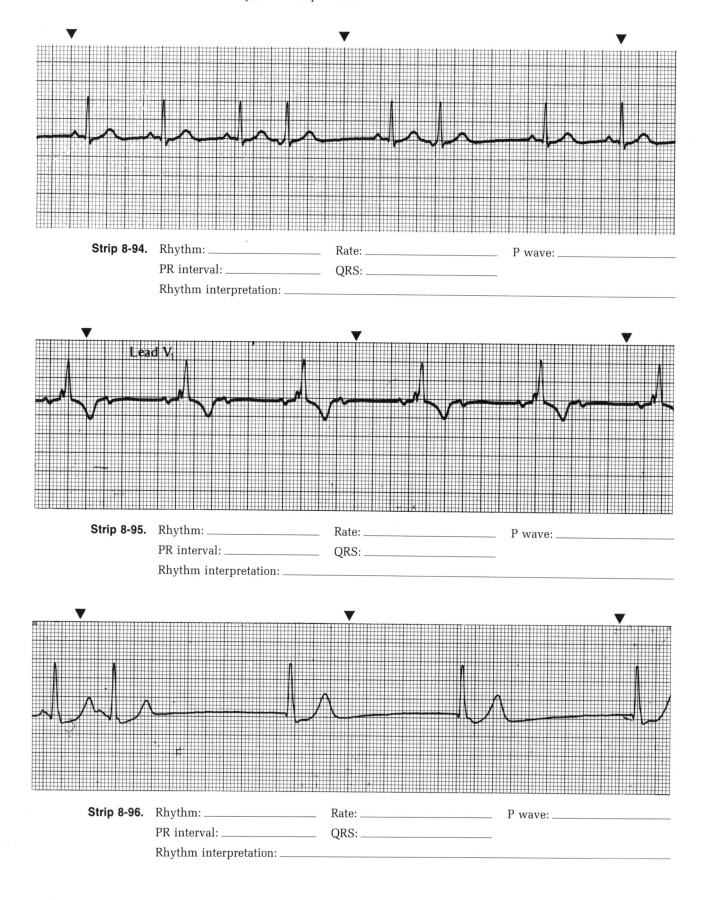

Strip 8-94. Rhythm: _____ Rate: _____ P wave: _____

PR interval: _____ QRS: _____

Rhythm interpretation: _____

Lead V₁

Strip 8-95. Rhythm: _____ Rate: _____ P wave: _____

PR interval: _____ QRS: _____

Rhythm interpretation: _____

Strip 8-96. Rhythm: _____ Rate: _____ P wave: _____

PR interval: _____ QRS: _____

Rhythm interpretation: _____

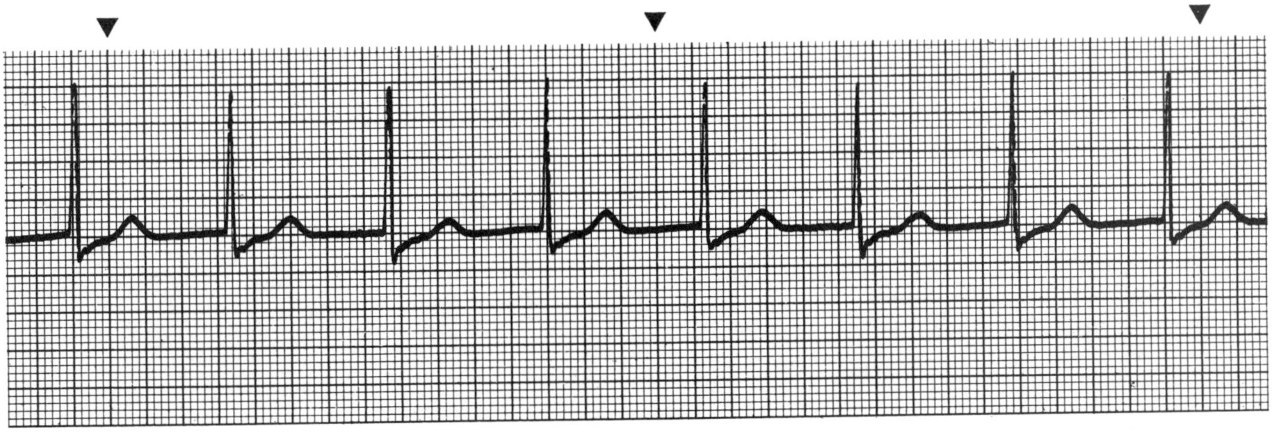

Strip 8-97. Rhythm: _____ Rate: _____ P wave: _____

PR interval: _____ QRS: _____

Rhythm interpretation: _____

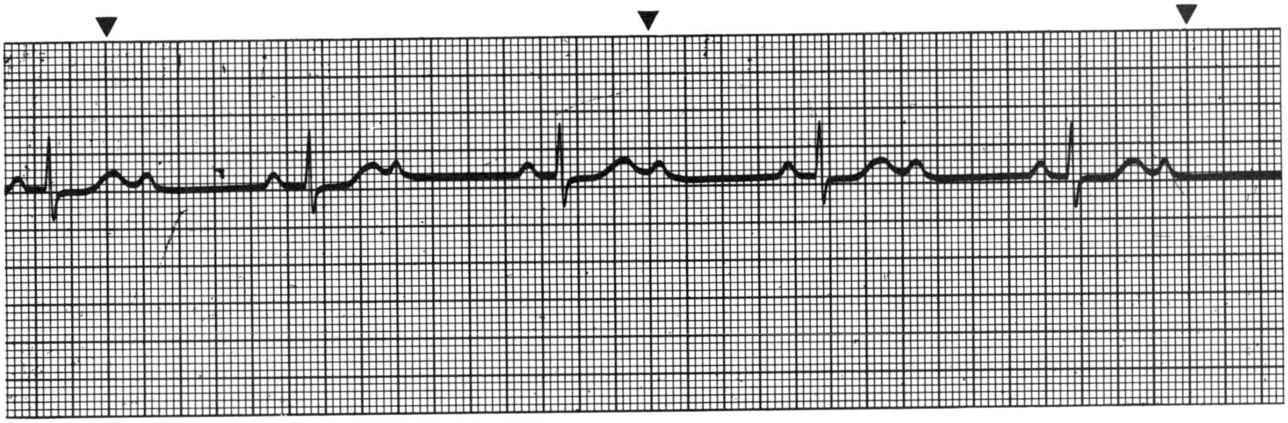

Strip 8-98. Rhythm: _____ Rate: _____ P wave: _____

PR interval: _____ QRS: _____

Rhythm interpretation: _____

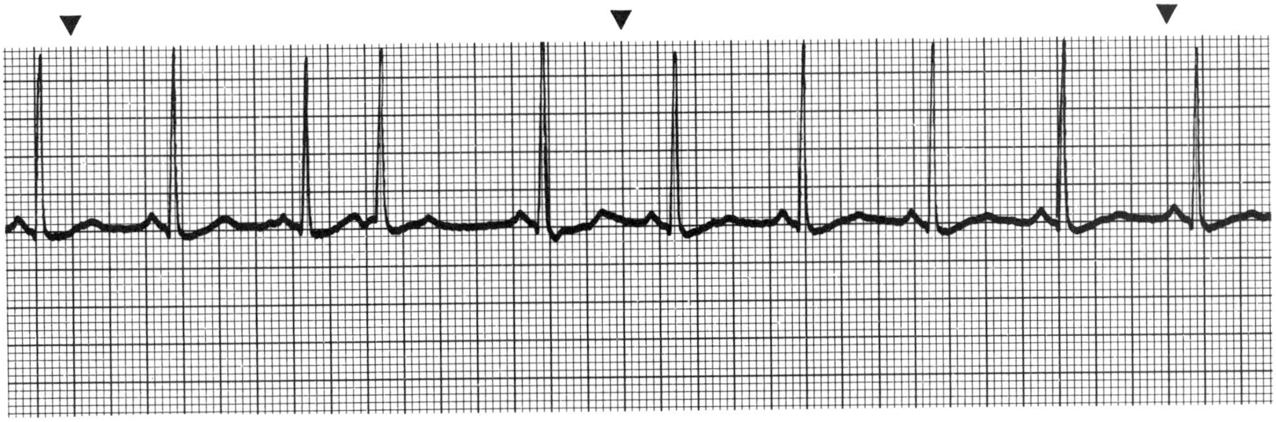

Strip 8-99. Rhythm: _____ Rate: _____ P wave: _____

PR interval: _____ QRS: _____

Rhythm interpretation: _____

9

Ventricular Rhythms and Bundle Branch Block

Huff J, Doernbach DP, White RD: *ECG WORKOUT: EXERCISES IN ARRHYTHMIA INTERPRETATION*, 2nd ed. © 1993 J.B. Lippincott Company.

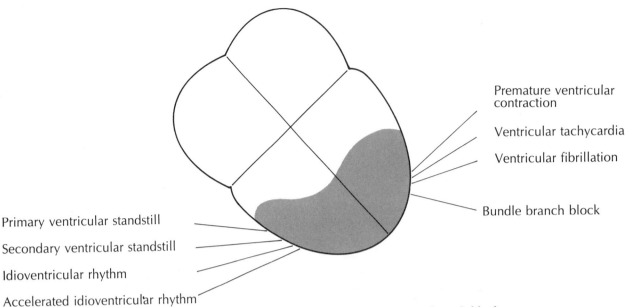

Premature ventricular
contraction

Ventricular tachycardia

Ventricular fibrillation

Bundle branch block

Primary ventricular standstill

Secondary ventricular standstill

Idioventricular rhythm

Accelerated idioventricular rhythm

Figure 9-1. Ventricular rhythms and bundle branch block.

Ventricular rhythms originate in the ventricles below the branching portion of the bundle of His and take the form of premature ventricular contractions (PVCs), ventricular tachycardia, ventricular fibrillation, idioventricular rhythm, accelerated idioventricular rhythm, and ventricular standstill (Figure 9-1). All of these rhythms are associated with a wide QRS (except ventricular fibrillation and primary ventricular standstill). The impulse focus in bundle branch block does not originate in ventricular tissue but is included in this rhythm group because of the location of the block within the intraventricular system and the resulting wide QRS complex.

Some of the rhythms (PVCs, ventricular tachycardia, ventricular fibrillation) result from ventricular irritability secondary to myocardial ischemia. Idioventricular rhythm usually appears as an escape rhythm as a result of momentary slowing of the sinoatrial node. An automatic focus in the ventricles is responsible for accelerated idioventricular rhythm. Bundle branch block results from an obstruction in one of the bundle branches. Primary ventricular standstill usually is associated with some form of heart block, whereas secondary ventricular standstill occurs from advanced circulatory failure.

Most of these rhythms are, or have the potential to be, life-threatening and demand prompt recognition and intervention.

BUNDLE BRANCH BLOCK

A bundle branch block refers to an obstruction in one of the branches of the bundle of His. Normally, the sinus impulses traverse the atrioventricular and His bundles, are conducted down the left and right bundle branches, and stimulate the ventricles simultaneously. Depolarization of both ventricles normally takes 0.10 seconds or less. When one of the bundle branches is blocked, impulses travel through the intact branch and stimulate the ventricle it supplies on schedule. The ventricle affected by the bundle branch block is stimulated indirectly by impulses crossing through the septum from the unaffected side. The time required for complete depolarization of both ventricles is delayed and is reflected on the electrocardiogram (ECG) as a wide QRS complex (0.12 seconds or more).

The presence of a bundle branch block can be recognized by a single monitoring lead by the presence of a wide QRS complex. However, the type of block (right or left bundle) can be determined only by the 12-lead ECG. A left bundle branch block obscures the ECG signs of acute myocardial infarction. The diagnosis of acute infarction in this situation depends primarily on the patient's history and enzyme studies. A right bundle branch block does not affect the ECG signs of infarction.

Bundle branch block causes no symptoms because the heart rate and rhythm are not affected. Acute bundle branch block generally reflects ischemic damage secondary to acute myocardial infarction. Chronic bundle branch block results from chronic degeneration or fibrotic scarring of the intraventricular conduction system. Chronic bundle branch block usually requires no treatment. Bundle branch block that develops as a result of acute myocardial infarction usually reflects extensive myocardial damage to the intraventricular system and bundle branches. A temporary transvenous

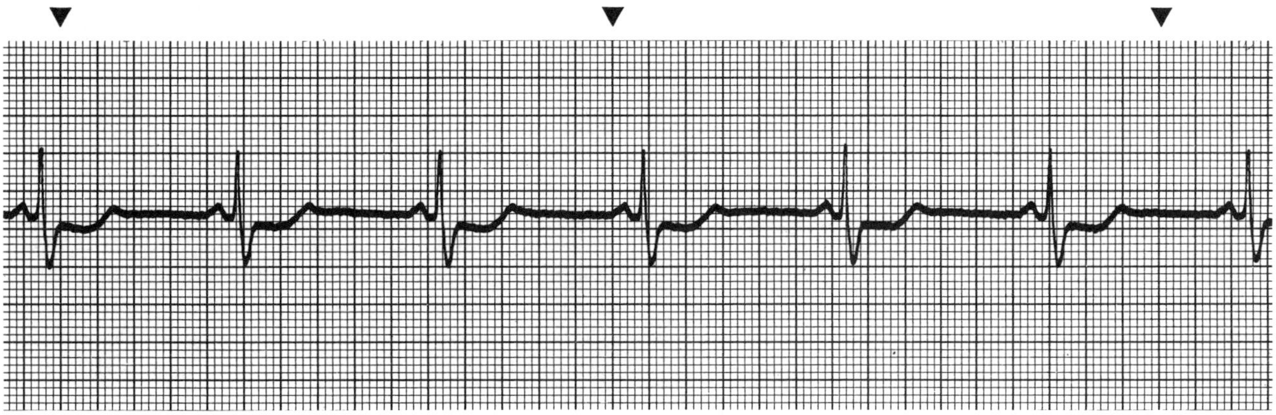

Figure 9-2. **Sinus Bradycardia with Bundle Branch Block**

Rhythm:	Regular
Rate:	54
P waves:	Sinus P waves are present
PR:	0.14 to 0.16 seconds
QRS:	0.12 seconds
Comment:	ST segment depression is present.

[handwritten: QRS is longer]

[handwritten: re-entry]

pacemaker is usually inserted prophylactically in this situation should sudden third-degree AV block or ventricular standstill develop (Box 9-1) (Figure 9-2).

Box 9-1. **Bundle Branch Block—Identifying ECG Features**

Rhythm:	Regular
Rate:	Usually normal; sometimes BBB is rate-related, appearing and disappearing with changes in heart rate.
P waves:	Sinus P waves are present
PR:	Normal
QRS:	Wide (0.12 seconds or greater)

PVC

A PVC results from the premature discharge of an ectopic ventricular focus. The PVC is characterized by a premature, wide, distorted QRS with no related P wave and is followed by a pause.

As a rule, the sinus node is not affected by the PVC (in contrast to the premature atrial contraction and premature junctional contraction) and it will continue to discharge on schedule. These sinus P waves usually are lost in the wide QRS complex of the PVC but can sometimes be seen before or after the QRS. The T wave associated with the PVC is usually directly opposite the main QRS deflection. If the QRS is dominantly upright, the T wave will be inverted; if the QRS is dominantly downward, the T wave will be upright. The pause following the PVC is usually fully compensatory. A fully compensatory pause means that the interval between the beat preceding the PVC and the beat following the PVC is exactly equal to two cardiac cycles.

PVCs do not constitute a basic rhythm but occur in conjunction with other rhythms (normal sinus rhythm, sinus bradycardia, sinus tachycardia, atrial fibrillation, and so on). PVCs may occur as a single beat, every other beat (bigeminal PVCs), every third beat (trigeminal PVCs), in pairs, in runs, or sandwiched between two sinus beats (interpolated PVCs). When PVCs occur in runs of three or more, the rhythm is called ventricular tachycardia. PVCs that arise from the same focus in the ventricle are uniform in size and shape and are called uniform or unifocal PVCs. PVCs that arise from different foci will differ in size and shape and are called multiform or multifocal PVCs.

PVCs are the most common of all arrhythmias associated with acute myocardial infarction. They reflect ventricular irritability and in the setting of myocardial ischemia are more likely to provoke ventricular tachycardia or ventricular fibrillation. Although the relationship between PVCs, ventricular tachycardia, and ventricular fibrillation has been clearly established, it should not be assumed that all PVCs are dangerous and need treatment. Many individuals without evidence of heart disease display PVCs that pose no threat at all. PVCs are considered dangerous if they occur in the following forms:

1. When PVCs occur frequently (more than 6 per minute).

2. When PVCs occur every other beat (bigeminy).

3. When the PVC strikes on the T wave of the preceding beat (the "R on T" pattern).

4. When PVCs originate from more than one focus (multiform or multifocal).

5. When there are two consecutive PVCs (pairs or couplets).

Lidocaine is the primary drug used to control PVCs. Lidocaine is initially administered intravenously in a bolus dose of 1 to 1.5 mg/kg, followed by half the initial dose every 5 minutes until PVCs are controlled or a total of 3 mg/kg has been given. If adequate doses of lidocaine fail to suppress PVCs, procainamide can be given intravenously at a rate of 20 mg/min until the arrhythmia is controlled, hypotension ensues, the QRS complex is widened by 50% of its original width, or a total of 17 mg/kg of the drug has been given. For PVCs refractory to lidocaine or procainamide, bretylium can be administered intravenously in a dose of 5 to 10 mg/kg over 8 to 10 minutes until PVCs are resolved or a total of 30 to 35 mg/kg dose has been given. If procainamide or bretylium is used, the blood pressure should be monitored carefully owing to the hypotensive effects of these drugs. Once PVCs are resolved, begin drip infusion of the antiarrhythmic agent that aided resolu-

tion. Lidocaine, procainamide, and bretylium can be mixed as 2 g in 500 mL D₅W and administered at 1 to 4 mg/min. PVCs accompanying slow ventricular rates can be best abolished by increasing the basic rate with atropine or overdrive pacing.

On some occasions a ventricular beat may occur late instead of early. These beats are called ventricular escape beats. The characteristics of the late beats will be the same as the PVC. Ventricular escape beats require no treatment. It is important, however, to identify the cause of the pause so that appropriate interventions can be initiated, if necessary (Box 9-2) (Figures 9-3 through 9-11).

Box 9-2. PVCs—Identifying Features

Rhythm:	Irregular owing to premature beat and pause
Rate:	Can occur with a variety of rhythms
P wave:	No P waves associated with PVC; however sinus P waves can sometimes be seen before or after the QRS
PR:	Not measurable
QRS:	Wide (0.12 seconds or more)

(text continues on page 171)

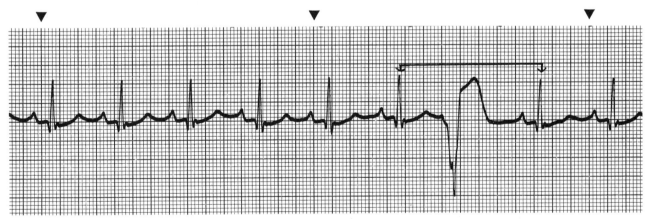

Figure 9-3. Normal Sinus Rhythm with One PVC

Rhythm:	Basic rhythm regular; irregular with PVC
Rate:	Basic rhythm rate 79
P waves:	Sinus P waves with basic rhythm
PR:	0.16 to 0.20 seconds (basic rhythm)
QRS:	0.08 to 0.10 seconds (basic rhythm) 0.14 to 0.16 seconds (PVC)
Comment:	The interval between the beat preceding the PVC and the beat following the PVC is equal to the time of two normal beats and represents a full compensatory pause.

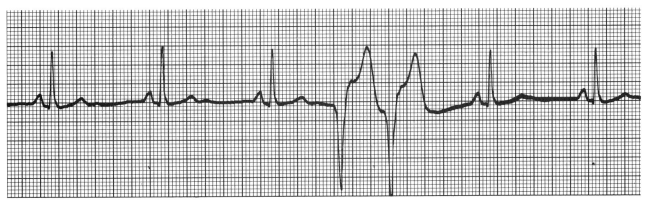

Figure 9-4. Paired PVCs.

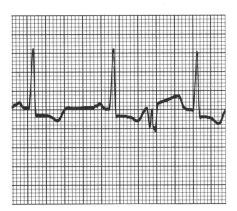

Figure 9-5. Interpolated PVCs.

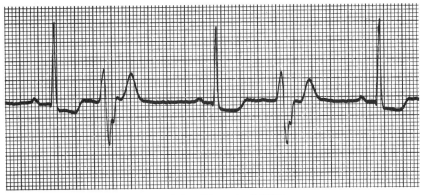

Figure 9-6. Bigeminal PVCs.

there is some CO

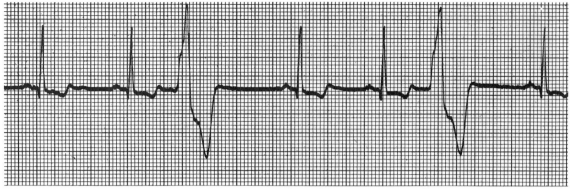

Figure 9-7. Trigeminal PVCs.

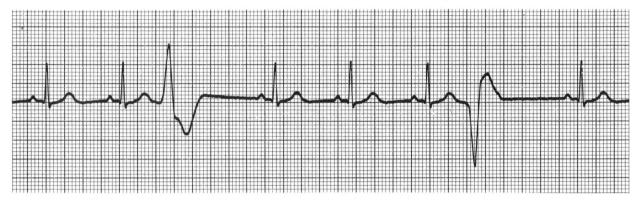

Figure 9-8. Multifocal PVCs.

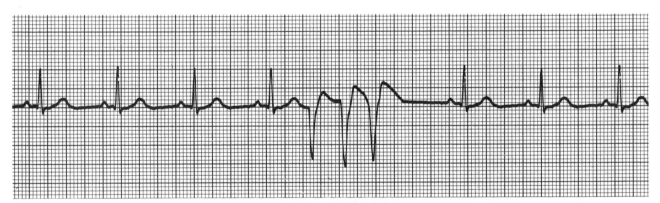

Figure 9-9. Run of PVCs (a paroxysm of ventricular tachycardia).

Run of V tach

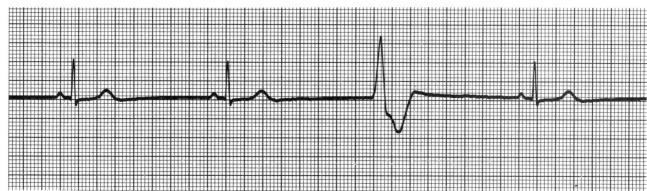

Figure 9-10. Ventricular escape beat.

Tx for PVC first
Ignore them ?
caffeine, aspirin
Lidocaine, quinidine, [bathuan cephan that don't respond] given on code
pronestyl,

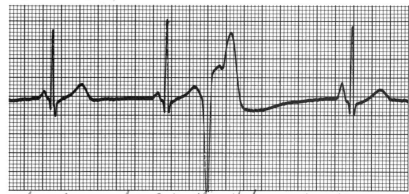

Figure 9-11. R-ON-T PVC.

3 mg = 45 cc/h   S/S Lidocaine: slurred speech, CNS stimulation, twitching, seizure
2 mg = 30 cc/h   10 mg = 1500/hr   short ½ life 2°   1-4 mg/min drip /kg
4 mg = 1 cc   60 cc/hr

VENTRICULAR TACHYCARDIA

Ventricular tachycardia is caused by a rapid discharge of an ectopic focus in the ventricles occurring at a rate of 140 to 250 per minute and usually reflects marked myocardial irritability. On the ECG, the rhythm appears as a series of consecutive wide QRS complexes that resemble PVCs. Like the PVC, the ectopic focus stimulates the ventricles directly without affecting the sinus node discharge. The sinus node will continue to discharge impulses regularly, but in most instances, the sinus P wave will be obscured in the wide QRS complex. The rhythm is usually regular, but there may be a slight irregularity.

Ventricular tachycardia may develop without any warning signs but most often is preceded by frequent or dangerous forms of PVCs. Ventricular tachycardia may appear as a sustained rhythm or a short run (three or more consecutive PVCs).

The seriousness of ventricular tachycardia depends primarily on its duration. Short runs of ventricular tachycardia usually are not dangerous but can progress into sustained ventricular tachycardia. When ventricular tachycardia becomes an established rhythm there is a reduction in cardiac output, and the patient often becomes hypotensive. Myocar-

dial ischemia can be provoked or accentuated by the systemic hypotension. Sustained ventricular tachycardia can degenerate into ventricular fibrillation.

Priorities of treatment depend on the person's tolerance of the rhythm. If the patient is stable, lidocaine is administered intravenously in a bolus dose of 1 to 1.5 mg/kg followed by half the initial dose every 5 minutes until the rhythm resolves or a total of 3 mg/kg has been given. If adequate doses of lidocaine fail to suppress the rhythm, procainamide can be given intravenously slowly at a rate of 20 mg/min until ventricular tachycardia resolves, hypotension ensues, the QRS complex is widened by 50% of its original width, or a total of 17 mg/kg has been given. If the rhythm is refractory to lidocaine and procainamide, bretylium can be administered intravenously in a dose of 5 to 10 mg/kg over 8 to 10 minutes until the rhythm is resolved or a total of 30 to 35 mg/kg has been given.

Once the rhythm resolves, begin drip infusion of the agent that aided resolution. Patients who fail to respond to drug therapy should be treated with synchronized electric shock. Owing to the hypotensive effects of procainamide and bretylium, some physicians prefer to administer lidocaine intravenously to a total of 3 mg/kg if necessary and then use car-

sustained PVC's   precordial thumb
CO ↓ minimal   deteriorate into Vent. fib

dioversion if the rhythm has not resolved. Cardioversion is the initial treatment in patients who are hemodynamically unstable (Box 9-3) (Figures 9-12 and 9-13).

VENTRICULAR FIBRILLATION

In ventricular fibrillation, an extraordinary electrical focus from the ventricles takes over so rapidly that the muscle fibers do not contract synchronously but twitch in a chaotic manner. The ECG tracing shows a series of wave deflections that are extremely irregular and of varying height, width, and shape.

Box 9-3. Ventricular Tachycardia—Identifying ECG Features

Rhythm:	Usually regular—may be slightly irregular
Rate:	140 to 250
P wave:	No P waves are produced by ventricular tissue. However, the SA node continues to discharge independently during ventricular tachycardia and sinus P waves may be seen, but usually the P waves are buried in the wide QRS complex.
PR:	Not measurable
QRS:	Wide (0.12 seconds or greater)

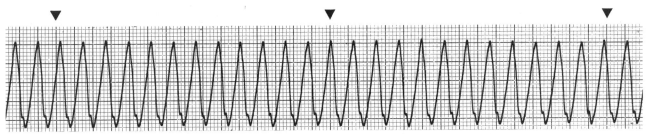

Figure 9-12. Ventricular Tachycardia

Rhythm:	Regular
Rate:	250
P wave:	Not identified
PR:	Not measurable
QRS:	0.16 seconds

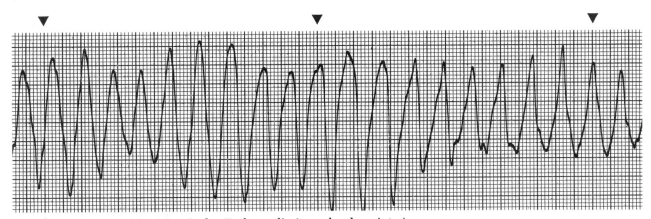

Figure 9-13. Ventricular Tachycardia (torsades de pointes)

Rhythm:	Regular
Rate:	188
P wave:	Not identified
PR:	Not measurable
QRS:	0.20 to 0.24 seconds
Comment:	This type of ventricular tachycardia is called torsades de pointes (twists of points). The QRS changes from negative to positive polarity and appears to twist around the isoelectric line. It is associated with a prolonged QT interval and is refractory to lidocaine and procainamide. Intravenous magnesium or temporary pacing has been successful in the treatment of this rhythm.

Ventricular fibrillation is the most common cause of death in patients with coronary heart disease. In most instances, this rhythm is triggered by PVCs or ventricular tachycardia, but it can occur spontaneously without preceding signs of ventricular irritability.

The muscle twitching in ventricular fibrillation is completely ineffective in propelling blood from the ventricles. Seconds after the onset of ventricular fibrillation, the patient becomes unconscious, peripheral pulses cease, and convulsions frequently occur owing to cerebral anoxia. Death occurs after several minutes unless the rhythm is terminated. Successful resuscitation is best accomplished within the first 2 minutes.

Ventricular fibrillation should be distinguished from primary and secondary ventricular standstill because all will present the same bedside picture. If ventricular fibrillation is witnessed, a precordial thump should be delivered because it can occasionally cause resumption of the heartbeat. If the blow to the chest is unsuccessful, defibrillation should be performed immediately at 200 joules. If the initial shock does not terminate the rhythm, a second shock of 300 joules and a third shock of 360 joules should follow rapidly. If ventricular fibrillation persists, cardiopulmonary resuscitation should be started, an IV line should be established, and the patient should be intubated. Epinephrine 1 mg IV is then given, followed by defibrillation at 360 joules. Epinephrine must be repeated every 3 to 5 minutes. If the rhythm persists, lidocaine is administered IV in a bolus dose of 1 to 1.5 mg/kg, followed by defibrillation at 360 joules. IV lidocaine can be repeated at half-dose increments every 5 minutes, followed by defibrillation at 360 joules, until a total dose of 3 mg/kg has been given. If adequate doses of lidocaine are unsuccessful in terminating the rhythm, bretylium 5 to 10 mg/kg can be administered IV, followed by defibrillation at 360 joules. IV bretylium can be repeated, followed by defibrillation, until a total dose of 30 to 35 mg/kg has been given. If the cardiac arrest persists, sodium bicarbonate 1 mEq/kg can be administered IV initially, followed by half the initial dose every 10 minutes. Once ventricular fibrillation is resolved, begin drip infusion of the antiarrhythmic agent, which aids resolution (Box 9-4) (Figure 9-14).

Box 9-4. Ventricular Fibrillation—Identifying ECG Features

Rhythm:	Chaotic
Rate:	0
P waves:	None; wave deflections are disorganized, chaotic, and of varying height, size, and shape
PR:	Not measurable
QRS:	Absent

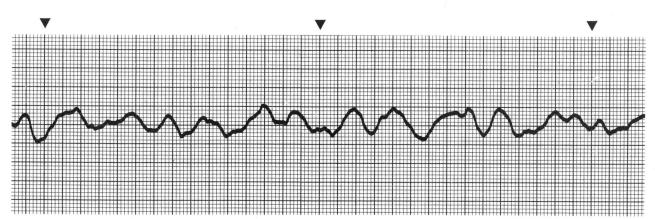

Figure 9-14. Ventricular Fibrillation

Rhythm:	Chaotic
Rate:	0
P waves:	None; wave deflections are chaotic and vary in height, size, and shape
PR:	Not measurable
QRS:	Absent

IDIOVENTRICULAR RHYTHM

An idioventricular rhythm occurs when the focus originates in the ventricles and discharges impulses at a rate of 30 to 40 per minute. The ECG tracing is characterized by an absence of P waves and wide QRS complexes occurring regularly at the inherent idioventricular rate of 30 to 40 per minute.

Idioventricular rhythm occurs when there is a failure of impulse formation or impulse blockage from higher pacemaker centers. The ventricle assumes control by default.

The rhythm may be transient, lasting only a few seconds, or continuous. Continuous idioventricular rhythm is dangerous, not only because of the slow rate but because the rhythm may develop into ventricular standstill or asystole. An external or temporary transvenous pacemaker should be used as soon as this rhythm is identified.

While preparations are being made for pacemaker placement, or if a pacemaker is not available, atropine 1 mg intravenously can be administered every 5 minutes until a total dose of 3 mg has been given. If atropine is refractory and hypotension is associated with the rhythm, dopamine in a dose of 5 to 20 μg/kg/min or epinephrine in a dose of 2 to 10 μg/min can be infused (Box 9-5) (Figure 9-15).

Box 9-5.	Idioventricular Rhythm—Identifying ECG Features
Rhythm:	Regular
Rate:	30 to 40
P waves:	Absent
PR:	Not measurable
QRS:	Wide (0.12 seconds or greater)

ACCELERATED IDIOVENTRICULAR RHYTHM

An accelerated idioventricular rhythm occurs when the focus originates in the ventricles and discharges impulses at a rate between 50 and 100 per minute. This rhythm is faster than the inherent idioventricular rate (30 to 40 per minute) but slower than ventricular tachycardia (140 to 250 per minute). The ECG tracing is characterized by an absence of P waves and wide QRS complexes occurring regularly at an accelerated idioventricular rate.

Accelerated idioventricular rhythm is common following acute inferior myocardial infarction and is frequently a reperfusion rhythm following thrombolytic therapy. It is a transient arrhythmia and usually produces no hemodynamic effects.

Most cardiologists do not treat accelerated idioventricular rhythm, especially if the rhythm occurs late (as an escape rhythm) and the patient remains asymptomatic. If the rhythm begins prematurely, some physicians choose to use lidocaine to suppress the rhythm.

Accelerated idioventricular rhythm that begins prematurely is more likely to lead to ventricular tachycardia (Box 9-6) (Figure 9-16).

Box 9-6.	Accelerated Idioventricular Rhythm—Identifying ECG Features
Rhythm:	Regular
Rate:	50 to 100
P waves:	Absent
PR:	Not measurable
QRS:	Wide (0.12 seconds or greater)

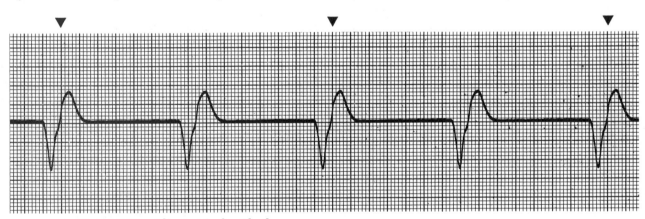

Figure 9-15. Idioventricular Rhythm

Rhythm: Regular

Rate: 41

P waves: Absent

PR: Not measurable

QRS: 0.16 to 0.18 seconds

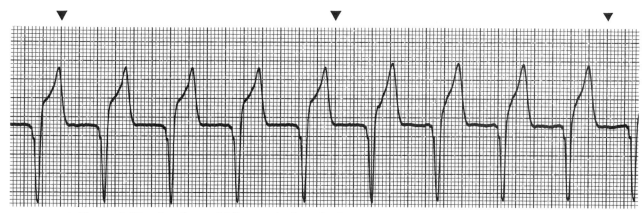

Figure 9-16.   Accelerated Idioventricular Rhythm

Rhythm: Regular

Rate: 84

P waves: Absent

PR: Not measurable

QRS: 0.12 seconds

PRIMARY VENTRICULAR STANDSTILL

In primary ventricular standstill, sinus impulses are discharged normally and produce P waves. Suddenly, all the impulses are blocked and none reach the ventricles. On the ECG tracing, QRS complexes disappear while P waves continue. Despite the seeming suddenness of the rhythm, primary ventricular standstill is a result of a conduction disorder and is preceded in practically all instances by some form of heart block, usually Mobitz II, third-degree AV block, or bundle branch block involving two or three fascicles of the bundle branches.

When primary ventricular standstill develops, ventricular contraction ceases, and there is a complete cessation of circulation. The patient becomes unconscious, peripheral pulses are absent, and cyanosis and convulsions may be present. Death occurs within a few minutes unless the rhythm is terminated.

The results of resuscitation are extremely poor. Consequently, prevention of ventricular standstill is of supreme importance. An external or temporary transvenous pacemaker should be placed prophylactically when serious conduction disorders are identified.

Primary ventricular standstill should be distinguished via ECG from ventricular fibrillation and secondary ventricular standstill because all will present the same bedside picture. If primary ventricular standstill is witnessed, a precordial thump can be delivered because it can occasionally cause resumption of the heartbeat. If the blow to the chest is unsuccessful, cardiopulmonary resuscitation should be started, an intravenous line should be established, and the patient should be intubated. Epinephrine 1 mg intravenously is then given and repeated every 3 to 5 minutes. If the rhythm persists, atropine 1 mg intravenously is given and repeated every 5 minutes until a total dose of 3 mg has been given. Sodium bicarbonate 1 mEq/kg can be administered intravenously initially followed by half the initial dose every 10 minutes. As soon as possible during the resuscitation attempt, an external or transvenous pacemaker should be placed (Box 9-7) (Figure 9-17).

Box 9-7.   Primary Ventricular Standstill—Identifying ECG Features

Rhythm: 0 (no QRS complexes)

Rate: 0 (no QRS complexes)

P waves: Sinus P waves present

PR: Not measurable

QRS: Absent

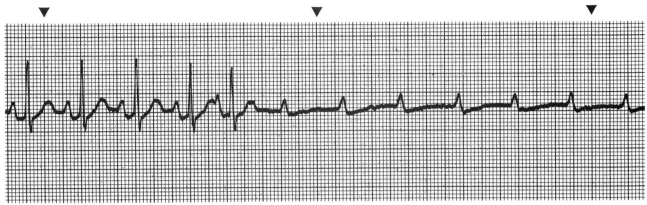

Figure 9-17. Normal Sinus Rhythm with One PAC Changing to Primary Ventricular Standstill

Rhythm:	Basic rhythm regular
Rate:	Basic rhythm 100
P waves:	Sinus P waves are present
PR:	0.16 to 0.18 seconds (basic rhythm)
QRS:	0.06 seconds (basic rhythm)

SECONDARY VENTRICULAR STANDSTILL

Like primary ventricular standstill, when secondary ventricular standstill develops, ventricular contraction ceases and there is a complete cessation of circulation. However, the cause of the rhythm and ECG pattern differs. Secondary ventricular standstill is caused by a hypoxic myocardium secondary to advanced heart failure and is usually a terminal rhythm. The ECG tracing will show wide QRS complexes at a slow rate of 10 to 30 per minute.

Secondary ventricular standstill should be distinguished via ECG from ventricular fibrillation and primary ventricular standstill because all will present the same bedside picture. Once secondary ventricular standstill is identified, cardiopulmonary re-

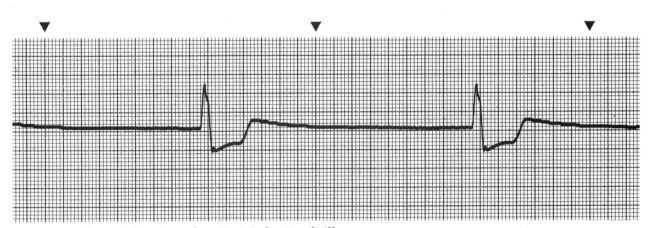

Figure 9-18. Secondary Ventricular Standstill

Rhythm:	Cannot be determined for sure; only one cardiac cycle
Rate:	About 20
P waves:	Absent
PR:	Not measurable
QRS:	0.12 seconds
Comment:	ST segment depression is present.

suscitation should be started, an intravenous line should be established, and the patient should be intubated. Epinephrine 1 mg intravenously is then given and repeated every 3 to 5 minutes. If the rhythm persists, atropine 1 mg intravenously is given and repeated every 5 minutes until a total dose of 3 mg has been given. To combat metabolic acidosis, sodium bicarbonate 1 mEq/kg can be administered intravenously followed by half the initial dose every 10 minutes. Secondary ventricular standstill seldom yields to resuscitative techniques (including cardiac pacing) because the oxygen-deprived myocardium is unable to respond to any stimulation (Box 9-8) (Figure 9-18).

Box 9-8.	Secondary Ventricular Standstill—Identifying ECG Features
Rhythm:	Regular, usually
Rate:	10 to 30
P waves:	Absent
PR:	Not measurable
QRS:	Wide (0.12 seconds or greater)

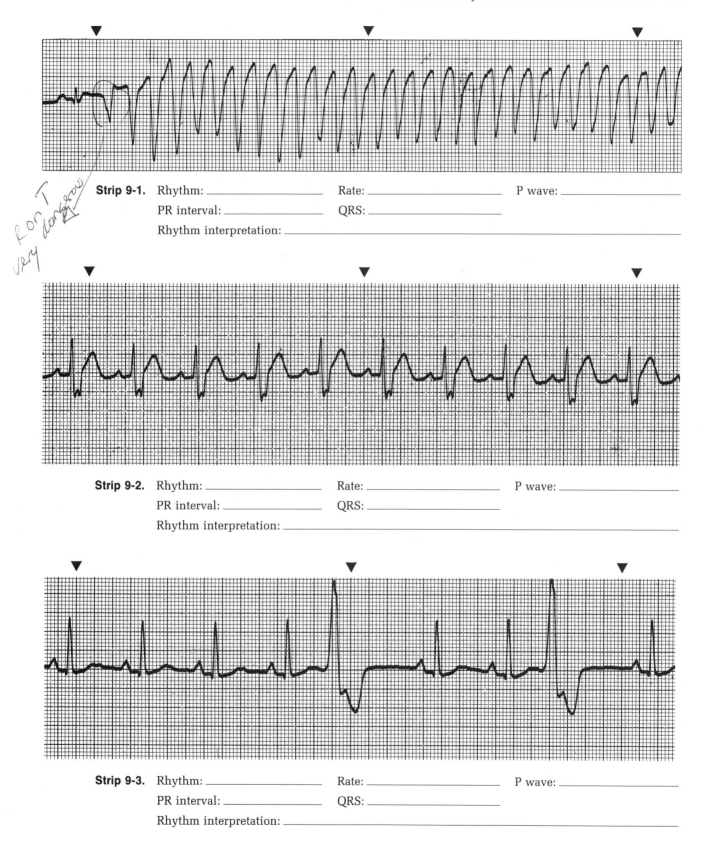

Strip 9-1. Rhythm: _____ Rate: _____ P wave: _____

PR interval: _____ QRS: _____

Rhythm interpretation: _____

Strip 9-2. Rhythm: _____ Rate: _____ P wave: _____

PR interval: _____ QRS: _____

Rhythm interpretation: _____

Strip 9-3. Rhythm: _____ Rate: _____ P wave: _____

PR interval: _____ QRS: _____

Rhythm interpretation: _____

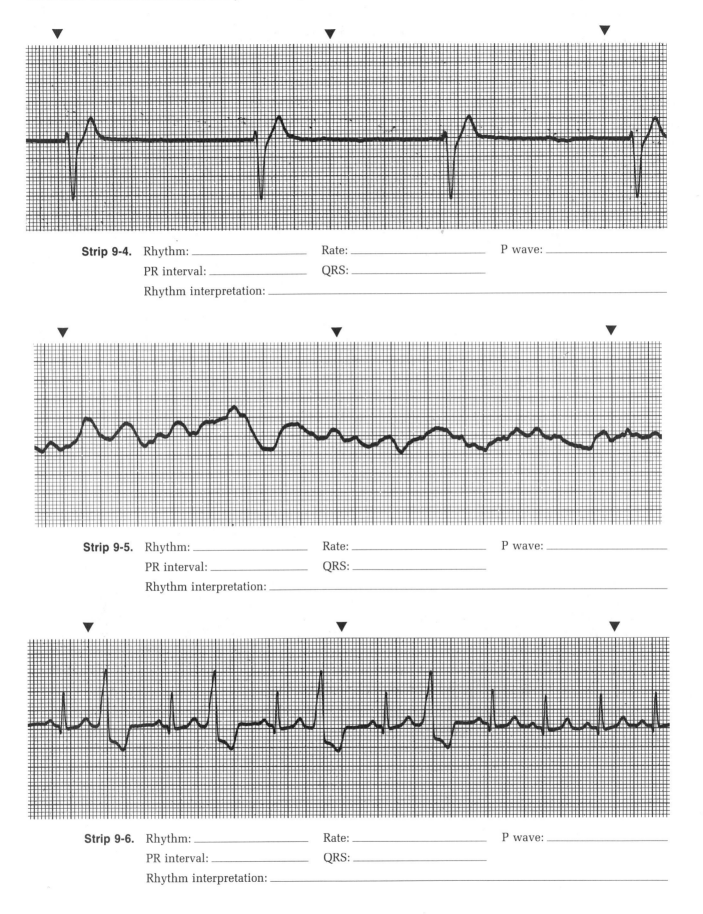

Strip 9-4. Rhythm: _____ Rate: _____ P wave: _____

PR interval: _____ QRS: _____

Rhythm interpretation: _____

Strip 9-5. Rhythm: _____ Rate: _____ P wave: _____

PR interval: _____ QRS: _____

Rhythm interpretation: _____

Strip 9-6. Rhythm: _____ Rate: _____ P wave: _____

PR interval: _____ QRS: _____

Rhythm interpretation: _____

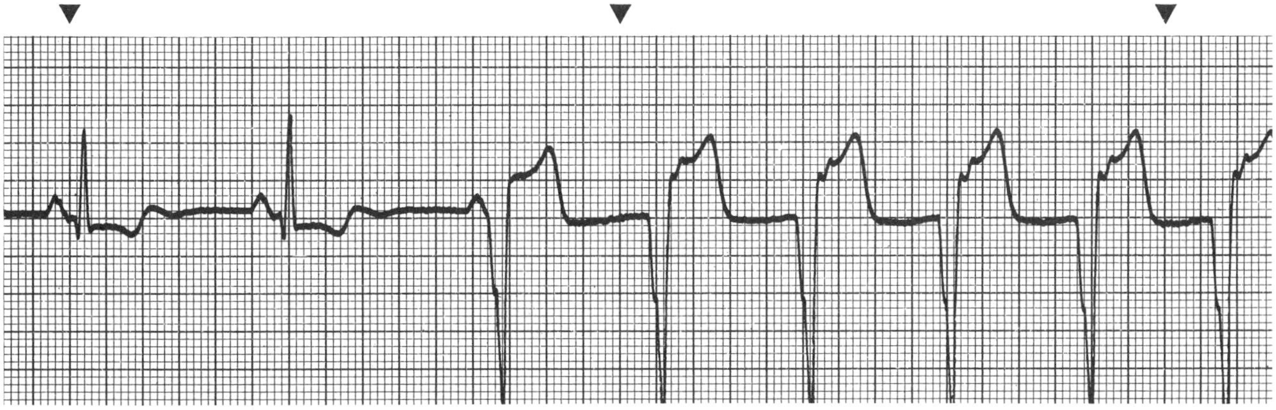

Strip 9-7. Rhythm: _____ Rate: _____ P wave: _____

PR interval: _____ QRS: _____

Rhythm interpretation: _____

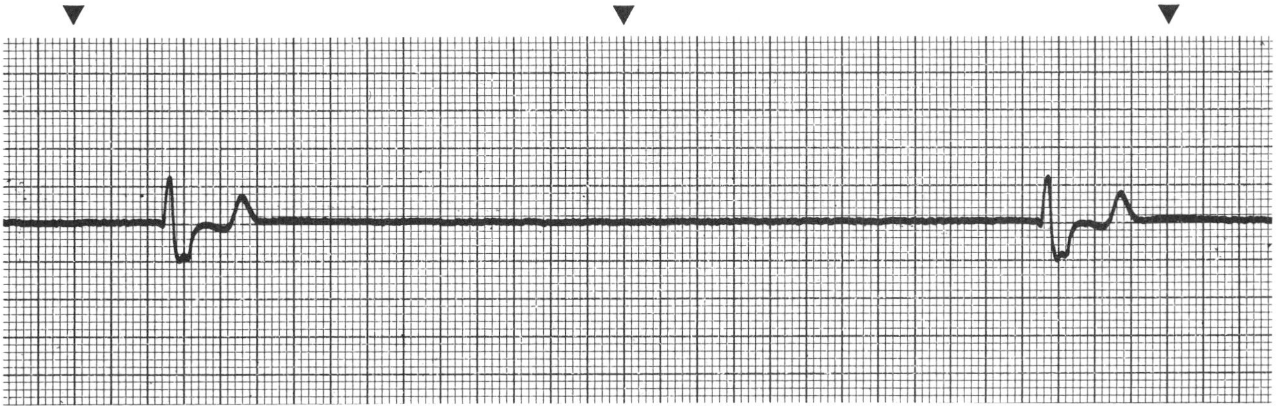

Strip 9-8. Rhythm: _____ Rate: _____ P wave: _____

PR interval: _____ QRS: _____

Rhythm interpretation: _____

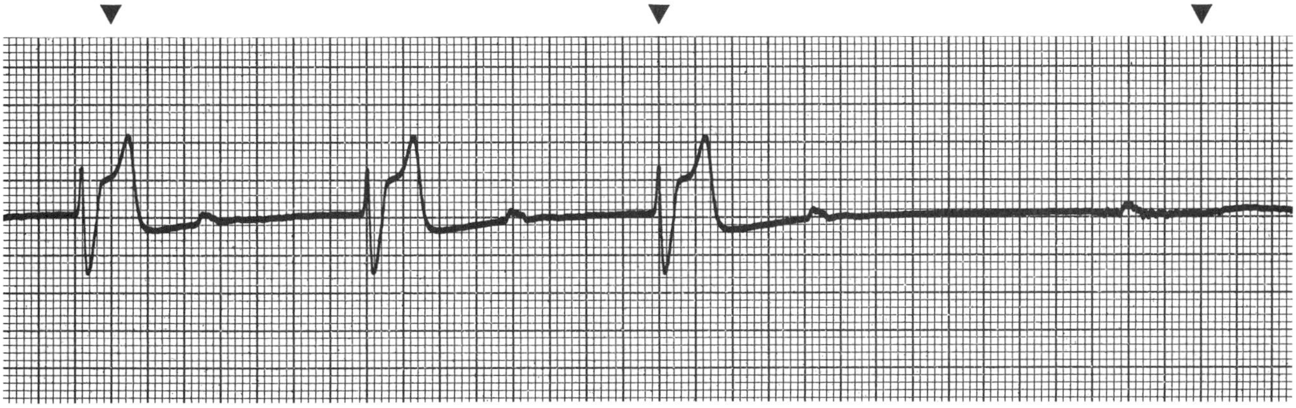

Strip 9-9. Rhythm: _____ Rate: _____ P wave: _____

PR interval: _____ QRS: _____

Rhythm interpretation: _____

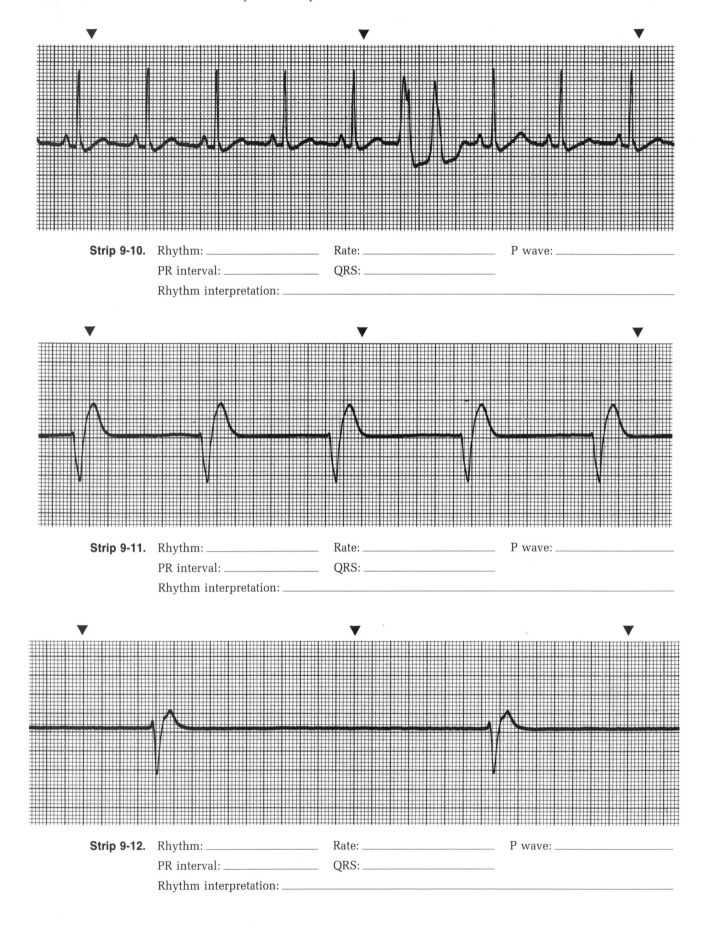

Strip 9-10. Rhythm: _____ Rate: _____ P wave: _____

PR interval: _____ QRS: _____

Rhythm interpretation: _____

Strip 9-11. Rhythm: _____ Rate: _____ P wave: _____

PR interval: _____ QRS: _____

Rhythm interpretation: _____

Strip 9-12. Rhythm: _____ Rate: _____ P wave: _____

PR interval: _____ QRS: _____

Rhythm interpretation: _____

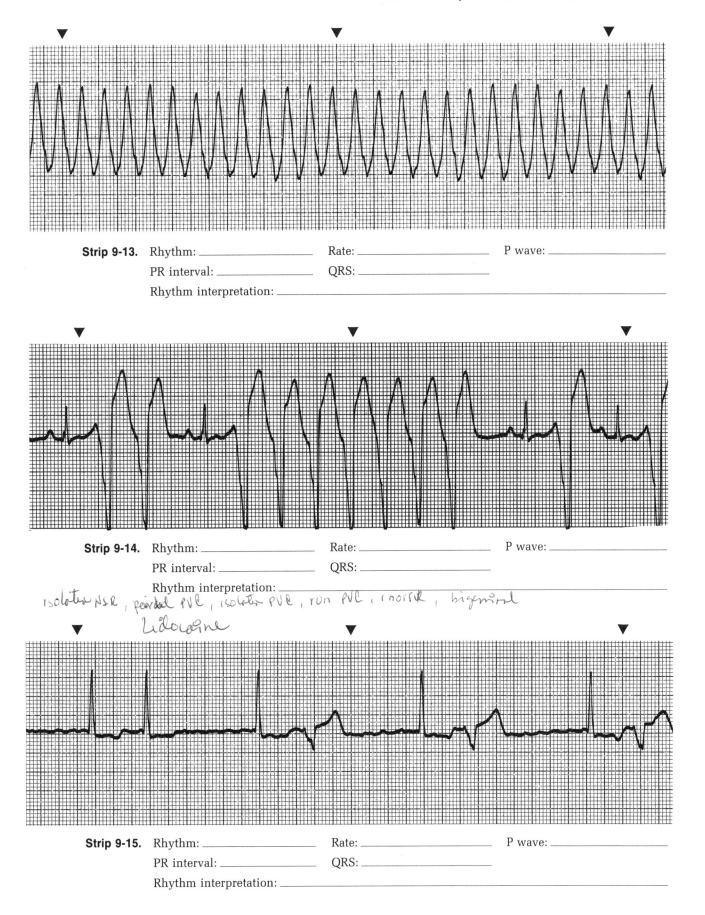

Strip 9-13. Rhythm: _____ Rate: _____ P wave: _____

PR interval: _____ QRS: _____

Rhythm interpretation: _____

Strip 9-14. Rhythm: _____ Rate: _____ P wave: _____

PR interval: _____ QRS: _____

Rhythm interpretation: _____

isolated NSR, paired PVC, isolated PVC, run PVC, nosrk, bigeminal

Lidocaine

Strip 9-15. Rhythm: _____ Rate: _____ P wave: _____

PR interval: _____ QRS: _____

Rhythm interpretation: _____

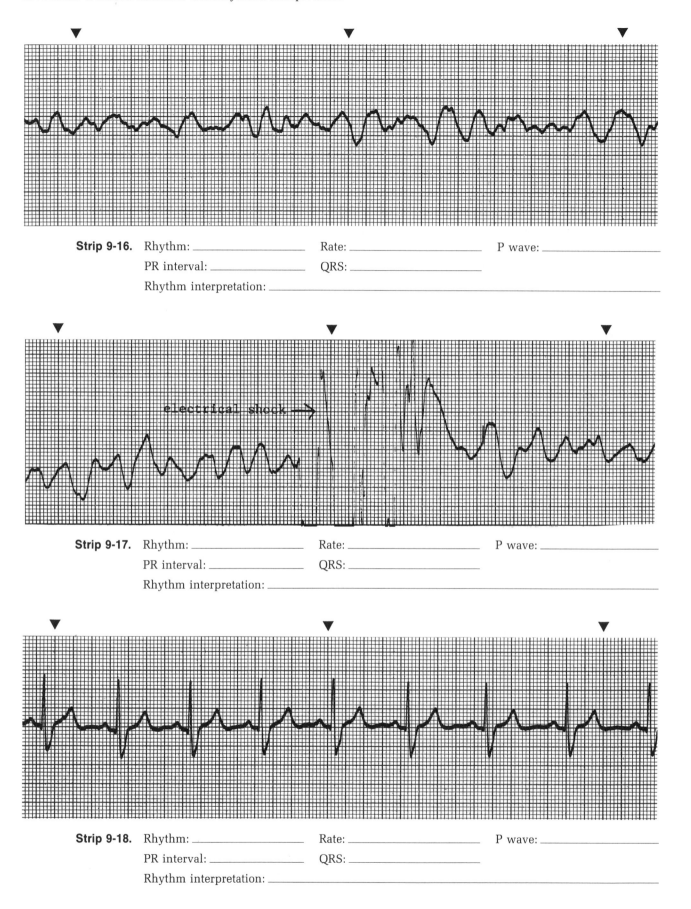

Strip 9-16. Rhythm: _____ Rate: _____ P wave: _____

PR interval: _____ QRS: _____

Rhythm interpretation: _____

Strip 9-17. Rhythm: _____ Rate: _____ P wave: _____

PR interval: _____ QRS: _____

Rhythm interpretation: _____

Strip 9-18. Rhythm: _____ Rate: _____ P wave: _____

PR interval: _____ QRS: _____

Rhythm interpretation: _____

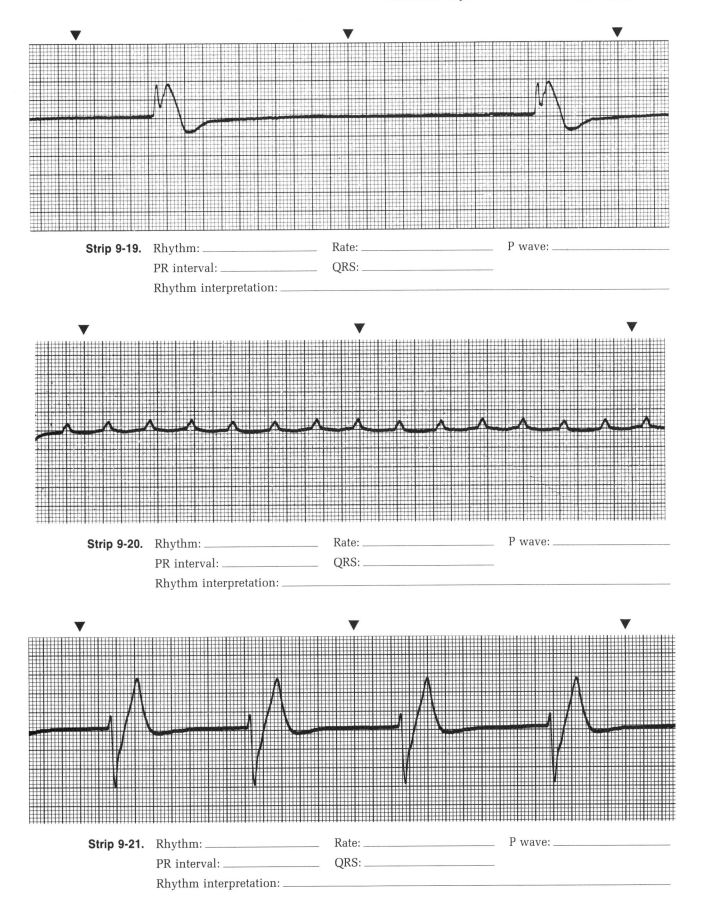

Strip 9-19. Rhythm: _____ Rate: _____ P wave: _____

PR interval: _____ QRS: _____

Rhythm interpretation: _____

Strip 9-20. Rhythm: _____ Rate: _____ P wave: _____

PR interval: _____ QRS: _____

Rhythm interpretation: _____

Strip 9-21. Rhythm: _____ Rate: _____ P wave: _____

PR interval: _____ QRS: _____

Rhythm interpretation: _____

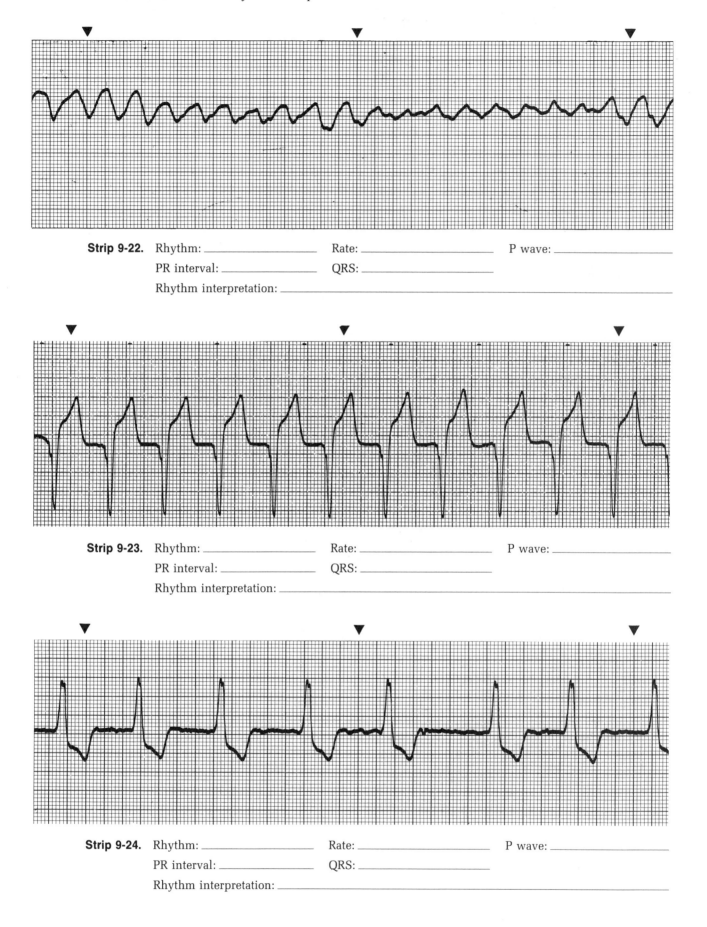

Strip 9-22. Rhythm: _____ Rate: _____ P wave: _____

PR interval: _____ QRS: _____

Rhythm interpretation: _____

Strip 9-23. Rhythm: _____ Rate: _____ P wave: _____

PR interval: _____ QRS: _____

Rhythm interpretation: _____

Strip 9-24. Rhythm: _____ Rate: _____ P wave: _____

PR interval: _____ QRS: _____

Rhythm interpretation: _____

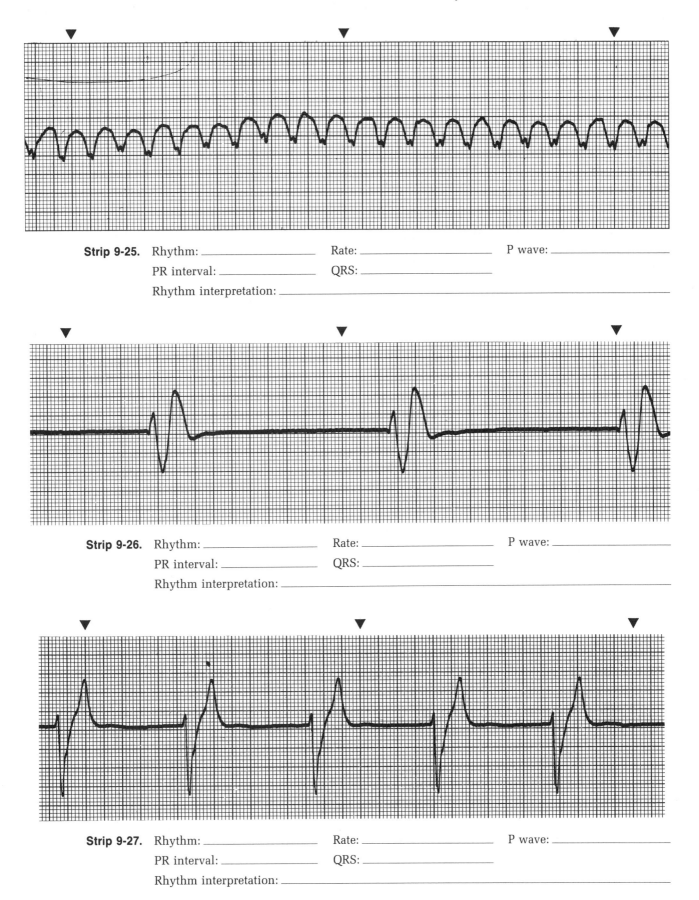

Strip 9-25. Rhythm: _____ Rate: _____ P wave: _____

PR interval: _____ QRS: _____

Rhythm interpretation: _____

Strip 9-26. Rhythm: _____ Rate: _____ P wave: _____

PR interval: _____ QRS: _____

Rhythm interpretation: _____

Strip 9-27. Rhythm: _____ Rate: _____ P wave: _____

PR interval: _____ QRS: _____

Rhythm interpretation: _____

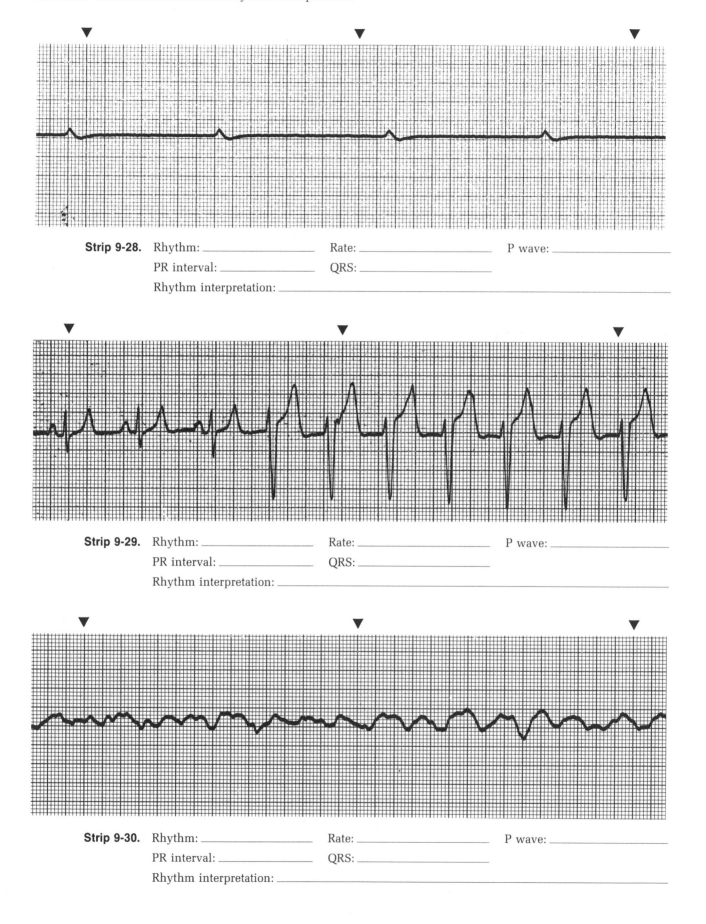

Strip 9-28. Rhythm: _____ Rate: _____ P wave: _____

PR interval: _____ QRS: _____

Rhythm interpretation: _____

Strip 9-29. Rhythm: _____ Rate: _____ P wave: _____

PR interval: _____ QRS: _____

Rhythm interpretation: _____

Strip 9-30. Rhythm: _____ Rate: _____ P wave: _____

PR interval: _____ QRS: _____

Rhythm interpretation: _____

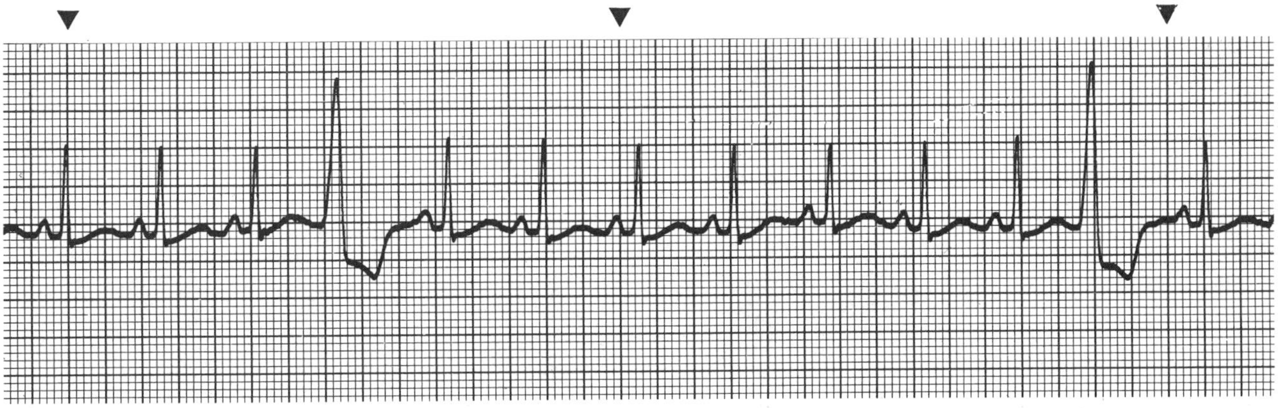

Strip 9-31. Rhythm: _____ Rate: _____ P wave: _____

PR interval: _____ QRS: _____

Rhythm interpretation: _____

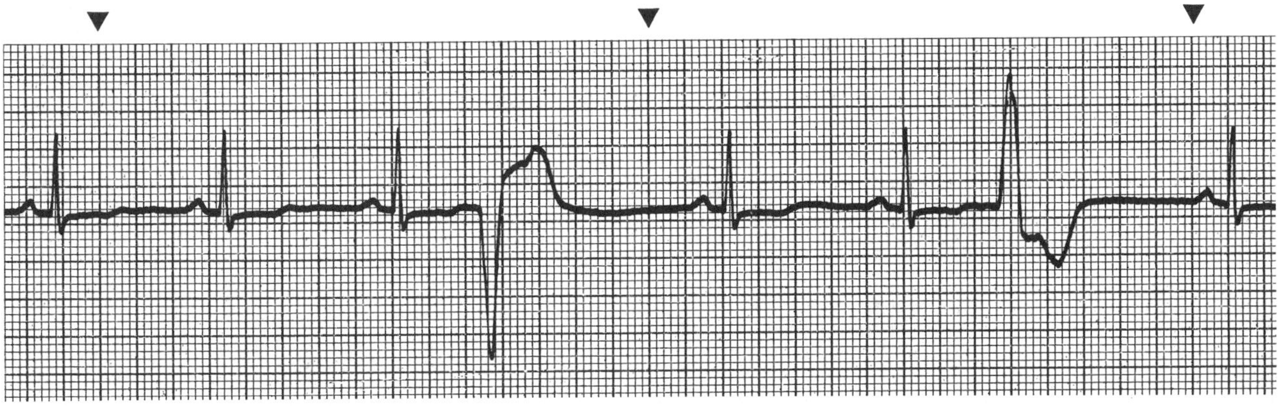

Strip 9-32. Rhythm: _____ Rate: _____ P wave: _____

PR interval: _____ QRS: _____

Rhythm interpretation: _____

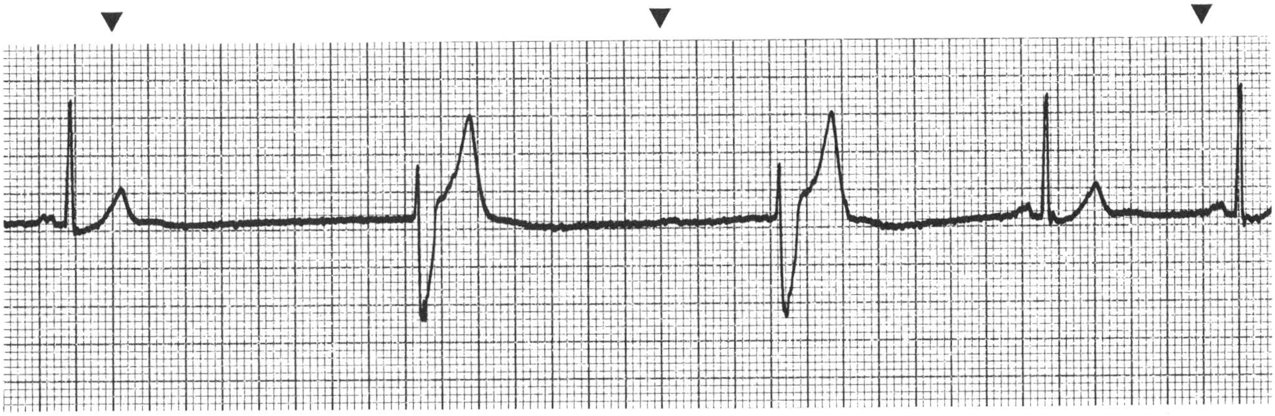

Strip 9-33. Rhythm: _____ Rate: _____ P wave: _____

PR interval: _____ QRS: _____

Rhythm interpretation: _____

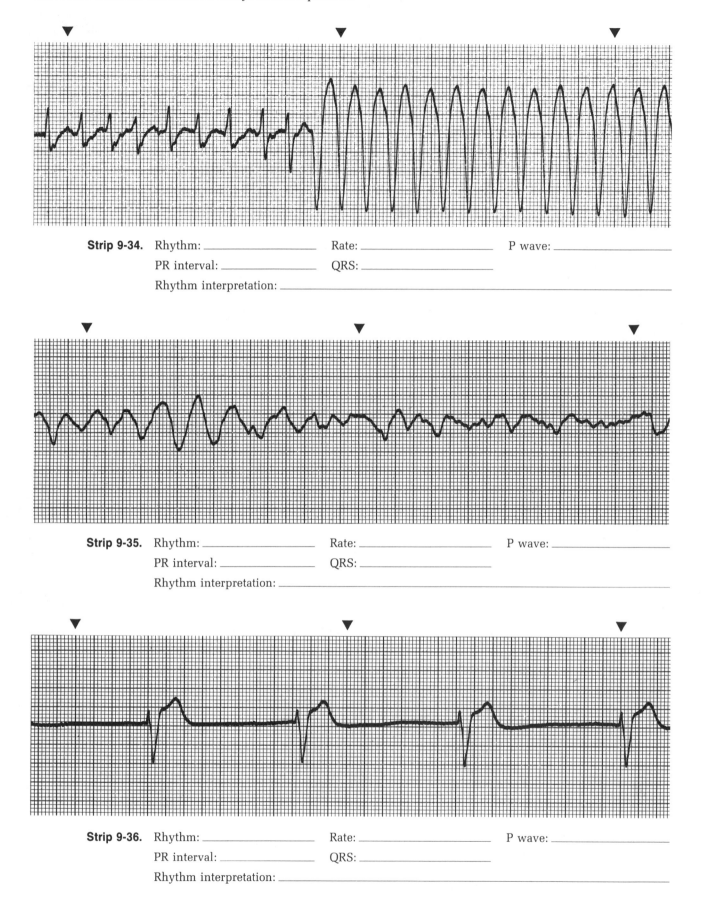

Strip 9-34. Rhythm: _____ Rate: _____ P wave: _____

PR interval: _____ QRS: _____

Rhythm interpretation: _____

Strip 9-35. Rhythm: _____ Rate: _____ P wave: _____

PR interval: _____ QRS: _____

Rhythm interpretation: _____

Strip 9-36. Rhythm: _____ Rate: _____ P wave: _____

PR interval: _____ QRS: _____

Rhythm interpretation: _____

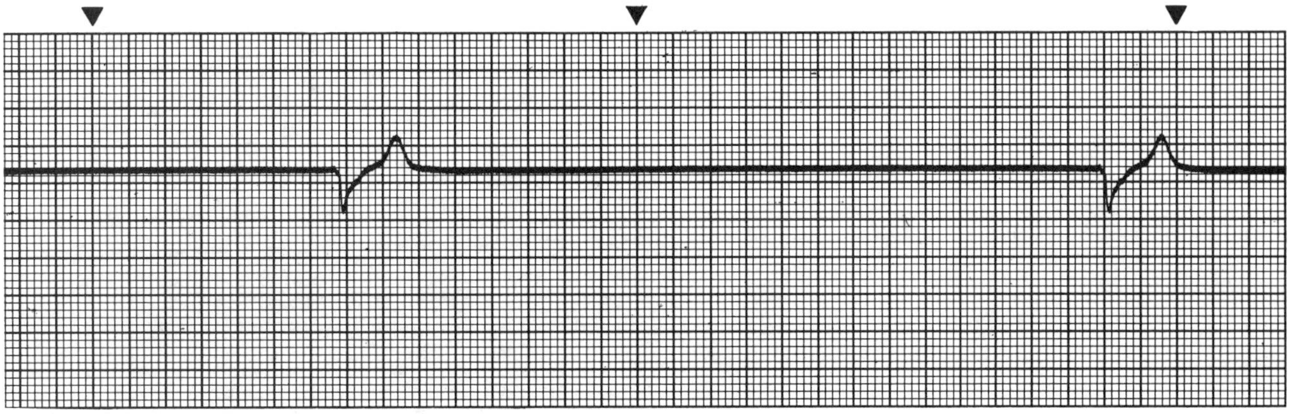

Strip 9-37. Rhythm: _____ Rate: _____ P wave: _____

PR interval: _____ QRS: _____

Rhythm interpretation: _____

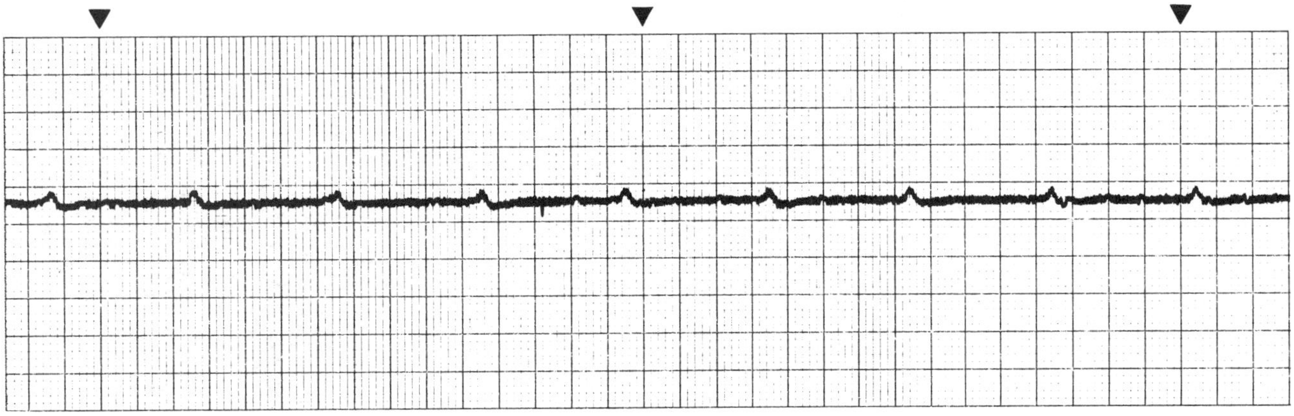

Strip 9-38. Rhythm: _____ Rate: _____ P wave: _____

PR interval: _____ QRS: _____

Rhythm interpretation: _____

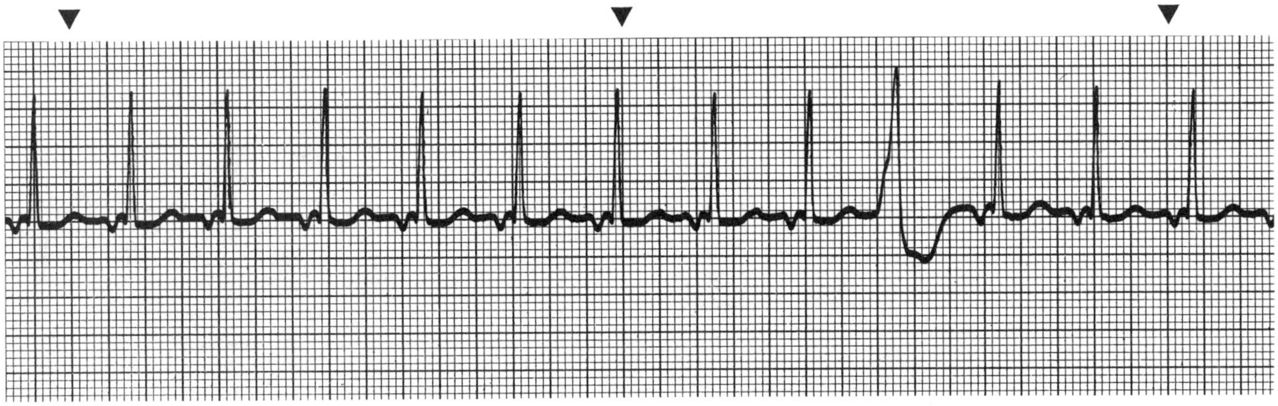

Strip 9-39. Rhythm: _____ Rate: _____ P wave: _____

PR interval: _____ QRS: _____

Rhythm interpretation: _____

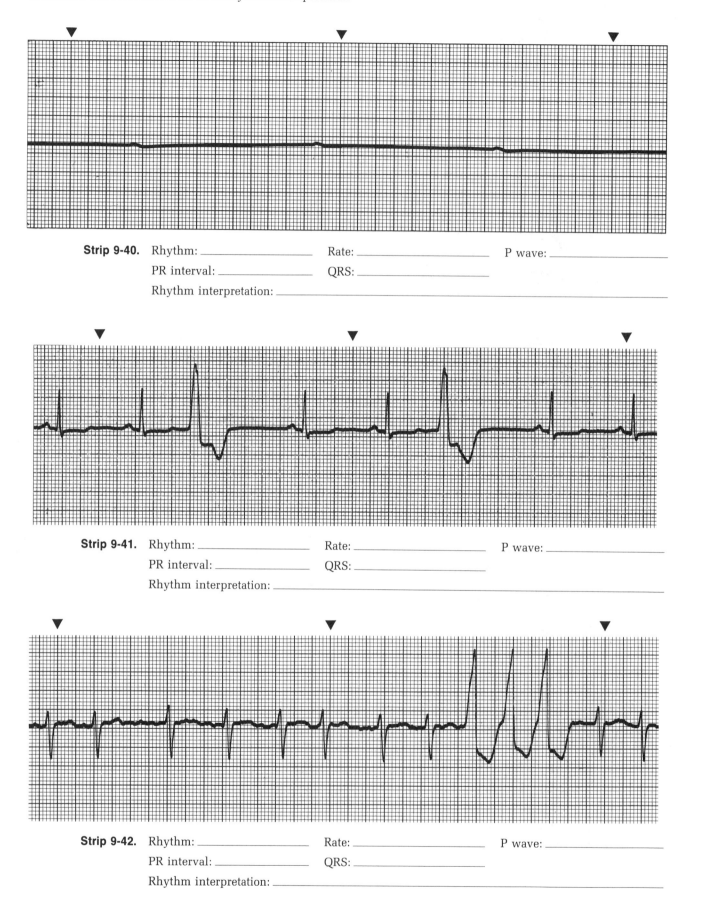

Strip 9-40. Rhythm: _____ Rate: _____ P wave: _____

PR interval: _____ QRS: _____

Rhythm interpretation: _____

Strip 9-41. Rhythm: _____ Rate: _____ P wave: _____

PR interval: _____ QRS: _____

Rhythm interpretation: _____

Strip 9-42. Rhythm: _____ Rate: _____ P wave: _____

PR interval: _____ QRS: _____

Rhythm interpretation: _____

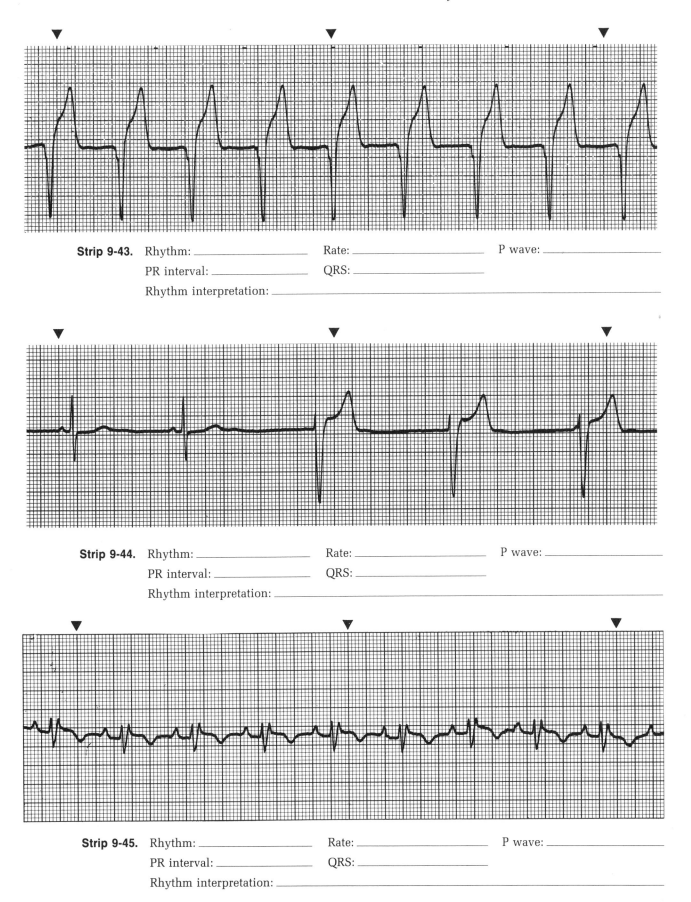

Strip 9-43. Rhythm: _____ Rate: _____ P wave: _____

PR interval: _____ QRS: _____

Rhythm interpretation: _____

Strip 9-44. Rhythm: _____ Rate: _____ P wave: _____

PR interval: _____ QRS: _____

Rhythm interpretation: _____

Strip 9-45. Rhythm: _____ Rate: _____ P wave: _____

PR interval: _____ QRS: _____

Rhythm interpretation: _____

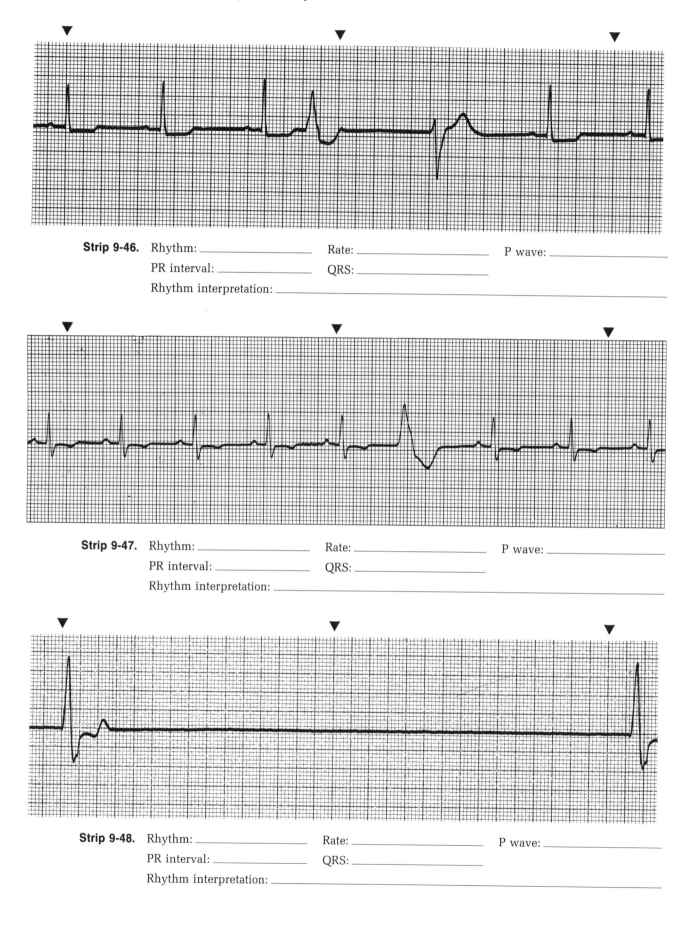

Strip 9-46. Rhythm: _____ Rate: _____ P wave: _____

PR interval: _____ QRS: _____

Rhythm interpretation: _____

Strip 9-47. Rhythm: _____ Rate: _____ P wave: _____

PR interval: _____ QRS: _____

Rhythm interpretation: _____

Strip 9-48. Rhythm: _____ Rate: _____ P wave: _____

PR interval: _____ QRS: _____

Rhythm interpretation: _____

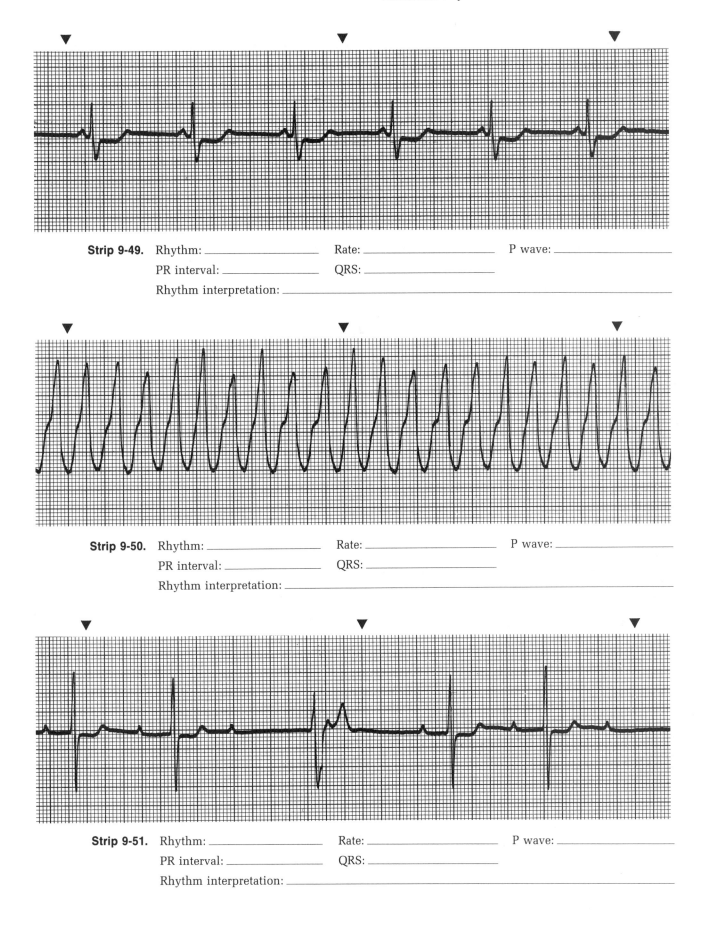

Strip 9-49. Rhythm: _____ Rate: _____ P wave: _____

PR interval: _____ QRS: _____

Rhythm interpretation: _____

Strip 9-50. Rhythm: _____ Rate: _____ P wave: _____

PR interval: _____ QRS: _____

Rhythm interpretation: _____

Strip 9-51. Rhythm: _____ Rate: _____ P wave: _____

PR interval: _____ QRS: _____

Rhythm interpretation: _____

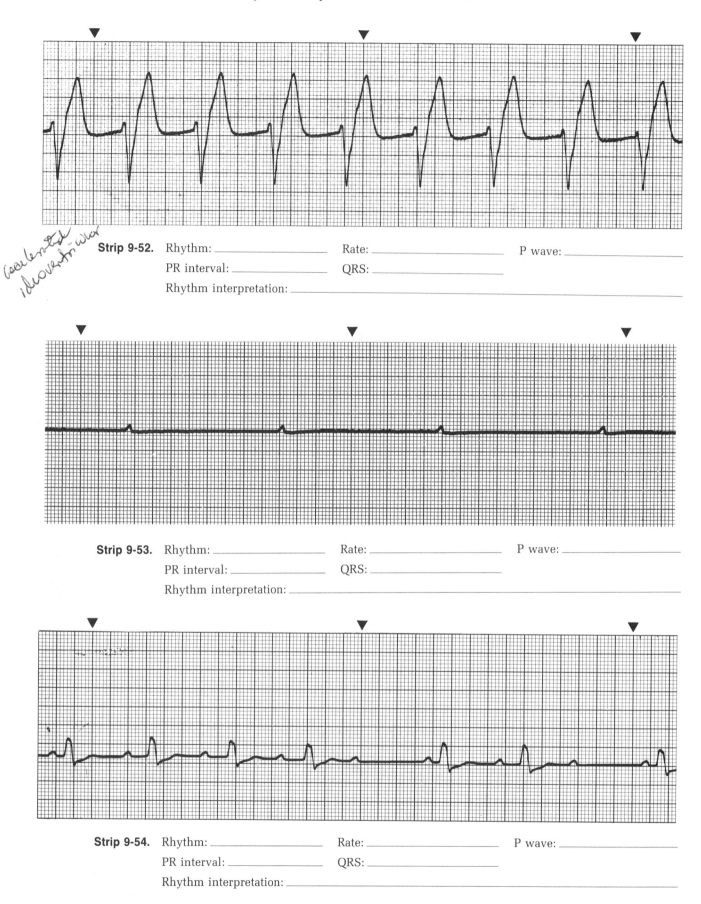

accelerated idioventricular

Strip 9-52. Rhythm: _____ Rate: _____ P wave: _____

PR interval: _____ QRS: _____

Rhythm interpretation: _____

Strip 9-53. Rhythm: _____ Rate: _____ P wave: _____

PR interval: _____ QRS: _____

Rhythm interpretation: _____

Strip 9-54. Rhythm: _____ Rate: _____ P wave: _____

PR interval: _____ QRS: _____

Rhythm interpretation: _____

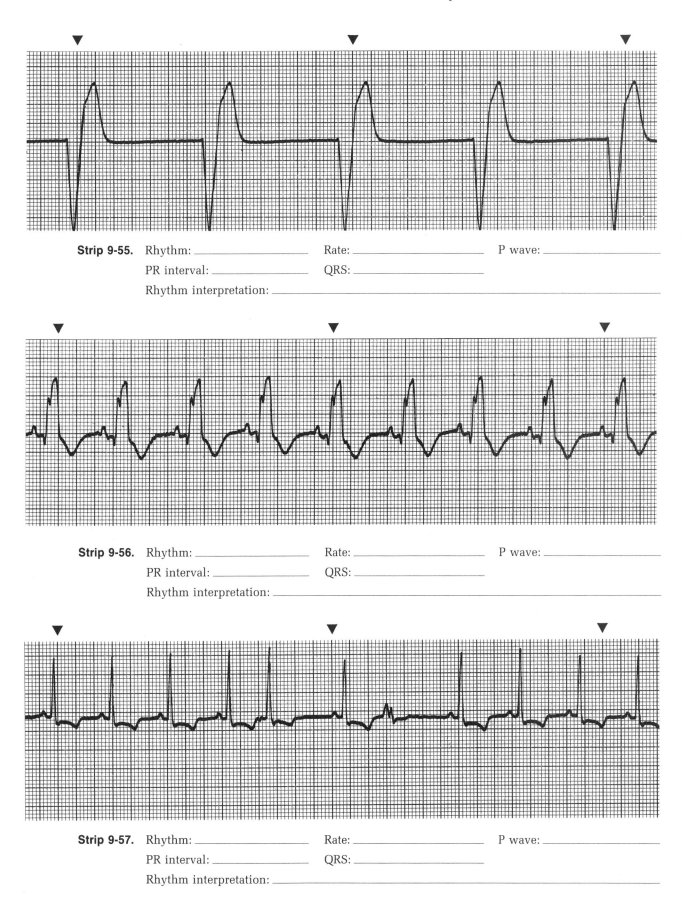

Strip 9-55. Rhythm: _____ Rate: _____ P wave: _____

PR interval: _____ QRS: _____

Rhythm interpretation: _____

Strip 9-56. Rhythm: _____ Rate: _____ P wave: _____

PR interval: _____ QRS: _____

Rhythm interpretation: _____

Strip 9-57. Rhythm: _____ Rate: _____ P wave: _____

PR interval: _____ QRS: _____

Rhythm interpretation: _____

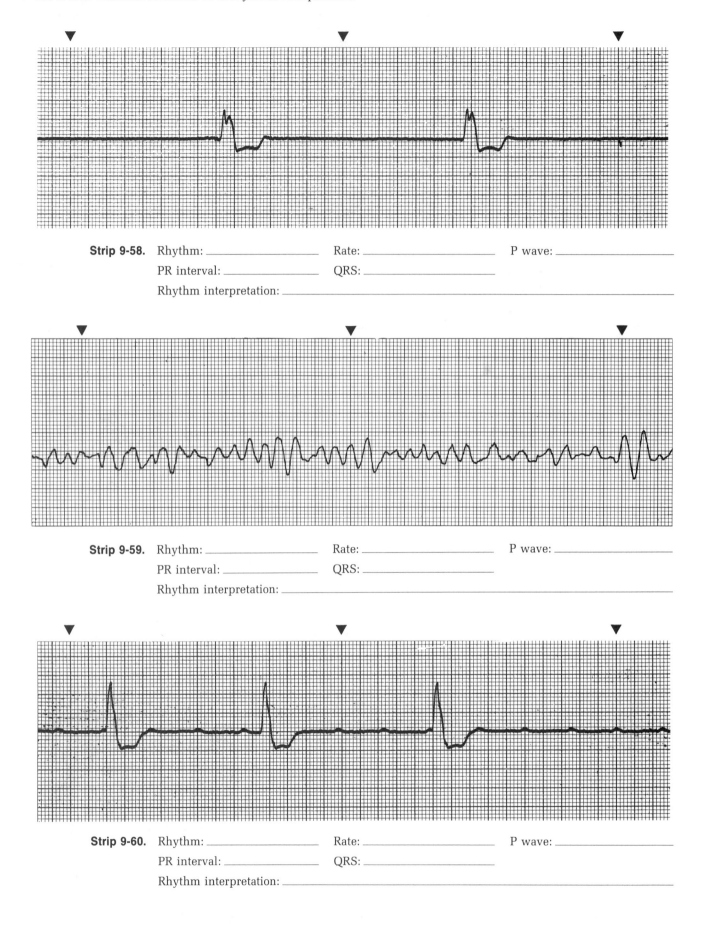

Strip 9-58. Rhythm: _____ Rate: _____ P wave: _____

PR interval: _____ QRS: _____

Rhythm interpretation: _____

Strip 9-59. Rhythm: _____ Rate: _____ P wave: _____

PR interval: _____ QRS: _____

Rhythm interpretation: _____

Strip 9-60. Rhythm: _____ Rate: _____ P wave: _____

PR interval: _____ QRS: _____

Rhythm interpretation: _____

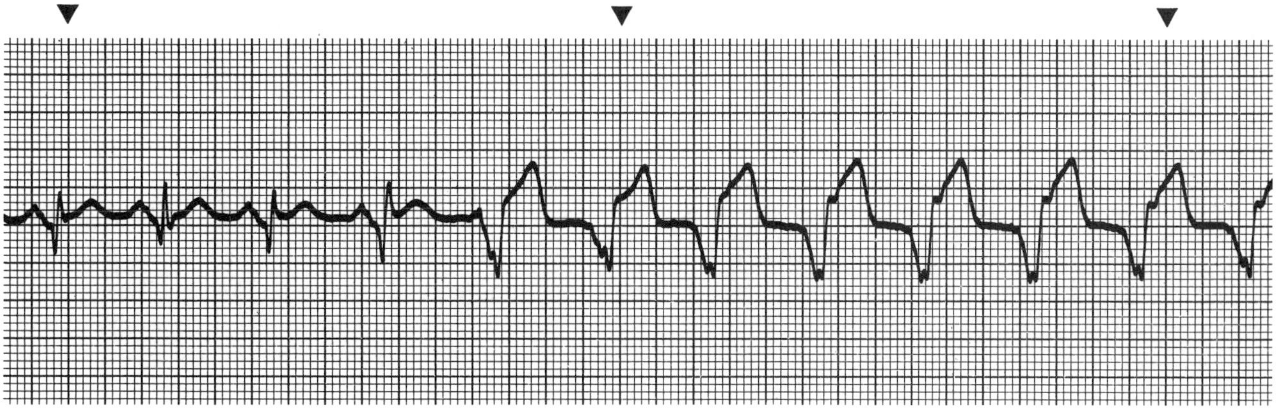

Strip 9-61. Rhythm: _____ Rate: _____ P wave: _____

PR interval: _____ QRS: _____

Rhythm interpretation: _____

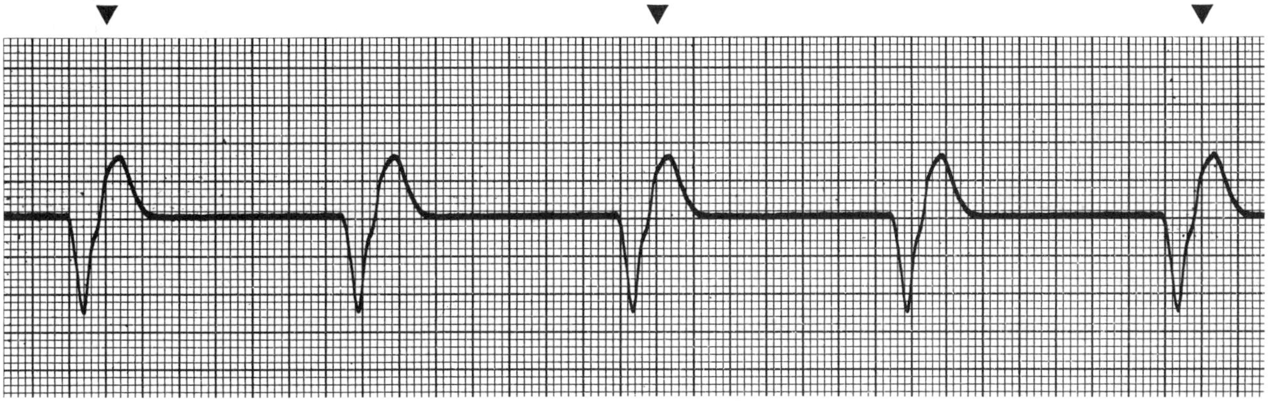

Strip 9-62. Rhythm: _____ Rate: _____ P wave: _____

PR interval: _____ QRS: _____

Rhythm interpretation: _____

electrical shock

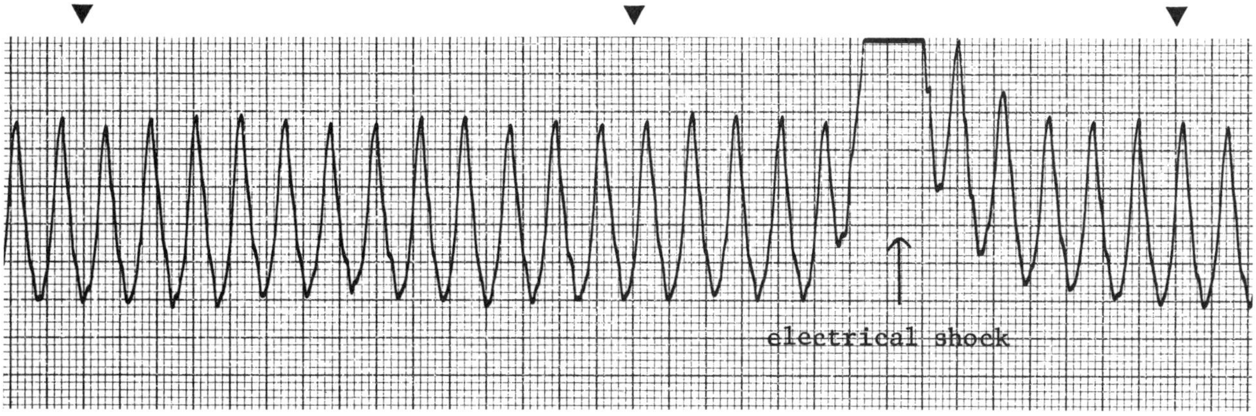

Strip 9-63. Rhythm: _____ Rate: _____ P wave: _____

PR interval: _____ QRS: _____

Rhythm interpretation: _____

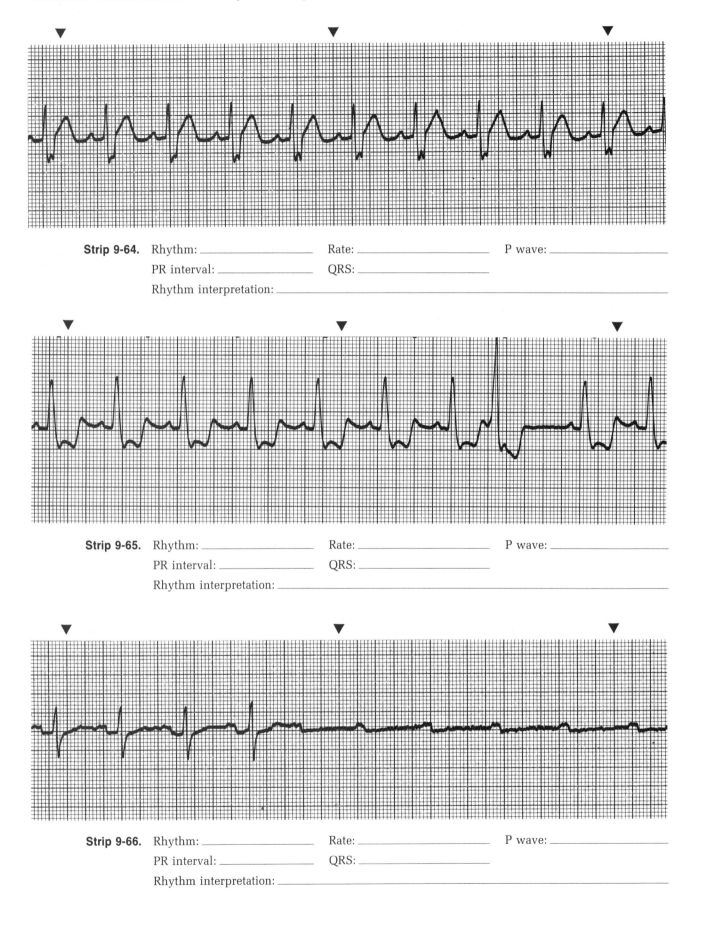

Strip 9-64. Rhythm: _____ Rate: _____ P wave: _____

PR interval: _____ QRS: _____

Rhythm interpretation: _____

Strip 9-65. Rhythm: _____ Rate: _____ P wave: _____

PR interval: _____ QRS: _____

Rhythm interpretation: _____

Strip 9-66. Rhythm: _____ Rate: _____ P wave: _____

PR interval: _____ QRS: _____

Rhythm interpretation: _____

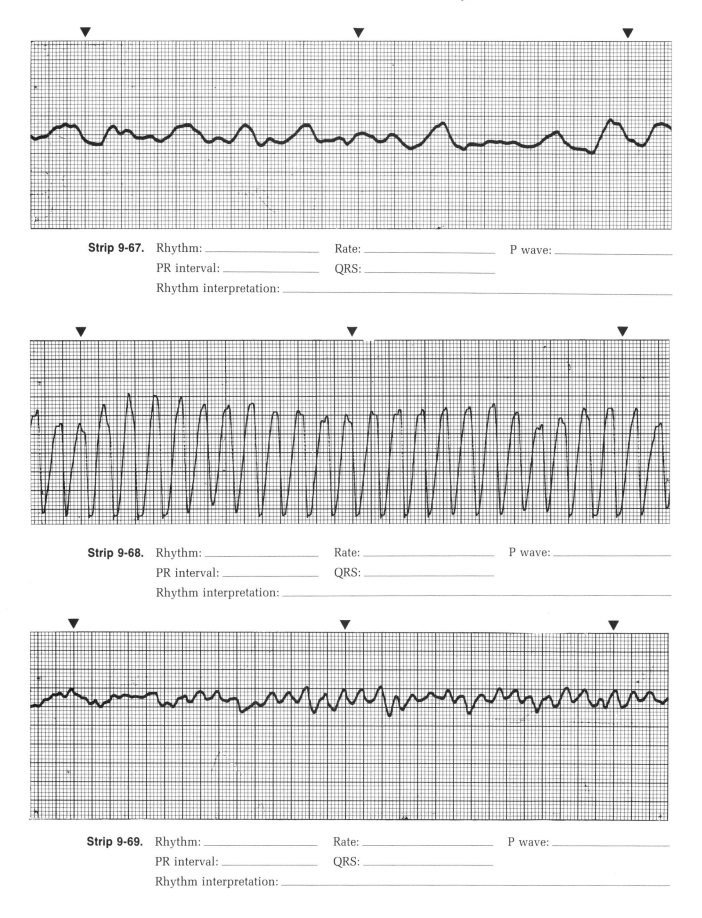

Strip 9-67. Rhythm: _____ Rate: _____ P wave: _____

PR interval: _____ QRS: _____

Rhythm interpretation: _____

Strip 9-68. Rhythm: _____ Rate: _____ P wave: _____

PR interval: _____ QRS: _____

Rhythm interpretation: _____

Strip 9-69. Rhythm: _____ Rate: _____ P wave: _____

PR interval: _____ QRS: _____

Rhythm interpretation: _____

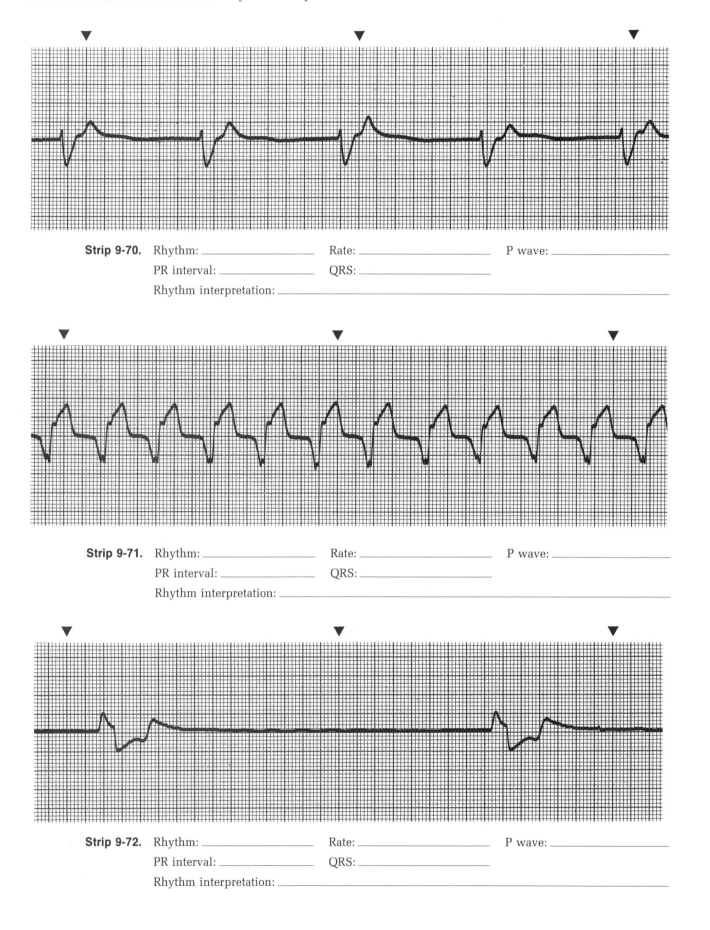

Strip 9-70. Rhythm: _____ Rate: _____ P wave: _____

PR interval: _____ QRS: _____

Rhythm interpretation: _____

Strip 9-71. Rhythm: _____ Rate: _____ P wave: _____

PR interval: _____ QRS: _____

Rhythm interpretation: _____

Strip 9-72. Rhythm: _____ Rate: _____ P wave: _____

PR interval: _____ QRS: _____

Rhythm interpretation: _____

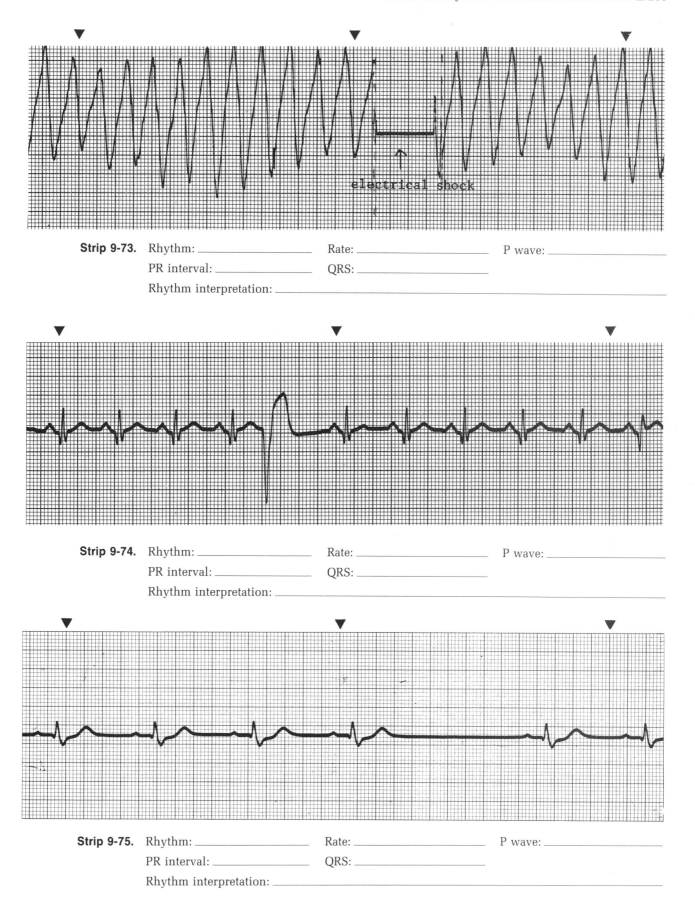

Strip 9-73. Rhythm: _____ Rate: _____ P wave: _____

PR interval: _____ QRS: _____

Rhythm interpretation: _____

Strip 9-74. Rhythm: _____ Rate: _____ P wave: _____

PR interval: _____ QRS: _____

Rhythm interpretation: _____

Strip 9-75. Rhythm: _____ Rate: _____ P wave: _____

PR interval: _____ QRS: _____

Rhythm interpretation: _____

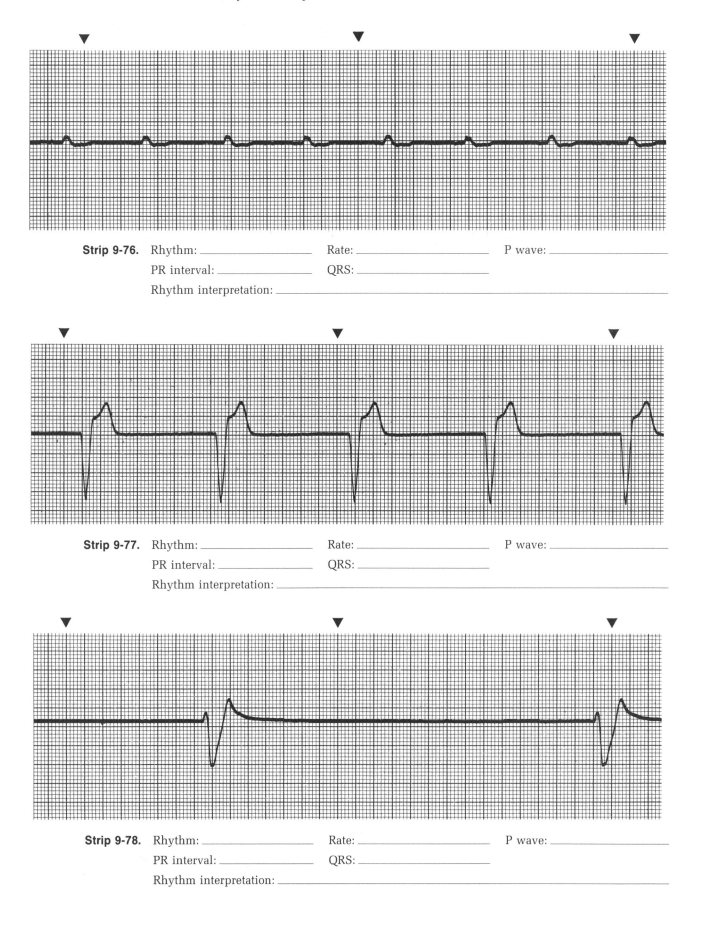

Strip 9-76. Rhythm: _____ Rate: _____ P wave: _____

PR interval: _____ QRS: _____

Rhythm interpretation: _____

Strip 9-77. Rhythm: _____ Rate: _____ P wave: _____

PR interval: _____ QRS: _____

Rhythm interpretation: _____

Strip 9-78. Rhythm: _____ Rate: _____ P wave: _____

PR interval: _____ QRS: _____

Rhythm interpretation: _____

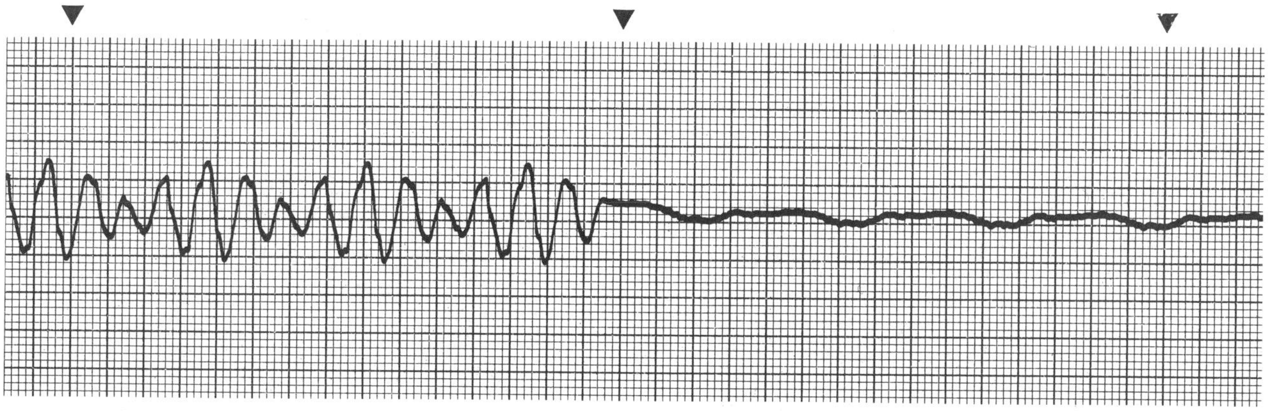

Strip 9-79. Rhythm: _____ Rate: _____ P wave: _____

PR interval: _____ QRS: _____

Rhythm interpretation: _____

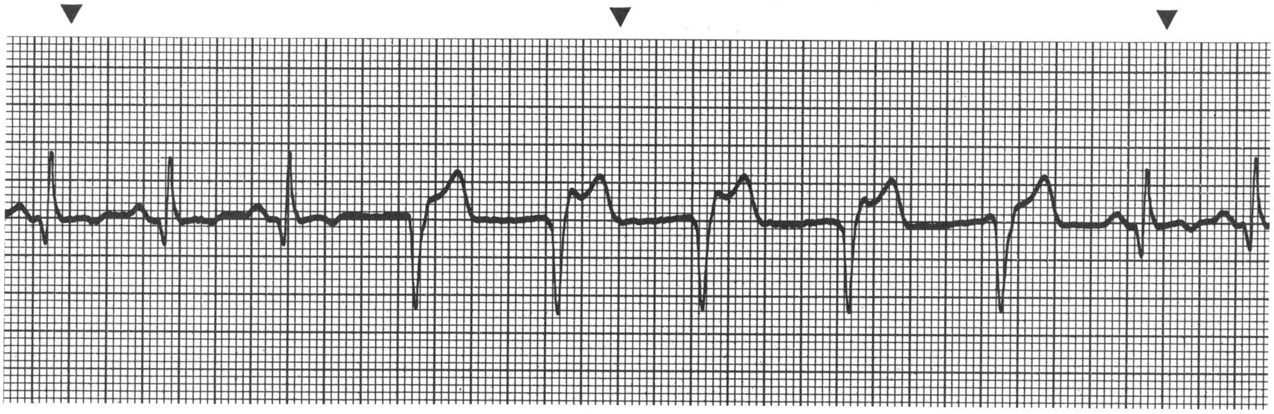

Strip 9-80. Rhythm: _____ Rate: _____ P wave: _____

PR interval: _____ QRS: _____

Rhythm interpretation: _____

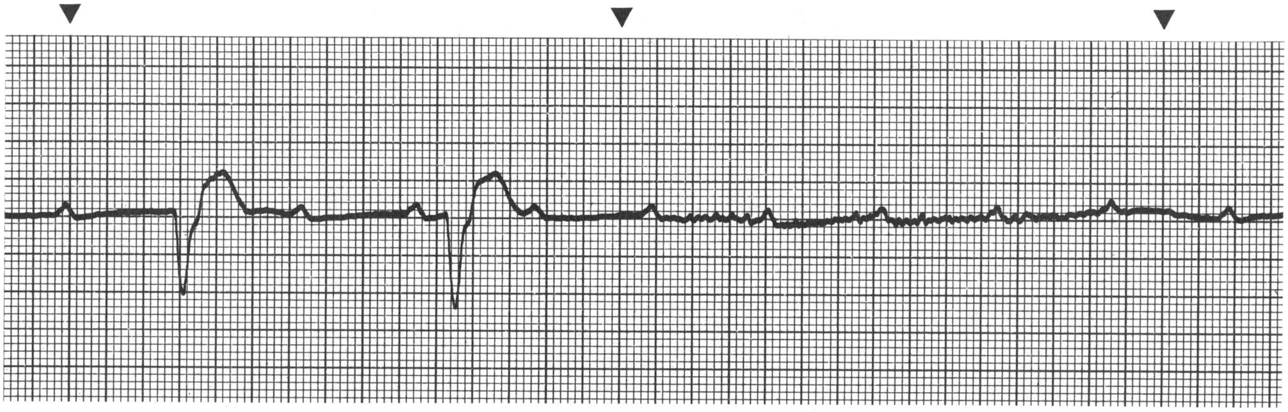

Strip 9-81. Rhythm: _____ Rate: _____ P wave: _____

PR interval: _____ QRS: _____

Rhythm interpretation: _____

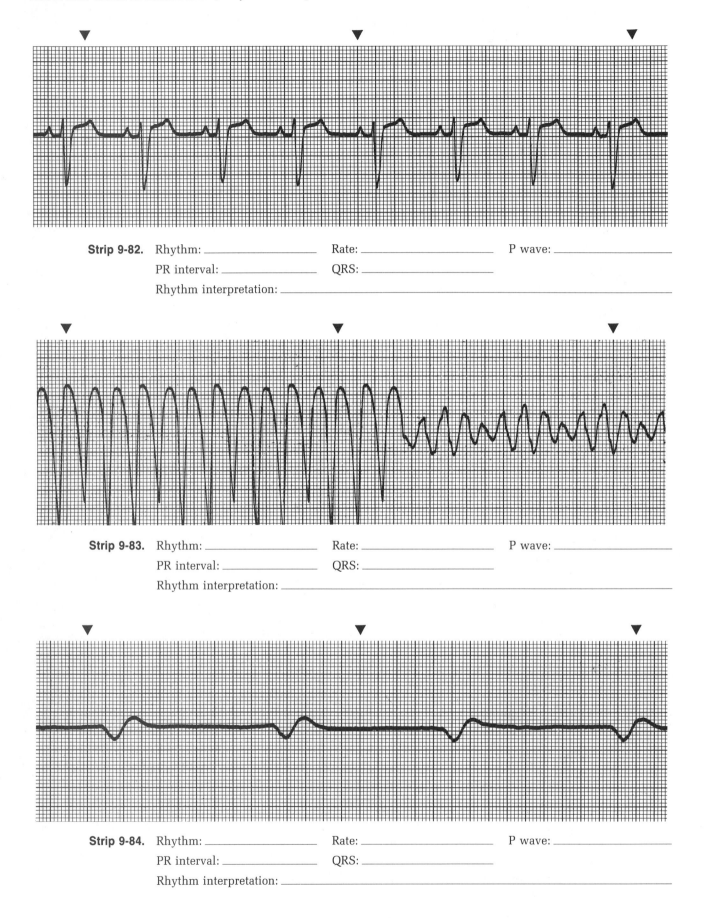

Strip 9-82. Rhythm: _____ Rate: _____ P wave: _____

PR interval: _____ QRS: _____

Rhythm interpretation: _____

Strip 9-83. Rhythm: _____ Rate: _____ P wave: _____

PR interval: _____ QRS: _____

Rhythm interpretation: _____

Strip 9-84. Rhythm: _____ Rate: _____ P wave: _____

PR interval: _____ QRS: _____

Rhythm interpretation: _____

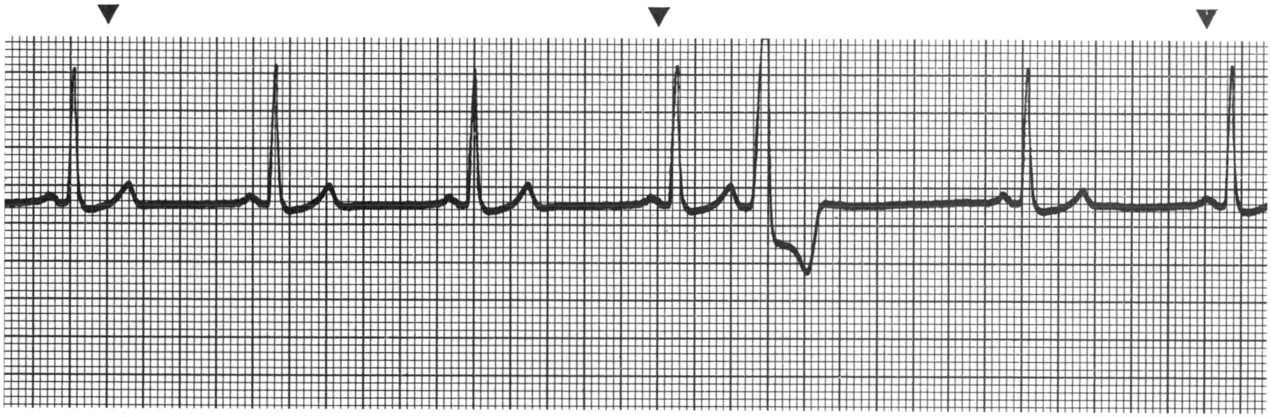

Strip 9-85. Rhythm: _____ Rate: _____ P wave: _____

PR interval: _____ QRS: _____

Rhythm interpretation: _____

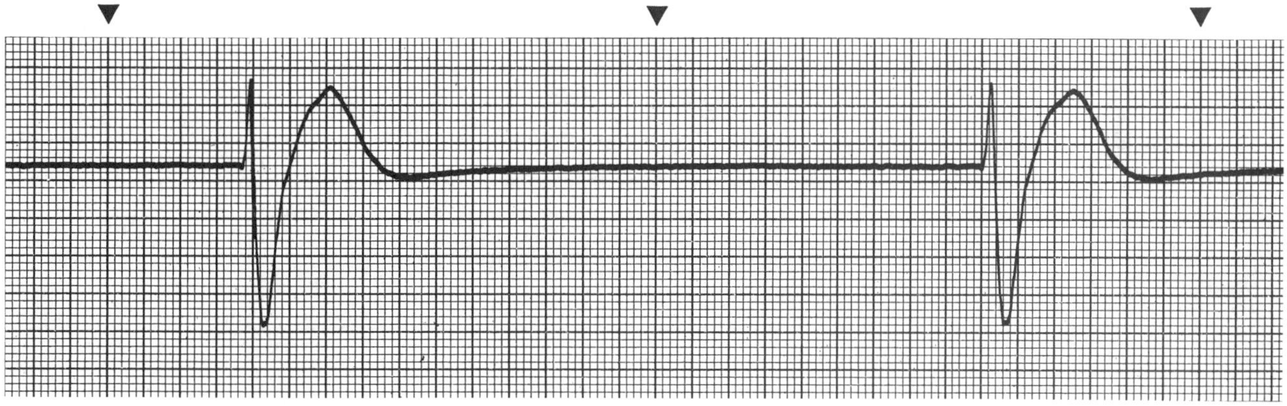

Strip 9-86. Rhythm: _____ Rate: _____ P wave: _____

PR interval: _____ QRS: _____

Rhythm interpretation: _____

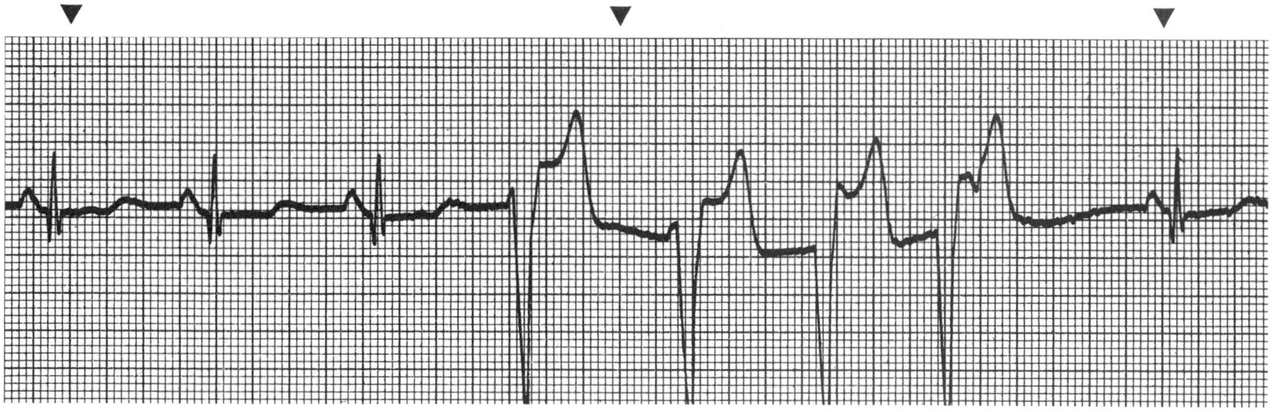

Strip 9-87. Rhythm: _____ Rate: _____ P wave: _____

PR interval: _____ QRS: _____

Rhythm interpretation: _____

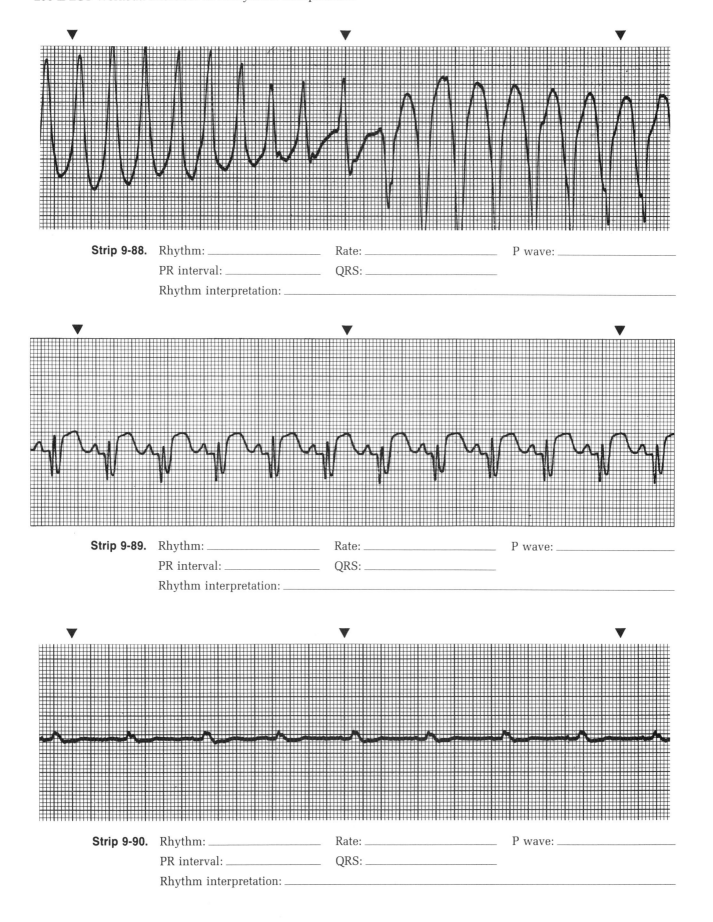

Strip 9-88. Rhythm: _____ Rate: _____ P wave: _____

PR interval: _____ QRS: _____

Rhythm interpretation: _____

Strip 9-89. Rhythm: _____ Rate: _____ P wave: _____

PR interval: _____ QRS: _____

Rhythm interpretation: _____

Strip 9-90. Rhythm: _____ Rate: _____ P wave: _____

PR interval: _____ QRS: _____

Rhythm interpretation: _____

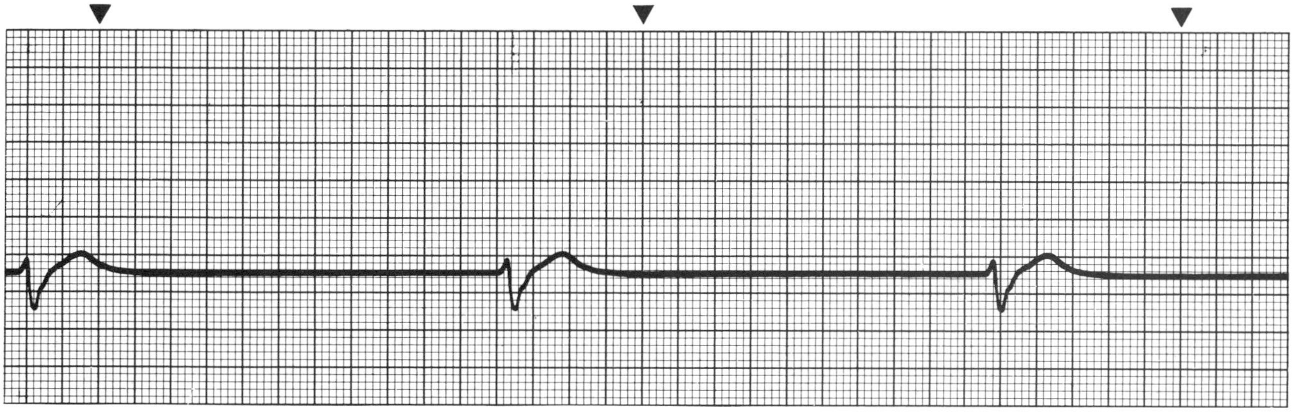

Strip 9-91. Rhythm: _____ Rate: _____ P wave: _____

PR interval: _____ QRS: _____

Rhythm interpretation: _____

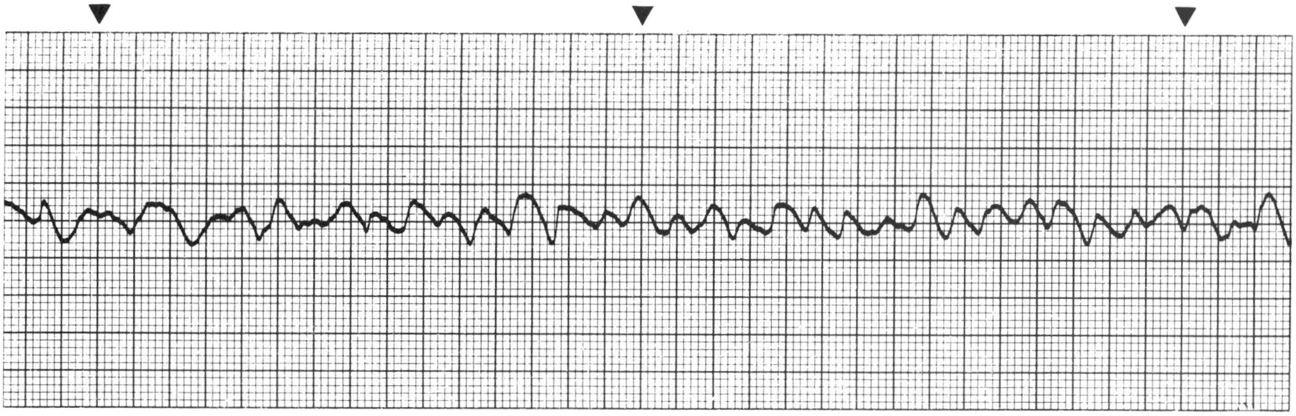

Strip 9-92. Rhythm: _____ Rate: _____ P wave: _____

PR interval: _____ QRS: _____

Rhythm interpretation: _____

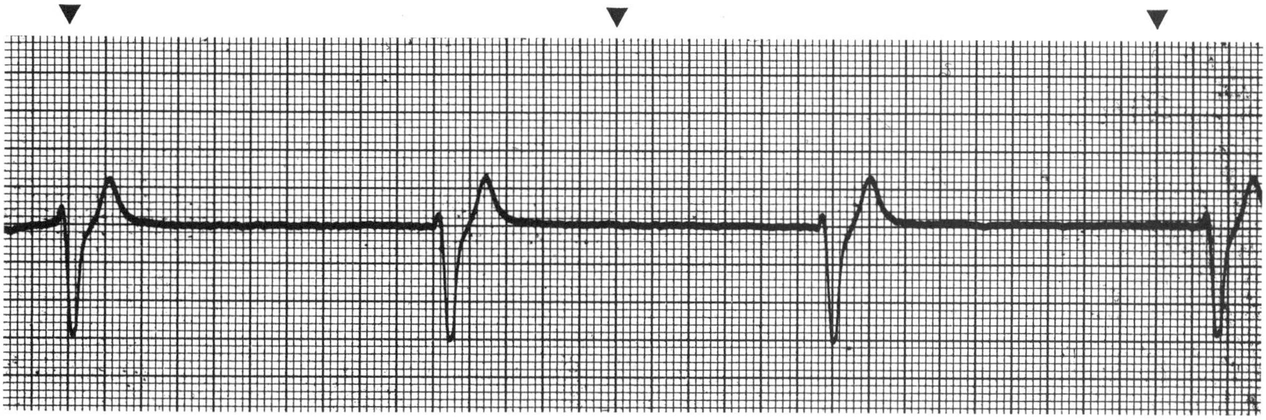

Strip 9-93. Rhythm: _____ Rate: _____ P wave: _____

PR interval: _____ QRS: _____

Rhythm interpretation: _____

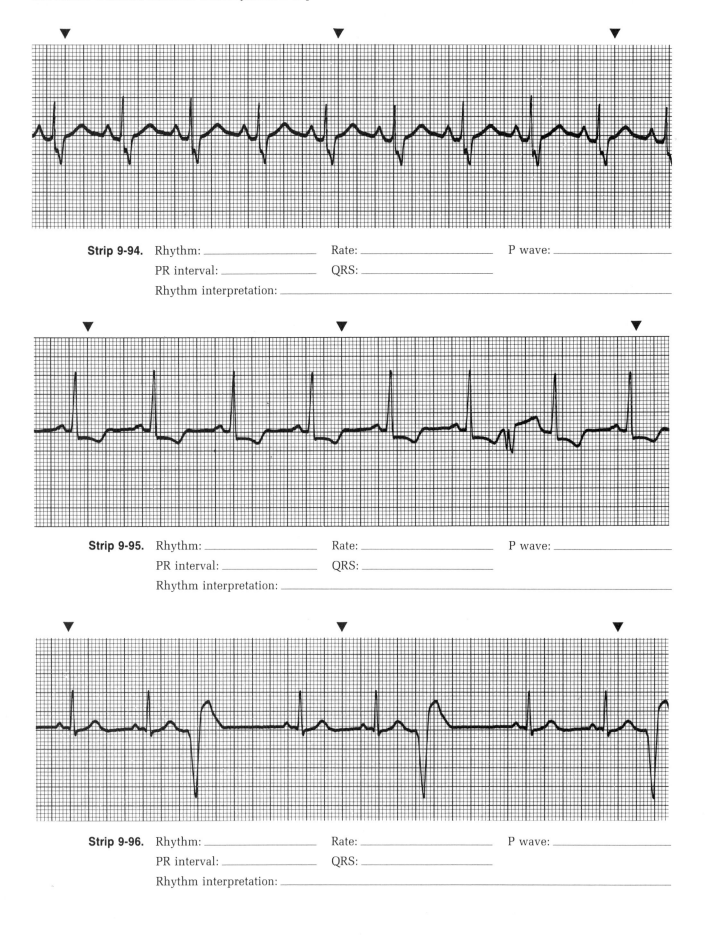

Strip 9-94. Rhythm: _____ Rate: _____ P wave: _____

PR interval: _____ QRS: _____

Rhythm interpretation: _____

Strip 9-95. Rhythm: _____ Rate: _____ P wave: _____

PR interval: _____ QRS: _____

Rhythm interpretation: _____

Strip 9-96. Rhythm: _____ Rate: _____ P wave: _____

PR interval: _____ QRS: _____

Rhythm interpretation: _____

Pacemakers

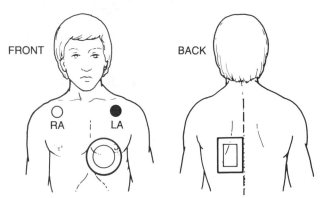

Figure 10-1. External pacemaker electrode placement.

A pacemaker is a battery-powered device that delivers an electrical stimulus to the myocardium, resulting in ventricular contraction. Pacemakers are used in patients whose inherent electrical system either does not generate impulses (sinus arrest) or generates impulses too slowly (bradycardia rhythms). Pacemakers are also used in high-grade conduction disorders (second-degree AV block, Mobitz II, and third-degree AV block) and in tachyarrhythmias (PVCs and ventricular tachycardia) that are refractory to drug therapy. Pacemakers may be external or internal.

With external pacing systems, large electrode pads are placed on the anterior and posterior chest (Figure 10-1), and the myocardium is stimulated indirectly by electric currents transmitted through the chest wall. External pacemakers are quick and easy to apply and are well tolerated. They are used in emergency situations where tranvenous access is not readily available.

There are two types of internal pacing systems—the temporary transvenous pacemaker and the permanent pacemaker. Both provide direct electrical stimulation either to the endocardial surface of the right ventricle or the epicardial surface of the heart.

Transient rhythm and conduction disorders are treated with a temporary transvenous pacemaker (Figure 10-2). With this type of pacemaker, the pacing electrode is inserted by transvenous route into the right ventricle and connected to an external pacemaker generator. Patients with chronic, irreversible rhythms or conduction disorders are treated with a permanent pacemaker (Figure 10-3). With this type of pacemaker, the pacing electrode is surgically inserted by the transvenous route (most common) or directly applied to the epicardial surface of the heart by thoracotomy. The pacing generator is then implanted in the subcutaneous tissue below the right or left clavicle.

Pacemakers function in one of two ways: as a fixed-rate pacemaker or as a demand pacemaker. Fixed-rate pacemakers initiate impulses at a set rate, irrespective of the patient's own heart rate. This type of pacemaker is potentially dangerous because the pacing stimulus may fall during the vulnerable period of the cardiac cycle and induce serious ventricular arrhythmias. Fixed-rate pacemakers are seldom used at the present time. Demand pacemakers sense the patient's own heart rate and discharge only when necessary (on demand). Many different types of demand pacemakers are available; some sense and pace in a single chamber (either atrium or ventricle), whereas others sense and pace dual chambers (both atrium and ventricle).

For a pacemaker to sense and pace appropriately, the electrode tip must be positioned properly in the right ventricle, be in contact with viable myocardium, and be able to detect electrical impulses transmitted by the heart. The pacing catheter serves to relay the information from the electrode tip to the pacing generator as well as send pacing im-

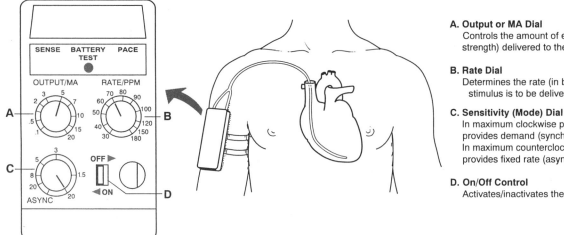

A. Output or MA Dial
Controls the amount of energy (stimulus strength) delivered to the endocarium.

B. Rate Dial
Determines the rate (in bpm) at which the stimulus is to be delivered.

C. Sensitivity (Mode) Dial
In maximum clockwise position, this provides demand (synchronous) pacing. In maximum counterclockwise position, this provides fixed rate (asynchronous) pacing.

D. On/Off Control
Activates/inactivates the pulse generator.

Figure 10-2. Temporary pacemaker.

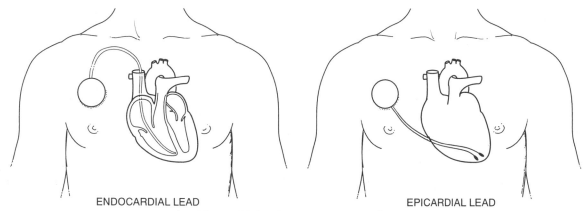

ENDOCARDIAL LEAD   EPICARDIAL LEAD

Figure 10-3. Permanent pacemaker.

pulses from the generator to the myocardium. Most difficulties encountered with cardiac pacing involve a failure of the pacemaker to sense intrinsic beats appropriately (undersensing) or a failure of the ventricle to respond to a pacing stimulus (loss of capture).

The temporary transvenous ventricular demand pacemaker is the most common mode of pacing used in the acute phase of myocardial infarction. This pacemaker paces and senses only in the ventricle and is inhibited only by ventricular activity. When ventricular activity is sensed, the pacemaker withholds a pacing impulse; if ventricular activity is not sensed, it will discharge impulses at a preset rate. Further discussion and electrocardiogram tracings focus on the temporary transvenous ventricular demand pacemaker.

PACEMAKER TERMS

Ventricular capture indicates that the ventricular chamber has responded to a pacing stimulus. This is evidenced on the electrocardiogram tracing by a pacemaker spike followed by a wide QRS complex (Figure 10-4, complex **A**).

A *native beat* is produced by the patient's own electrical network. These beats also are called intrinsic beats (see Figure 10-4, complex **B**).

A *fusion beat* occurs when the pacemaker fires an electrical impulse at the same time that the patient's normal electrical impulse has activated the ventricles. The two forces simultaneously depolarize the ventricles, resulting in a fusion beat. The fusion beat has the characteristics of both pacemaker and patient forces, resulting in a complex different in configuration and height from that caused by either of the forces alone. Fusion beats represent a normal manifestation of ventricular demand pacing (see Figure 10-4, complex **C**).

A *pseudofusion beat* is a pacemaker spike occurring within the QRS complex that does not

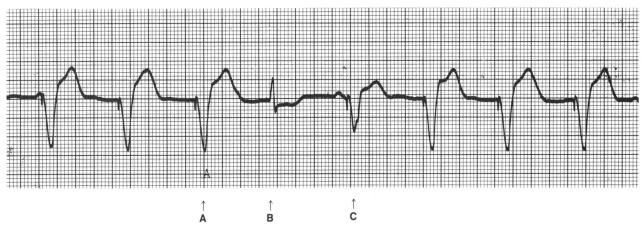

A   B   C

Figure 10-4. Ventricular capture (complex **A**), native beat (complex **B**), and fusion beat (complex **C**).

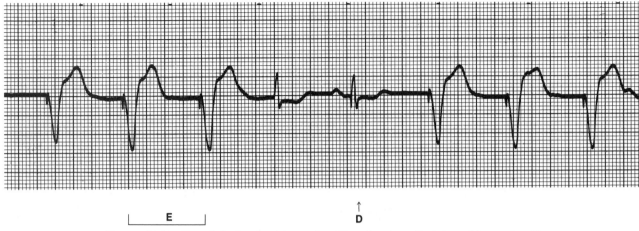

E   D

Figure 10-5. Pseudofusion beat (complex **D**) and automatic interval (complex **E**).

alter the height or configuration of the complex. Pseudofusion beats represent a normal manifestation of ventricular demand pacing (Figure 10-5, complex **D**).

The *automatic interval* is the heart rate at which the pacemaker is set. This interval is measured from one pacing spike to the next consecutive pacing spike (see Figure 10-5, interval **E**).

Pacemaker rhythm occurs when the heart's rhythm is controlled entirely by the pacemaker. This is evidenced by a tracing in

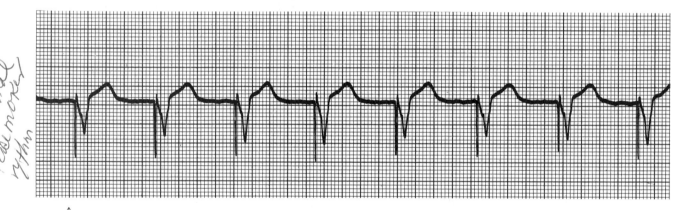

Figure 10-6. Pacemaker rhythm.

Table 10-1. Loss of capture

Causes	Actions
1. Electrical milliamps set too low*	1. Increase milliamps on generator
2. Loose connections between lead wire, cables, generator	2. Ensure secure connections between lead, bridging cable, and generator
3. Dislodgement of lead wire*	3. a. Reposition patient—lead may move to better position
	b. Obtain chest x-ray to determine electrode placement

* Most common causes

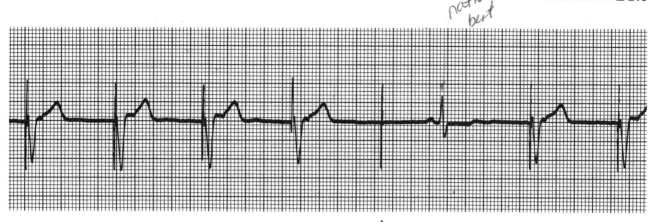

native beat

Figure 10-7. Loss of capture.

which no patient beats are seen and all QRS complexes are pacemaker induced (Figure 10-6).

PACEMAKER MALFUNCTIONS

Loss of Capture

Loss of capture is noted on the electrocardiogram by a lack of ventricular response to a pacing stimulus. This is evidenced by a pacemaker spike that occurs at the normal automatic interval rate but is not followed by a QRS complex (Table 10-1) (Figure 10-7).

Undersensing

Undersensing occurs when the pacemaker circuitry does not sense the patient's intrinsic beats. This is evidenced on the electrocardiogram tracing by a pacemaker spike that occurs too early (earlier than the automatic interval rate). Ventricular capture may or may not occur (Table 10-2) (Figure 10-8).

Table 10-2. Undersensing

Causes	Actions
1. Sensitivity threshold set too low	1. Increase sensitivity threshold on generator
2. Patient beats are of too low voltage and go undetected by pacemaker's sensing mechanism*	2. a. If patient's intrinsic rhythm is adequate, turn pacer off b. If patient's intrinsic rhythm is inadequate, increase pacing rate to overdrive intrinsic rate
3. Dislodgement of lead wire*	3. a. Reposition patient; lead may move to better position b. Obtain chest x-ray to determine electrode placement
4. Circuitry failure of pulse generator	
4. Change generators	

* Most common causes

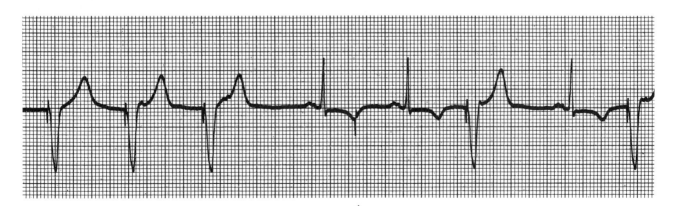

Figure 10-8. Undersensing.

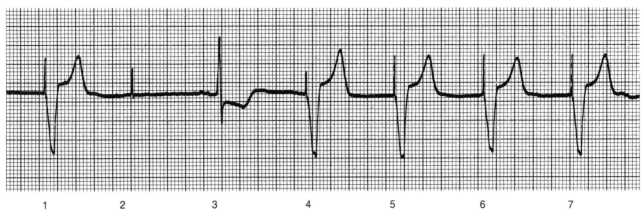

Figure 10-9. Pacemaker rhythm strip.
Automatic Interval—The automatic interval can be measured from Number 4 to Number 5. The rate is 63.
Analysis—Number 3 is a native beat. Numbers 1, 4, 5, 6, and 7 are ventricular capture beats (paced beats). Number 2 is a spike that occurs on time but doesn't capture the ventricles.
Interpretation—Loss of capture malfunction.

ANALYZING PACEMAKER RHYTHM STRIPS (VENTRICULAR DEMAND TYPE)

1. Identify patient complexes (native beats) (Figure 10-9).

2. Place an index card above two consecutive paced beats. Mark on index card the interval from one pacing spike to the next. This is the automatic interval and will be used to identify pacing malfunctions.

3. Starting at the left side of the rhythm strip, analyze each spike or beat with a spike. Place a left mark on the index card on the spike (or native QRS if no spike) preceding the spike to be analyzed. Observe the relationship of the spike in question to the right mark on the index card:

Question	Answer
a. Does the spike being analyzed match the right mark on the index card?	**i.** Ventricular capture beat
	ii. Fusion beat
	iii. Pseudofusion beat
b. Does the spike being analyzed occur earlier than the right mark on the index card?	**iv.** Loss of capture malfunction
	i. Undersensing malfunction

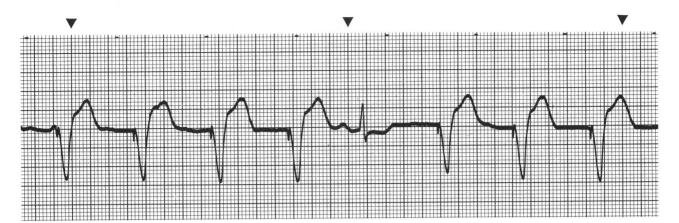

Strip 10-1. Automatic interval rate:
Analysis:

Interpretation:

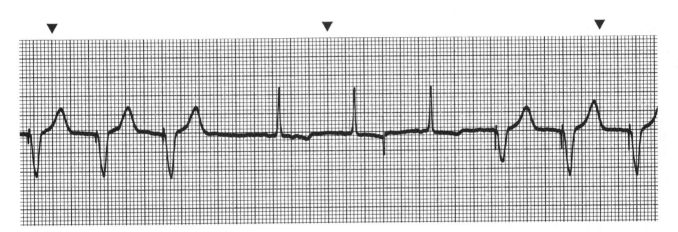

Strip 10-2. Automatic interval rate:
Analysis:

Interpretation:

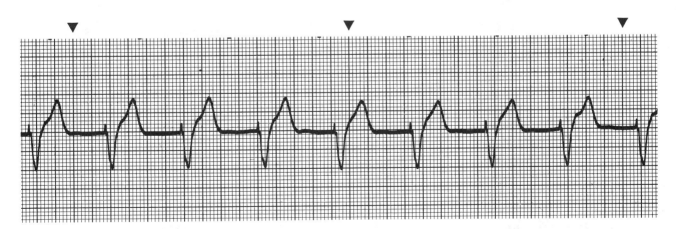

Strip 10-3. Automatic interval rate:
Analysis:

Interpretation:

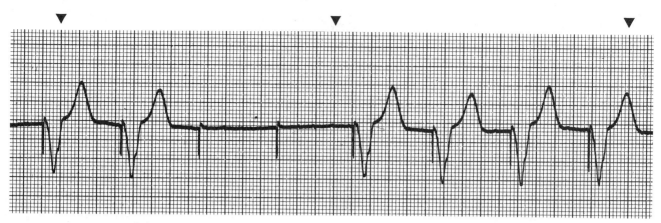

Strip 10-4. Automatic interval rate:

Analysis:

Interpretation:

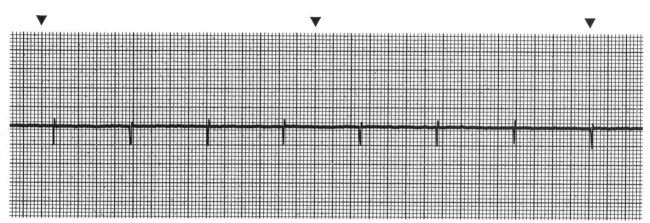

Strip 10-5. Automatic interval rate:

Analysis:

Interpretation:

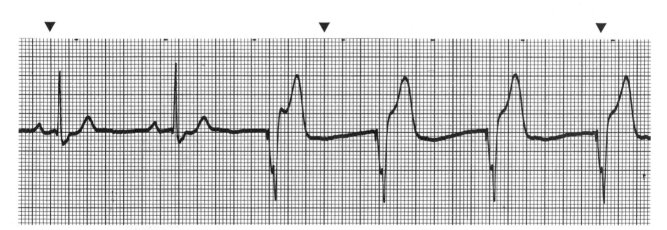

Strip 10-6. Automatic interval rate:

Analysis:

Interpretation:

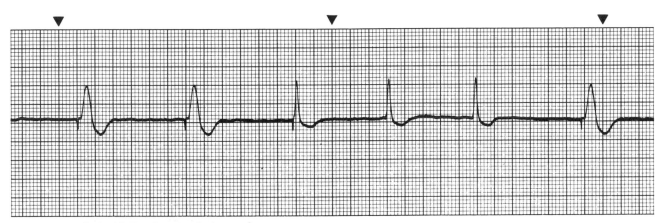

Strip 10-7.   Automatic interval rate:
Analysis:

Interpretation:

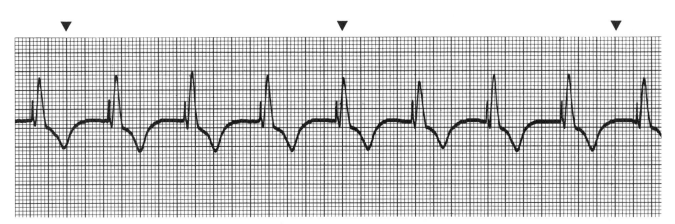

Strip 10-8.   Automatic interval rate:
Analysis:

Interpretation:

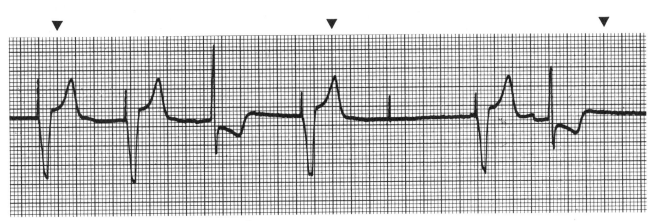

Strip 10-9.   Automatic interval rate:
Analysis:

Interpretation:

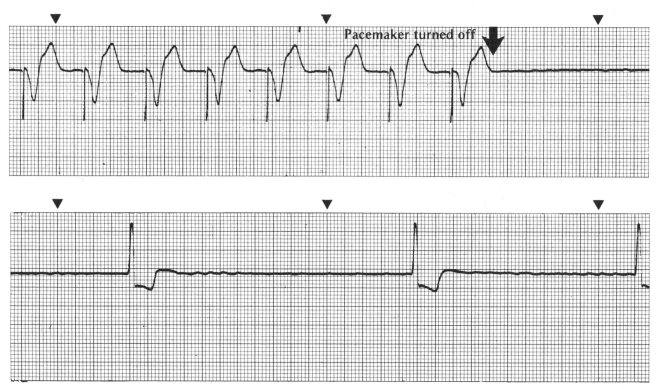

Pacemaker turned off

Strip 10-10. Automatic interval rate:
Analysis:

Interpretation:

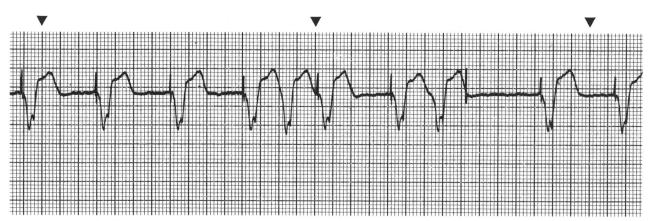

Strip 10-11. Automatic interval rate:
Analysis:

Interpretation:

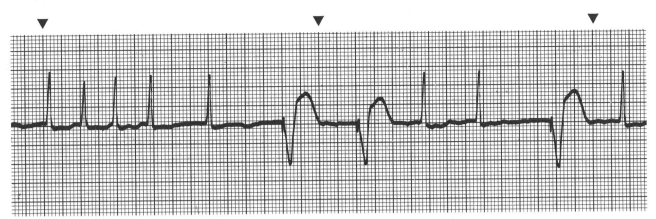

Strip 10-12. Automatic interval rate:
Analysis:

Interpretation:

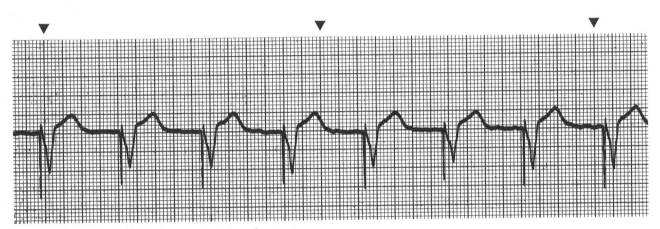

Strip 10-13. Automatic interval rate:
Analysis:

Interpretation:

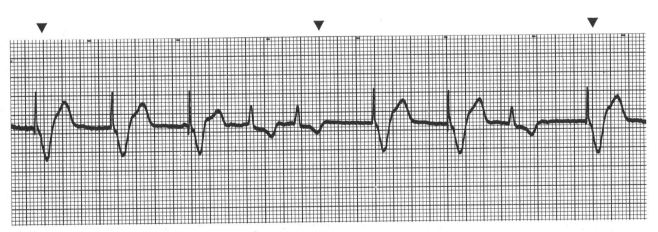

Strip 10-14. Automatic interval rate:
Analysis:

Interpretation:

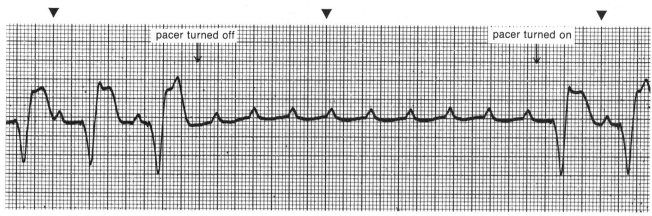

Strip 10-15. Automatic interval rate:
Analysis:

Interpretation:

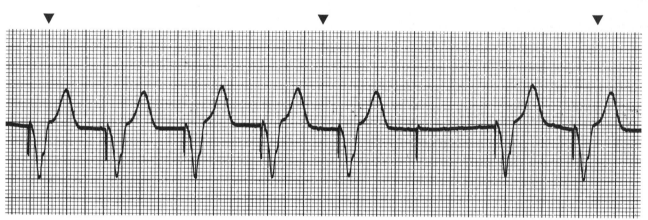

Strip 10-16. Automatic interval rate:
Analysis:

Interpretation:

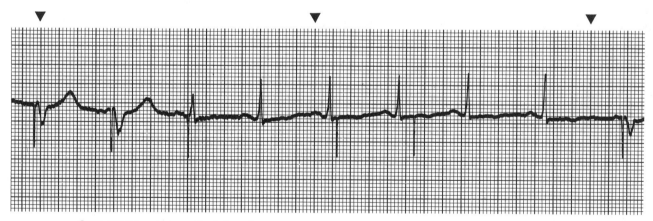

Strip 10-17. Automatic interval rate:
Analysis:

Interpretation:

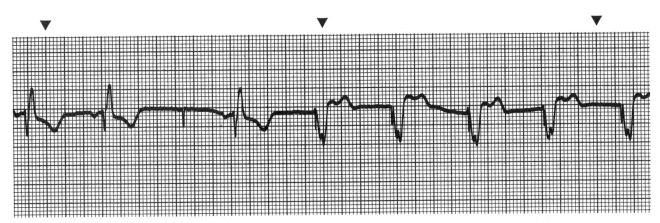

Strip 10-18. Automatic interval rate:
Analysis:

Interpretation:

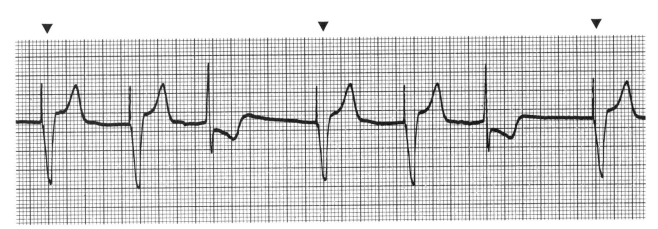

Strip 10-19. Automatic interval rate:
Analysis:

Interpretation:

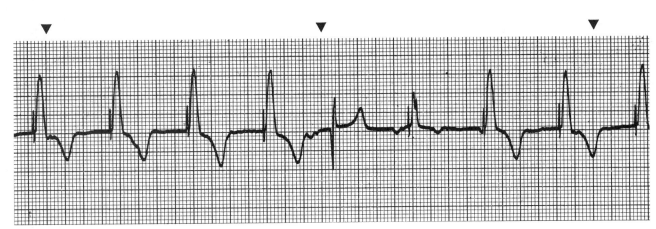

Strip 10-20. Automatic interval rate:
Analysis:

Interpretation:

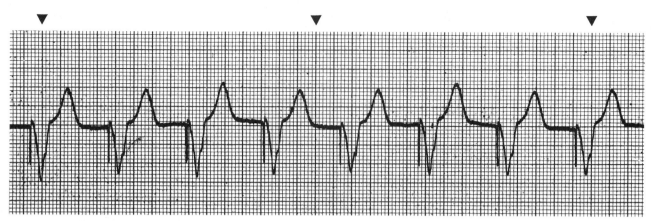

Strip 10-21. Automatic interval rate:
Analysis:

Interpretation:

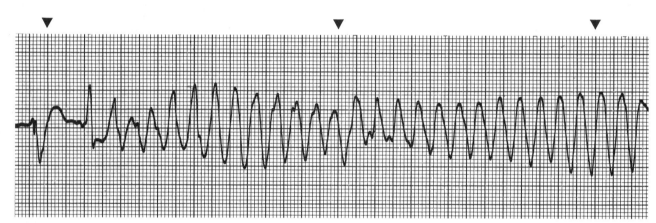

Strip 10-22. Automatic interval rate:
Analysis:

Interpretation:

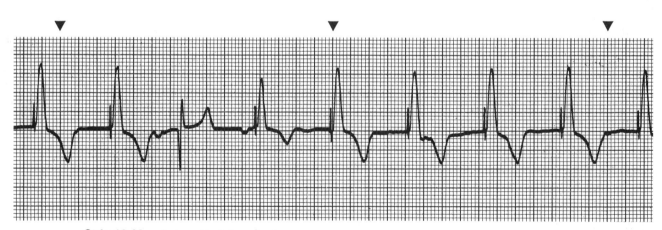

Strip 10-23. Automatic interval rate:
Analysis:

Interpretation:

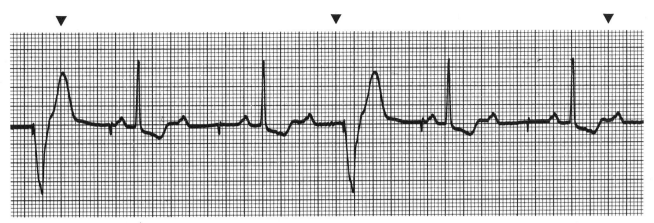

Strip 10-24. Automatic interval rate:
Analysis:

Interpretation:

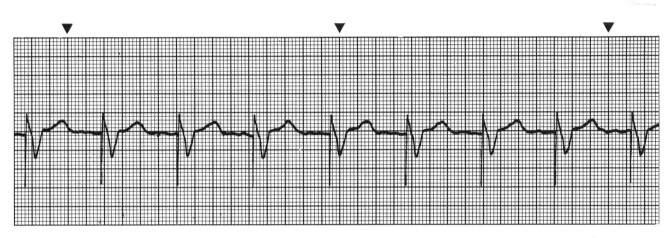

Strip 10-25. Automatic interval rate:
Analysis:

Interpretation:

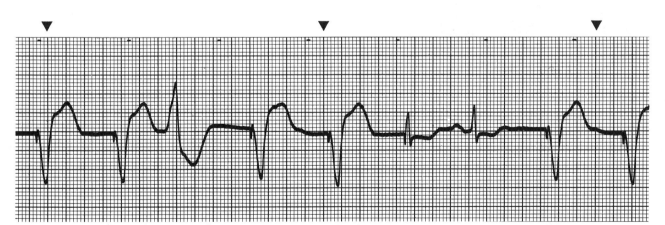

Strip 10-26. Automatic interval rate:
Analysis:

Interpretation:

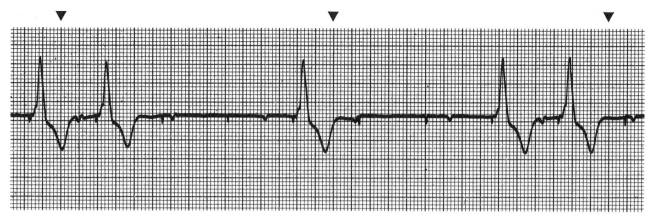

Strip 10-27. Automatic interval rate:

Analysis:

Interpretation:

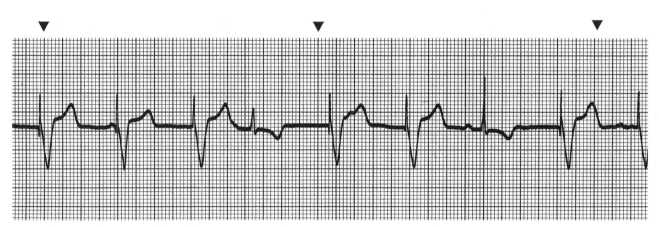

Strip 10-28. Automatic interval rate:

Analysis:

Interpretation:

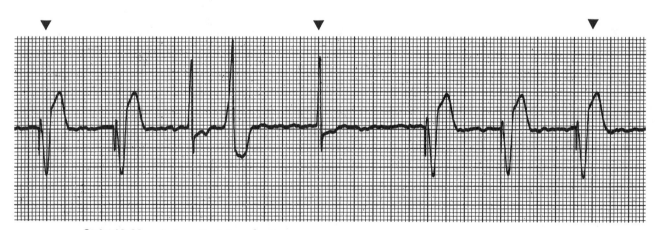

Strip 10-29. Automatic interval rate:

Analysis:

Interpretation:

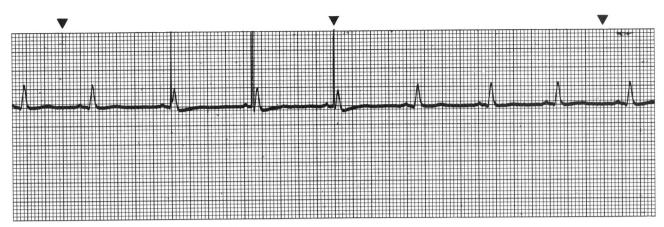

Strip 10-30. Automatic interval rate:
Analysis:

Interpretation:

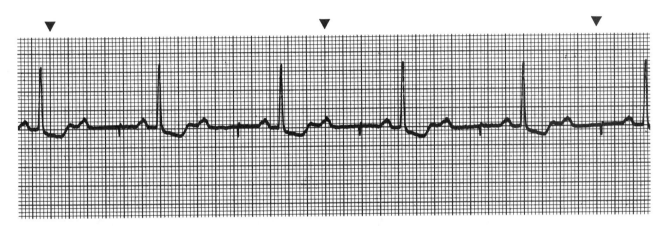

Strip 10-31. Automatic interval rate:
Analysis:

Interpretation:

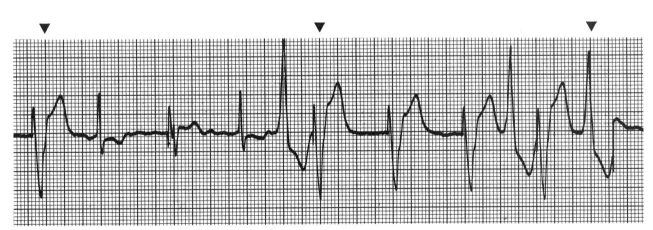

Strip 10-32. Automatic interval rate:
Analysis:

Interpretation:

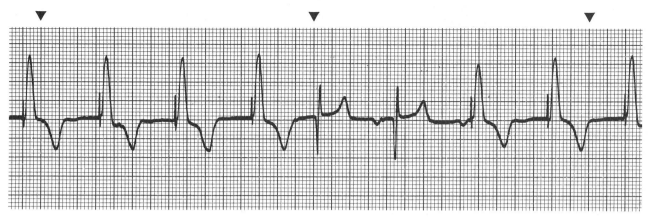

Strip 10-33.   Automatic interval rate:
                   Analysis:

                   Interpretation:

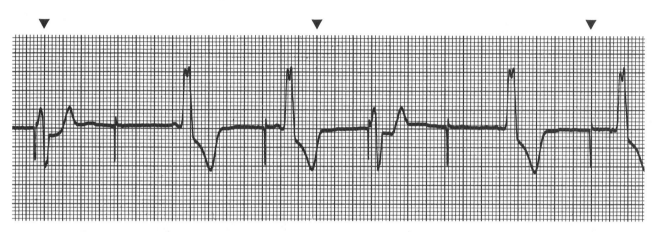

Strip 10-34.   Automatic interval rate:
                   Analysis:

                   Interpretation:

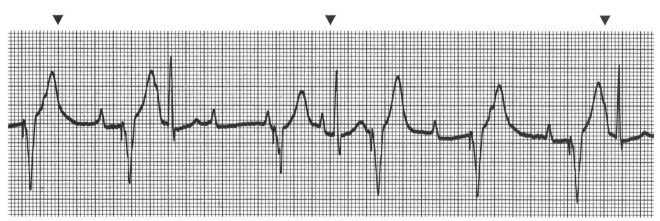

Strip 10-35.   Automatic interval rate:
                   Analysis:

                   Interpretation:

Post-test A

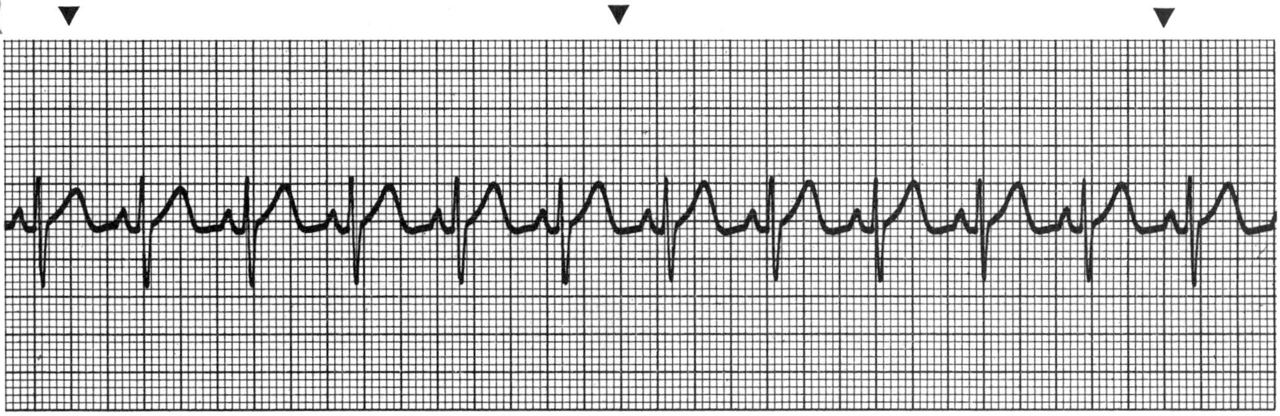

Sinus tachycardia

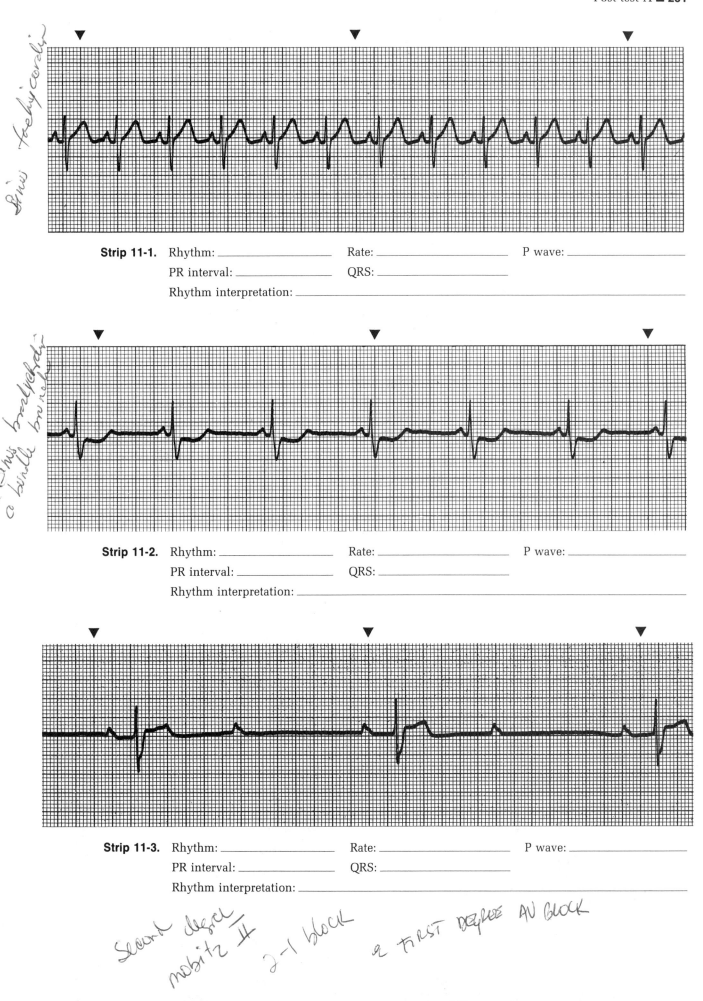

Strip 11-1. Rhythm: ____________ Rate: ____________ P wave: ____________
PR interval: ____________ QRS: ____________
Rhythm interpretation: ______________________________

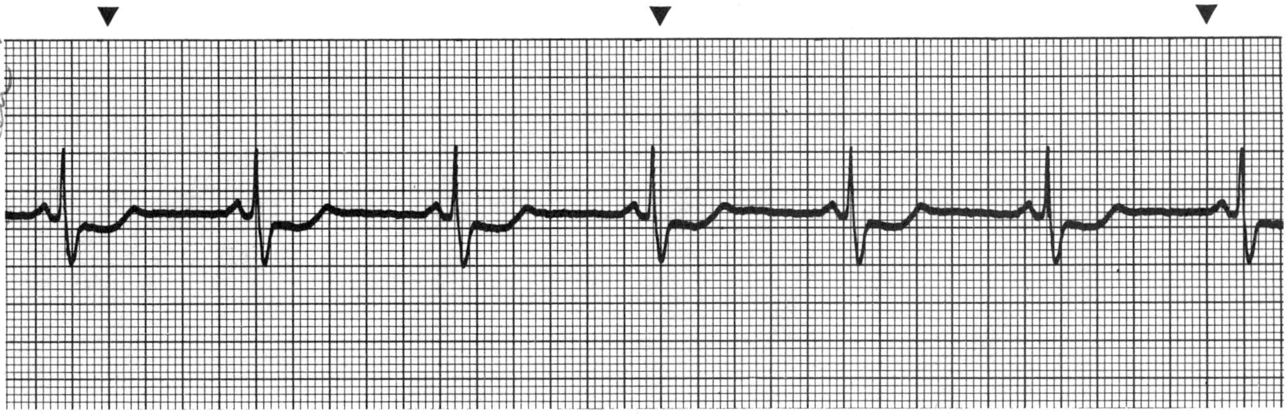

Sinus bradycardia c bundle branch

Strip 11-2. Rhythm: ____________ Rate: ____________ P wave: ____________
PR interval: ____________ QRS: ____________
Rhythm interpretation: ______________________________

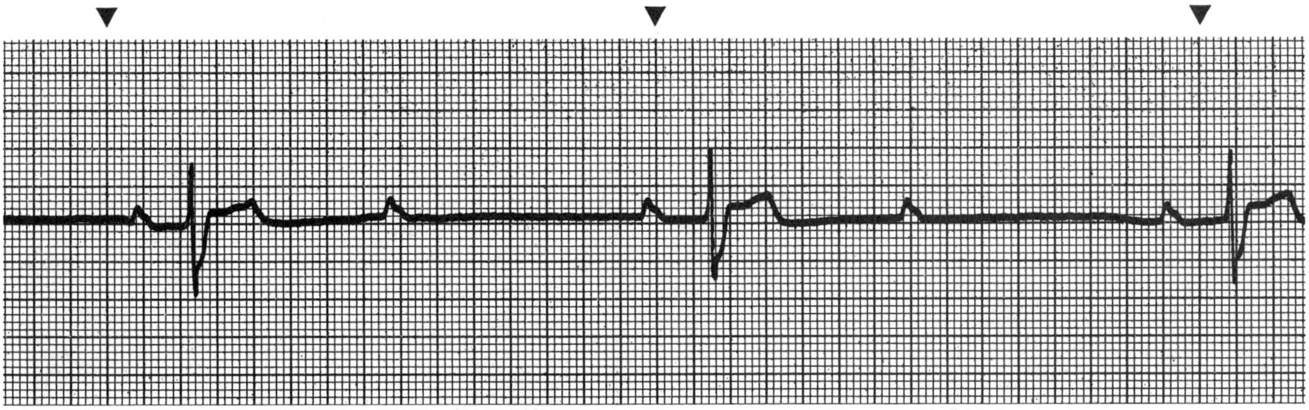

Strip 11-3. Rhythm: ____________ Rate: ____________ P wave: ____________
PR interval: ____________ QRS: ____________
Rhythm interpretation: ______________________________

Second degree mobitz II 2-1 block c FIRST DEGREE AV BLOCK

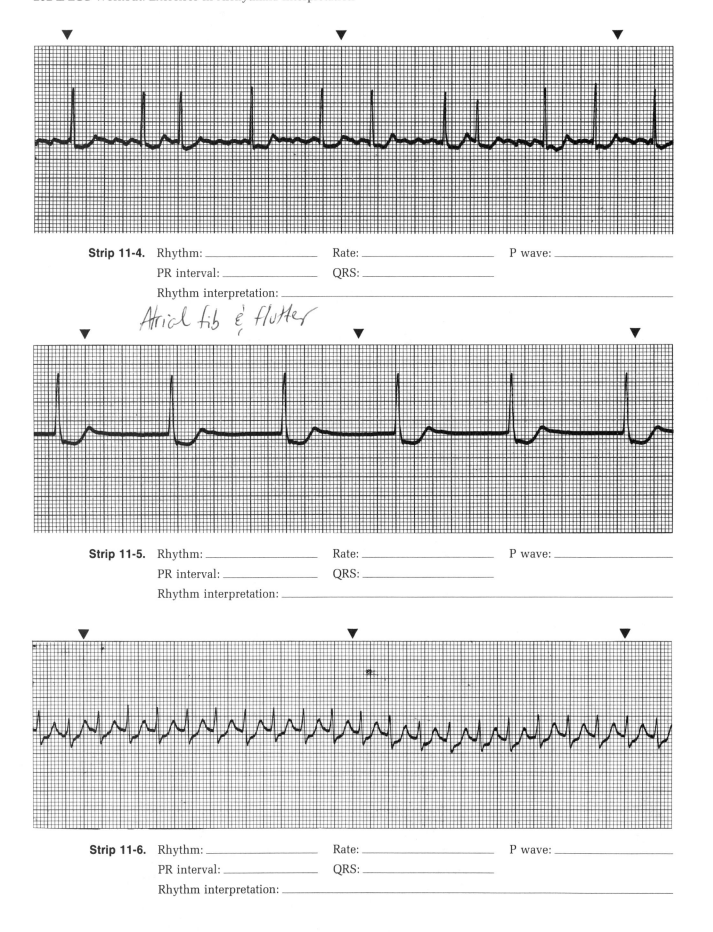

Strip 11-4. Rhythm: _____ Rate: _____ P wave: _____

PR interval: _____ QRS: _____

Rhythm interpretation: _____

Atrial fib č flutter

Strip 11-5. Rhythm: _____ Rate: _____ P wave: _____

PR interval: _____ QRS: _____

Rhythm interpretation: _____

Strip 11-6. Rhythm: _____ Rate: _____ P wave: _____

PR interval: _____ QRS: _____

Rhythm interpretation: _____

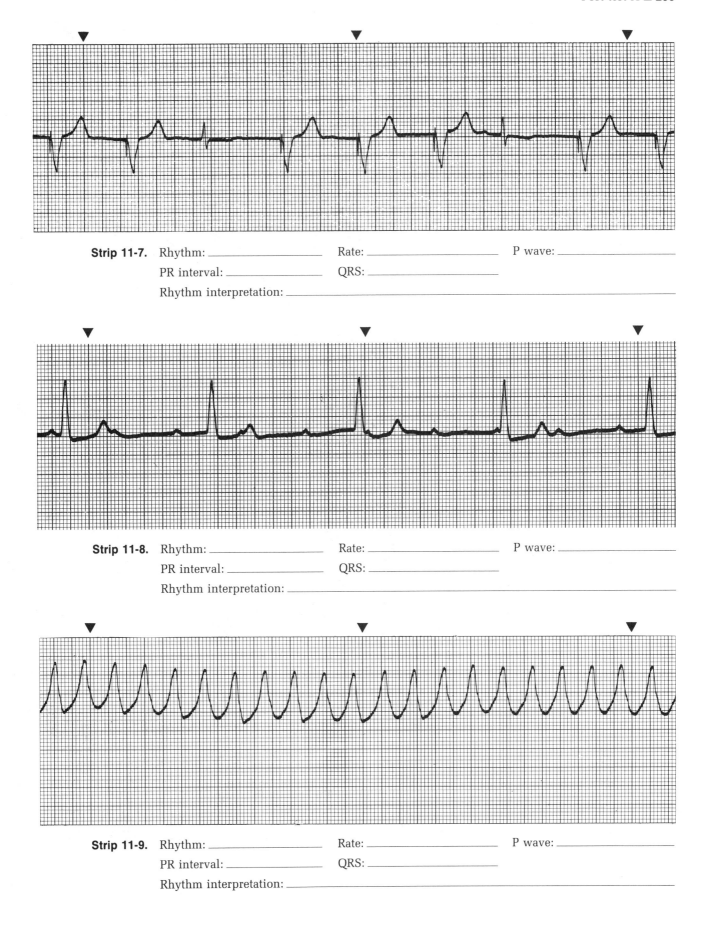

Strip 11-7. Rhythm: _____ Rate: _____ P wave: _____

PR interval: _____ QRS: _____

Rhythm interpretation: _____

Strip 11-8. Rhythm: _____ Rate: _____ P wave: _____

PR interval: _____ QRS: _____

Rhythm interpretation: _____

Strip 11-9. Rhythm: _____ Rate: _____ P wave: _____

PR interval: _____ QRS: _____

Rhythm interpretation: _____

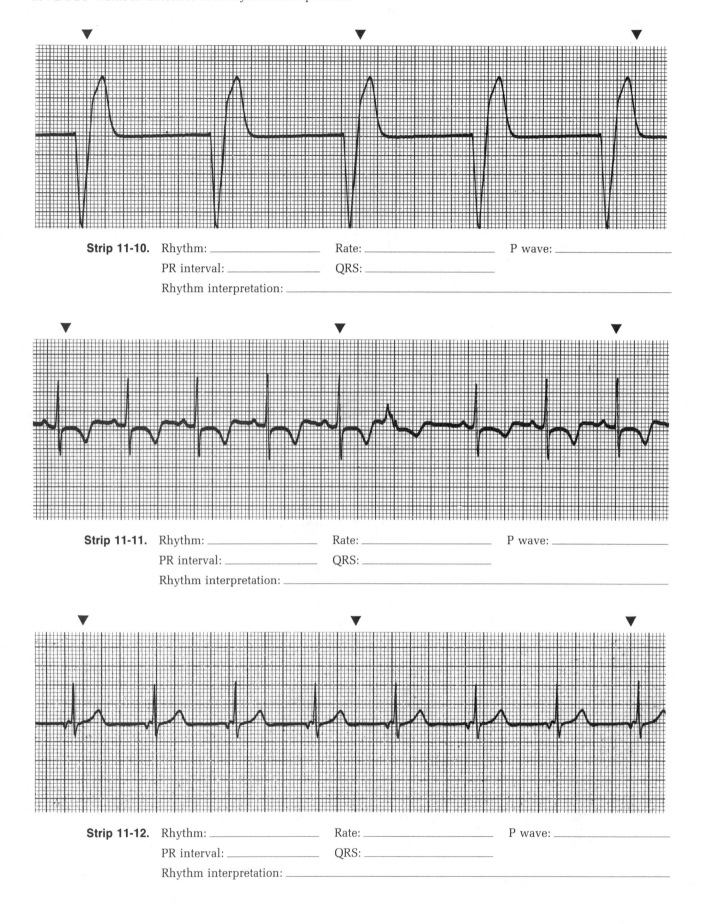

Strip 11-10. Rhythm: _____ Rate: _____ P wave: _____

PR interval: _____ QRS: _____

Rhythm interpretation: _____

Strip 11-11. Rhythm: _____ Rate: _____ P wave: _____

PR interval: _____ QRS: _____

Rhythm interpretation: _____

Strip 11-12. Rhythm: _____ Rate: _____ P wave: _____

PR interval: _____ QRS: _____

Rhythm interpretation: _____

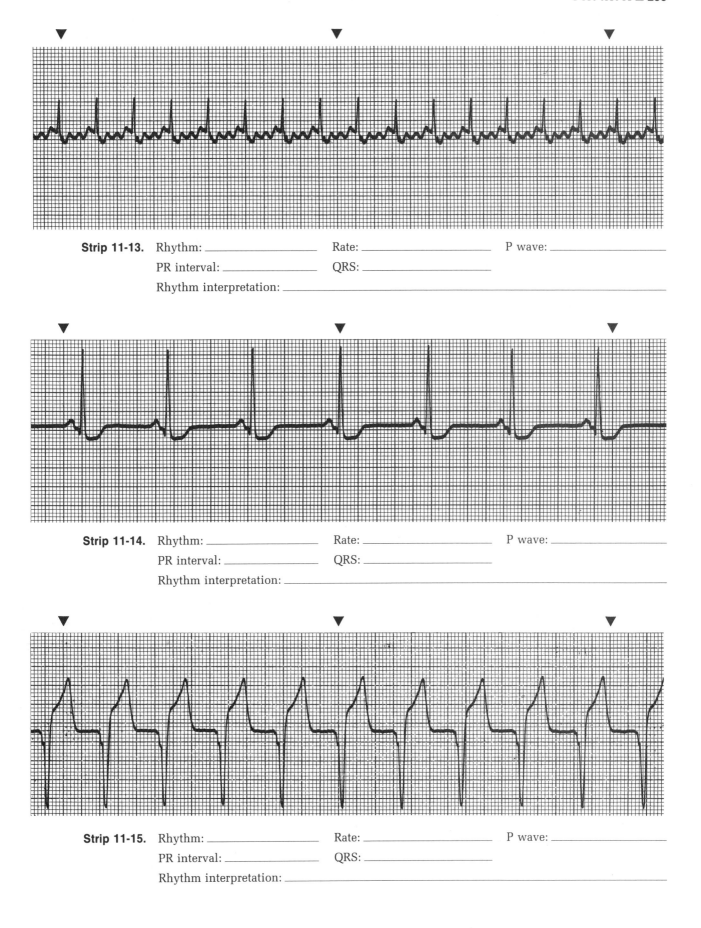

Strip 11-13. Rhythm: _____ Rate: _____ P wave: _____

PR interval: _____ QRS: _____

Rhythm interpretation: _____

Strip 11-14. Rhythm: _____ Rate: _____ P wave: _____

PR interval: _____ QRS: _____

Rhythm interpretation: _____

Strip 11-15. Rhythm: _____ Rate: _____ P wave: _____

PR interval: _____ QRS: _____

Rhythm interpretation: _____

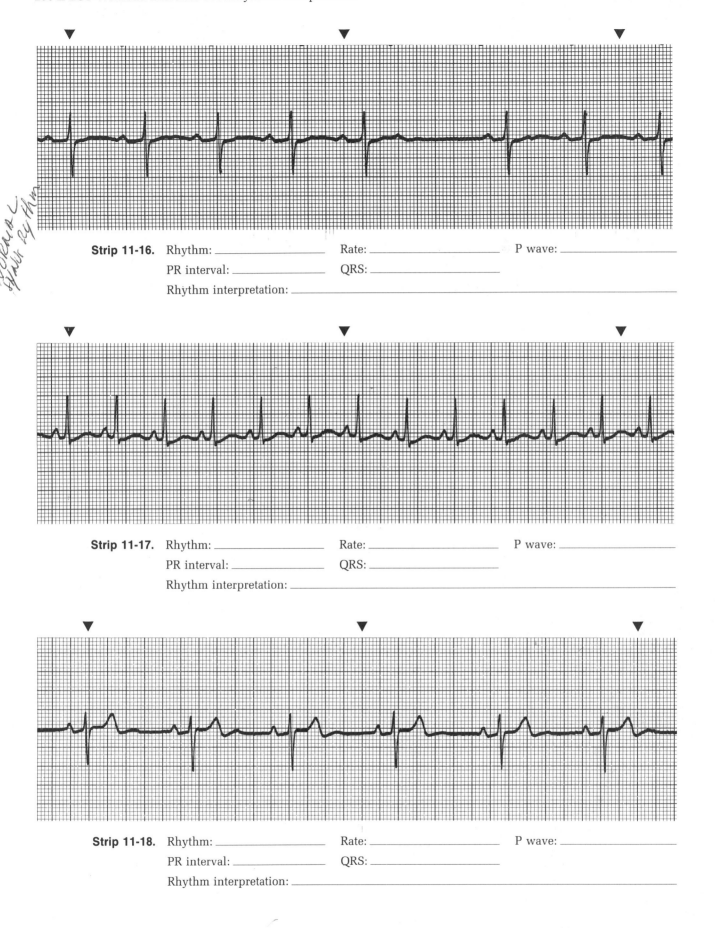

Normal
Sinus rhythm

Strip 11-16. Rhythm: _____ Rate: _____ P wave: _____

PR interval: _____ QRS: _____

Rhythm interpretation: _____

Strip 11-17. Rhythm: _____ Rate: _____ P wave: _____

PR interval: _____ QRS: _____

Rhythm interpretation: _____

Strip 11-18. Rhythm: _____ Rate: _____ P wave: _____

PR interval: _____ QRS: _____

Rhythm interpretation: _____

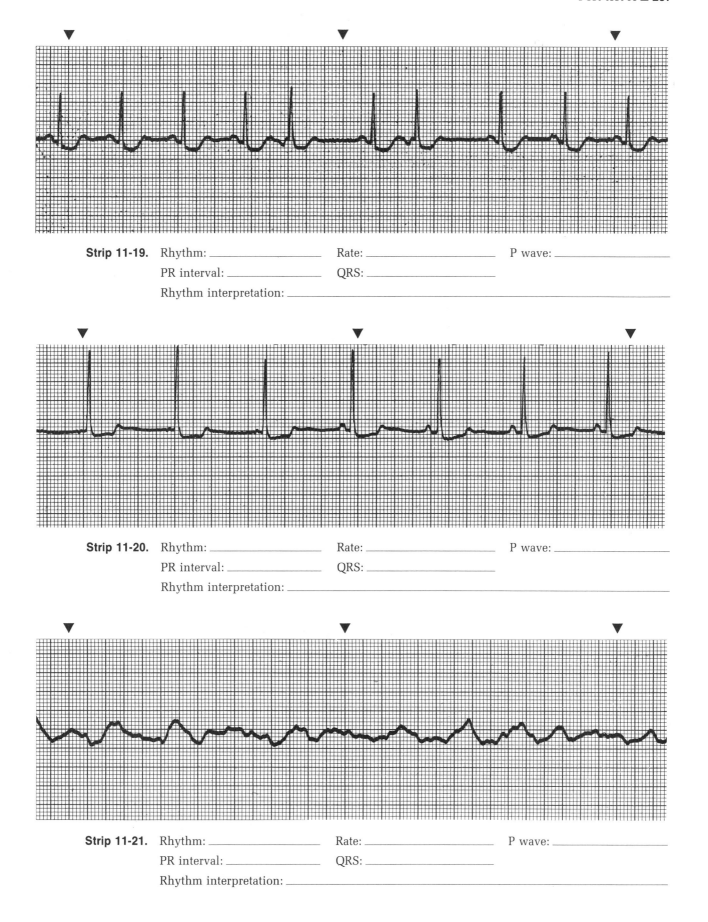

Strip 11-19. Rhythm: _____ Rate: _____ P wave: _____

PR interval: _____ QRS: _____

Rhythm interpretation: _____

Strip 11-20. Rhythm: _____ Rate: _____ P wave: _____

PR interval: _____ QRS: _____

Rhythm interpretation: _____

Strip 11-21. Rhythm: _____ Rate: _____ P wave: _____

PR interval: _____ QRS: _____

Rhythm interpretation: _____

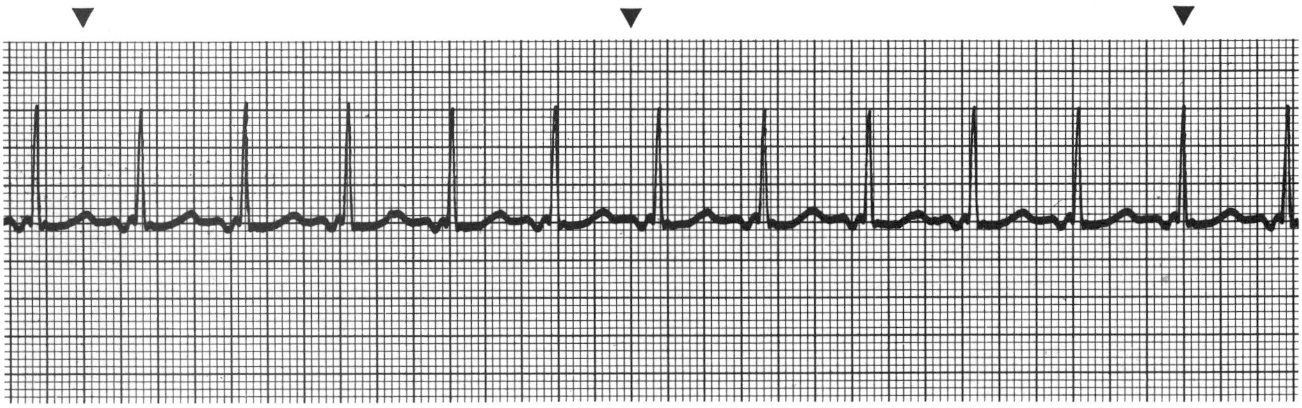

Strip 11-22. Rhythm: _____ Rate: _____ P wave: _____

PR interval: _____ QRS: _____

Rhythm interpretation: _____

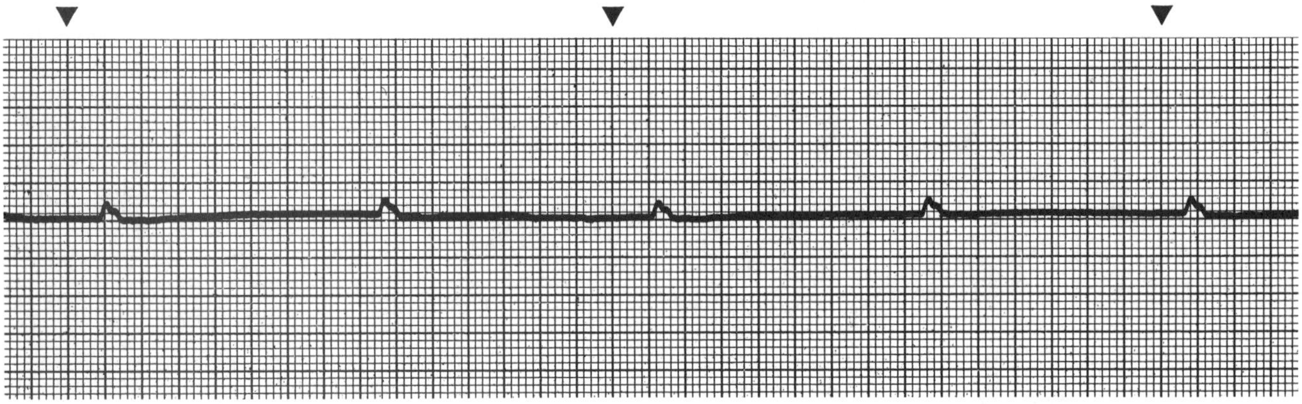

Strip 11-23. Rhythm: _____ Rate: _____ P wave: _____

PR interval: _____ QRS: _____

Rhythm interpretation: _____

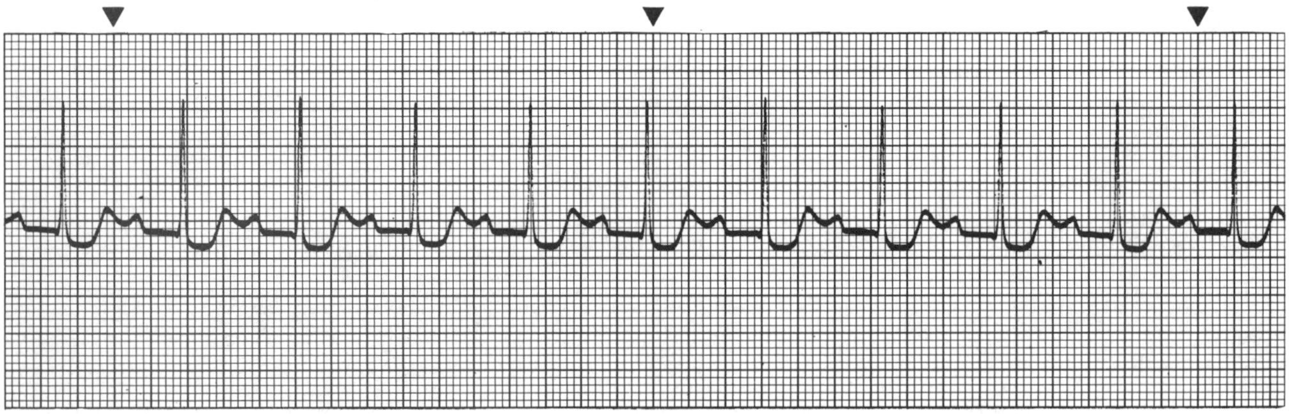

Strip 11-24. Rhythm: _____ Rate: _____ P wave: _____

PR interval: _____ QRS: _____

Rhythm interpretation: _____

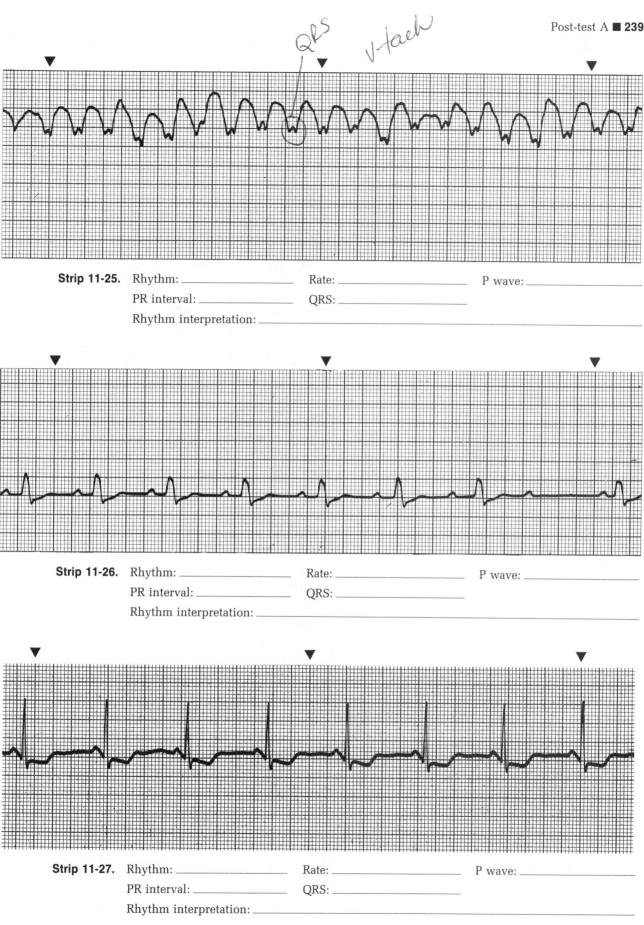

Strip 11-25. Rhythm: _____ Rate: _____ P wave: _____

PR interval: _____ QRS: _____

Rhythm interpretation: _____

Strip 11-26. Rhythm: _____ Rate: _____ P wave: _____

PR interval: _____ QRS: _____

Rhythm interpretation: _____

Strip 11-27. Rhythm: _____ Rate: _____ P wave: _____

PR interval: _____ QRS: _____

Rhythm interpretation: _____

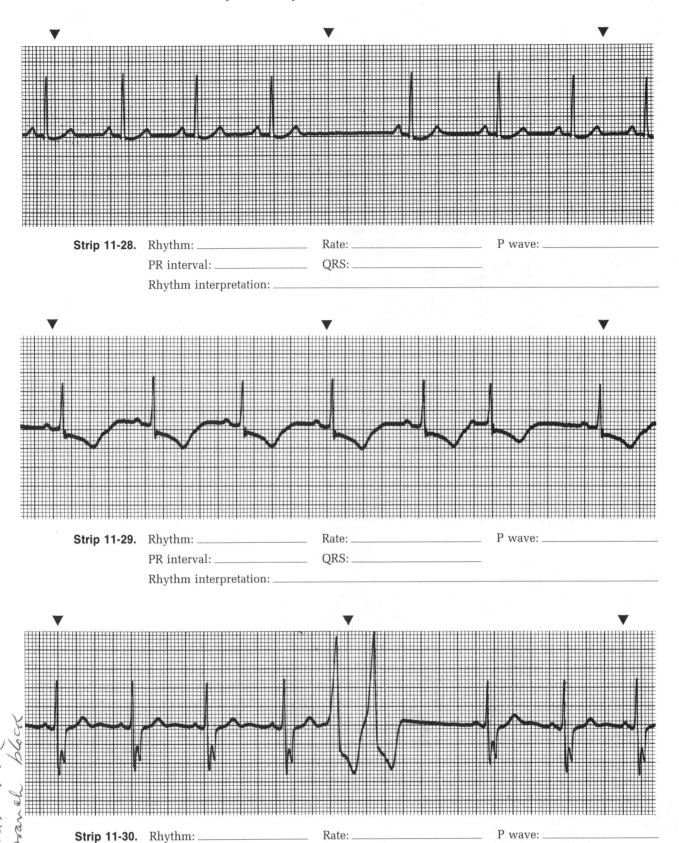

Strip 11-28. Rhythm: _____ Rate: _____ P wave: _____

PR interval: _____ QRS: _____

Rhythm interpretation: _____

Strip 11-29. Rhythm: _____ Rate: _____ P wave: _____

PR interval: _____ QRS: _____

Rhythm interpretation: _____

Strip 11-30. Rhythm: _____ Rate: _____ P wave: _____

PR interval: _____ QRS: _____

Rhythm interpretation: _____

Bundle branch block Pair PVC

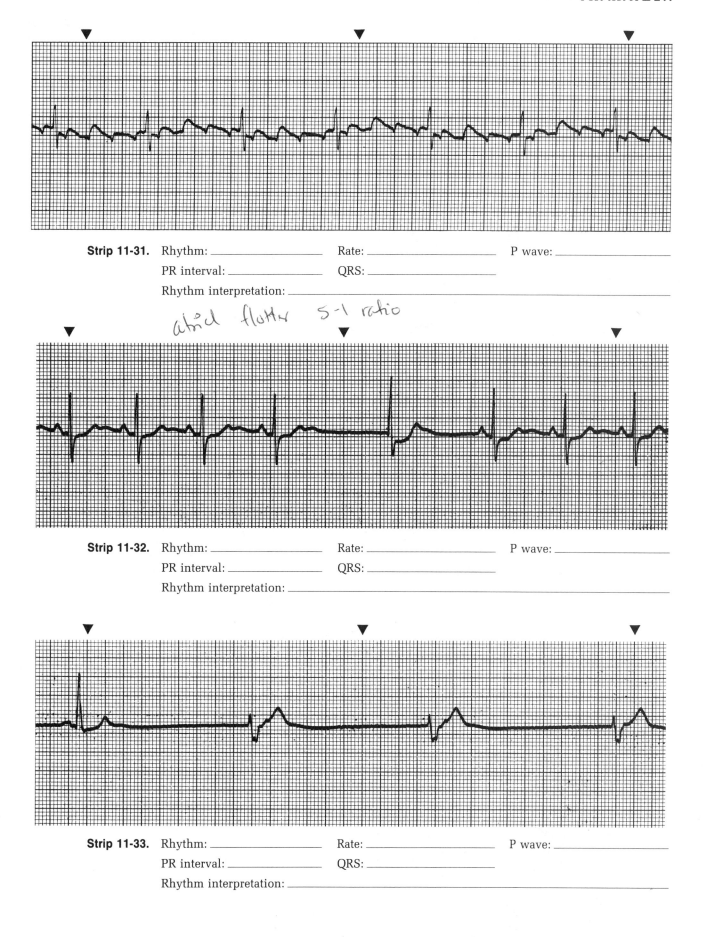

Strip 11-31. Rhythm: _____ Rate: _____ P wave: _____

PR interval: _____ QRS: _____

Rhythm interpretation: _____

atrial flutter 5-1 ratio

Strip 11-32. Rhythm: _____ Rate: _____ P wave: _____

PR interval: _____ QRS: _____

Rhythm interpretation: _____

Strip 11-33. Rhythm: _____ Rate: _____ P wave: _____

PR interval: _____ QRS: _____

Rhythm interpretation: _____

*Pacemaker
loss of capture
native beat*

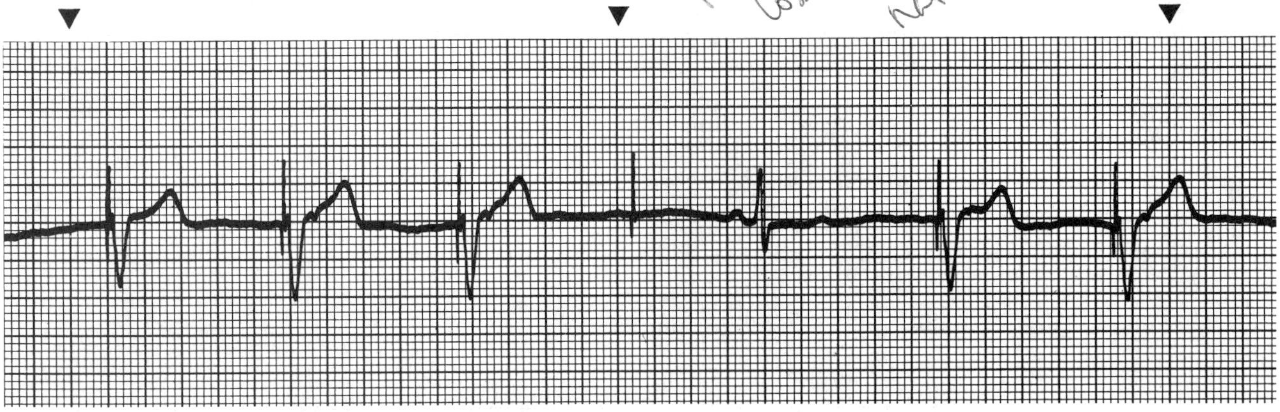

Strip 11-34. Rhythm: _____ Rate: _____ P wave: _____

PR interval: _____ QRS: _____

Rhythm interpretation: _____

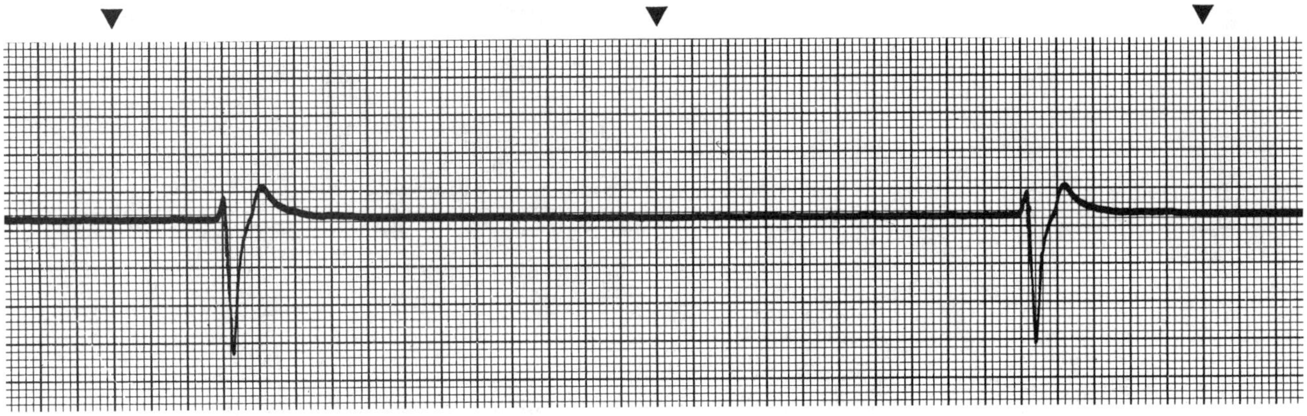

Strip 11-35. Rhythm: _____ Rate: _____ P wave: _____

PR interval: _____ QRS: _____

Rhythm interpretation: _____

electrical shock

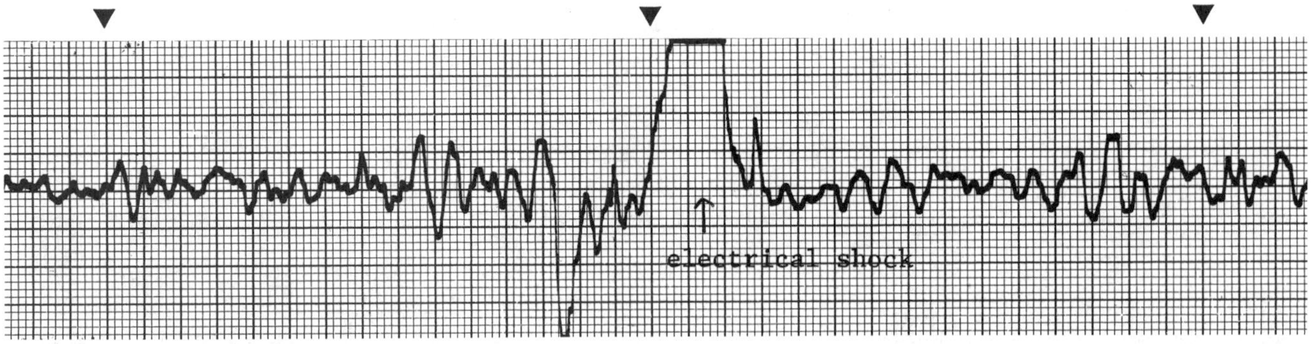

Strip 11-36. Rhythm: _____ Rate: _____ P wave: _____

PR interval: _____ QRS: _____

Rhythm interpretation: _____

*coarse
V fib
only*

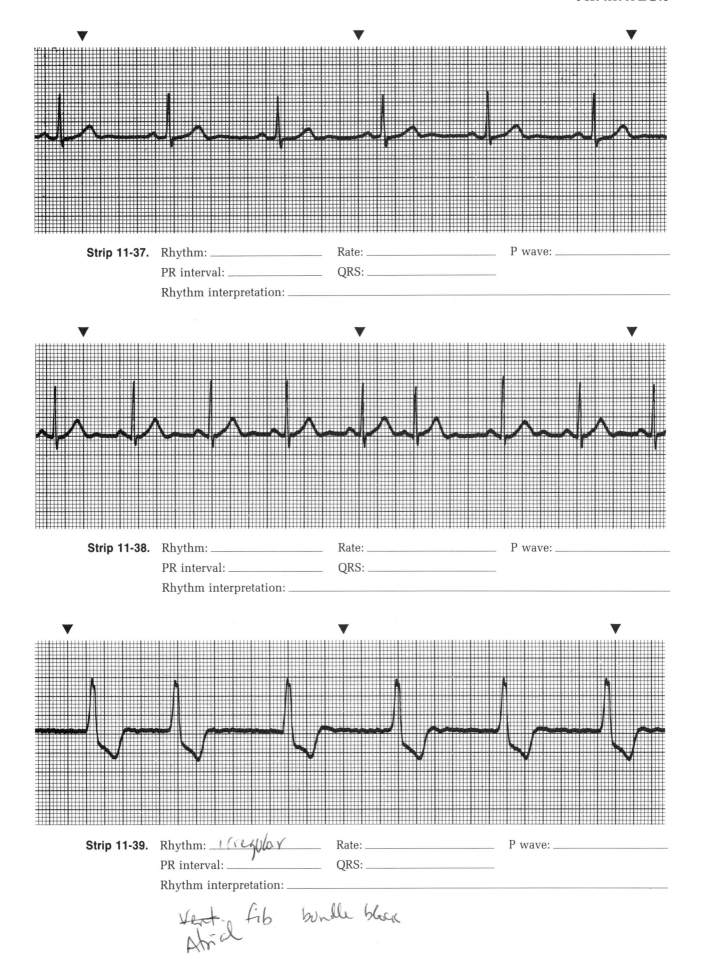

Strip 11-37. Rhythm: _____ Rate: _____ P wave: _____

PR interval: _____ QRS: _____

Rhythm interpretation: _____

Strip 11-38. Rhythm: _____ Rate: _____ P wave: _____

PR interval: _____ QRS: _____

Rhythm interpretation: _____

Strip 11-39. Rhythm: _irregular_ Rate: _____ P wave: _____

PR interval: _____ QRS: _____

Rhythm interpretation: _____

Vent. fib bundle block
Atrial

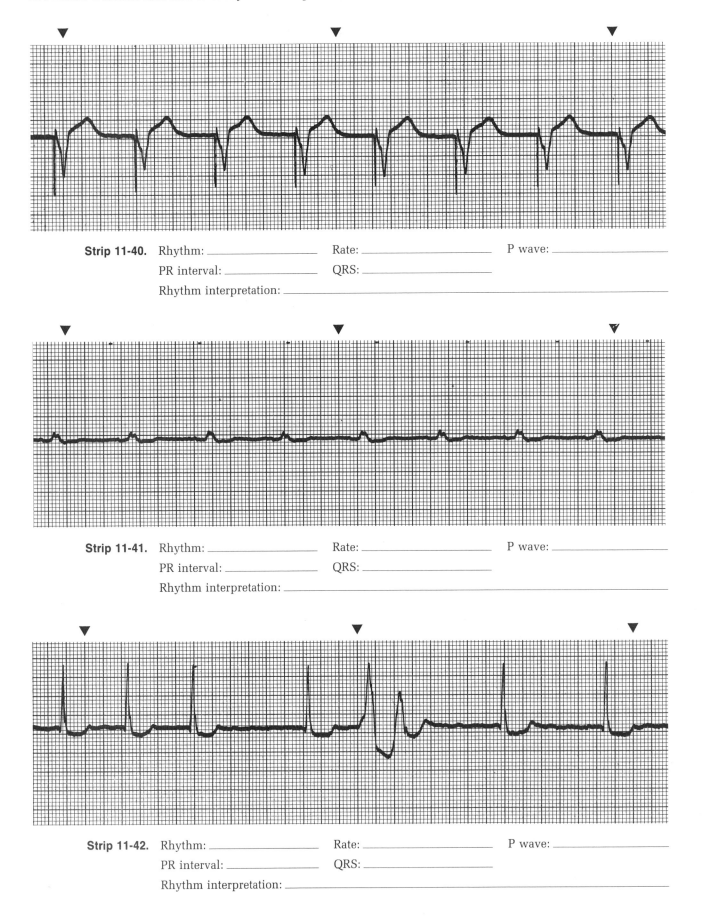

Strip 11-40. Rhythm: _____ Rate: _____ P wave: _____

PR interval: _____ QRS: _____

Rhythm interpretation: _____

Strip 11-41. Rhythm: _____ Rate: _____ P wave: _____

PR interval: _____ QRS: _____

Rhythm interpretation: _____

Strip 11-42. Rhythm: _____ Rate: _____ P wave: _____

PR interval: _____ QRS: _____

Rhythm interpretation: _____

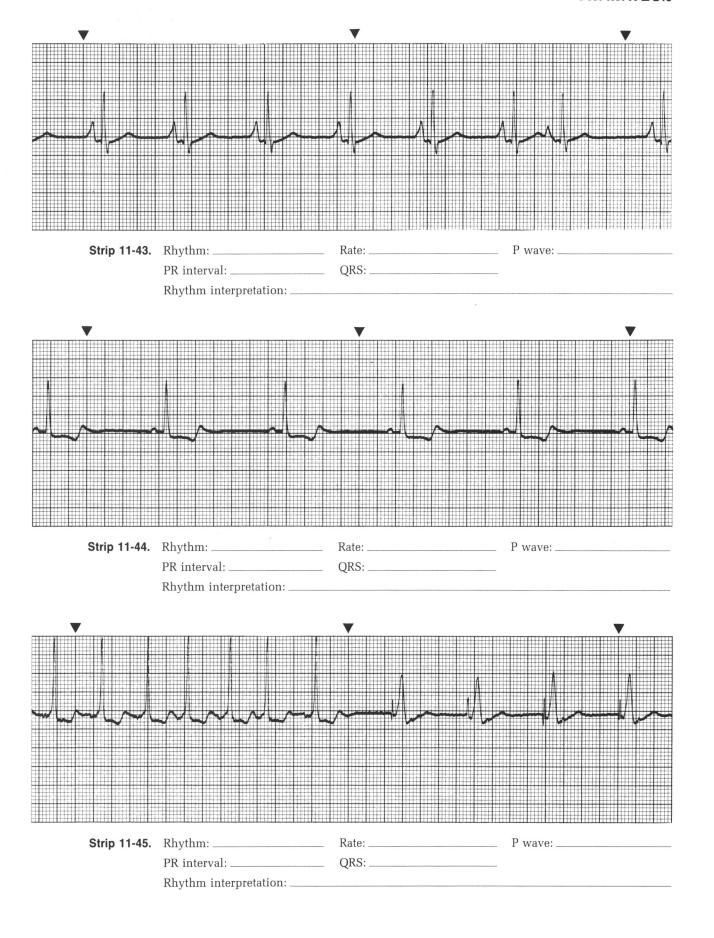

Strip 11-43. Rhythm: _____ Rate: _____ P wave: _____

PR interval: _____ QRS: _____

Rhythm interpretation: _____

Strip 11-44. Rhythm: _____ Rate: _____ P wave: _____

PR interval: _____ QRS: _____

Rhythm interpretation: _____

Strip 11-45. Rhythm: _____ Rate: _____ P wave: _____

PR interval: _____ QRS: _____

Rhythm interpretation: _____

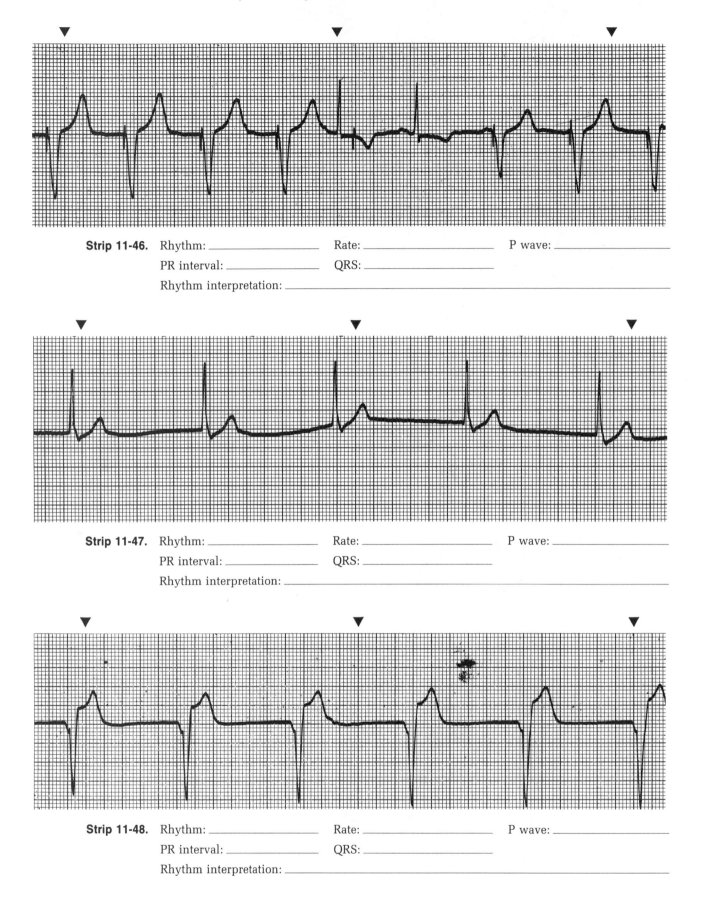

Strip 11-46. Rhythm: _____ Rate: _____ P wave: _____

PR interval: _____ QRS: _____

Rhythm interpretation: _____

Strip 11-47. Rhythm: _____ Rate: _____ P wave: _____

PR interval: _____ QRS: _____

Rhythm interpretation: _____

Strip 11-48. Rhythm: _____ Rate: _____ P wave: _____

PR interval: _____ QRS: _____

Rhythm interpretation: _____

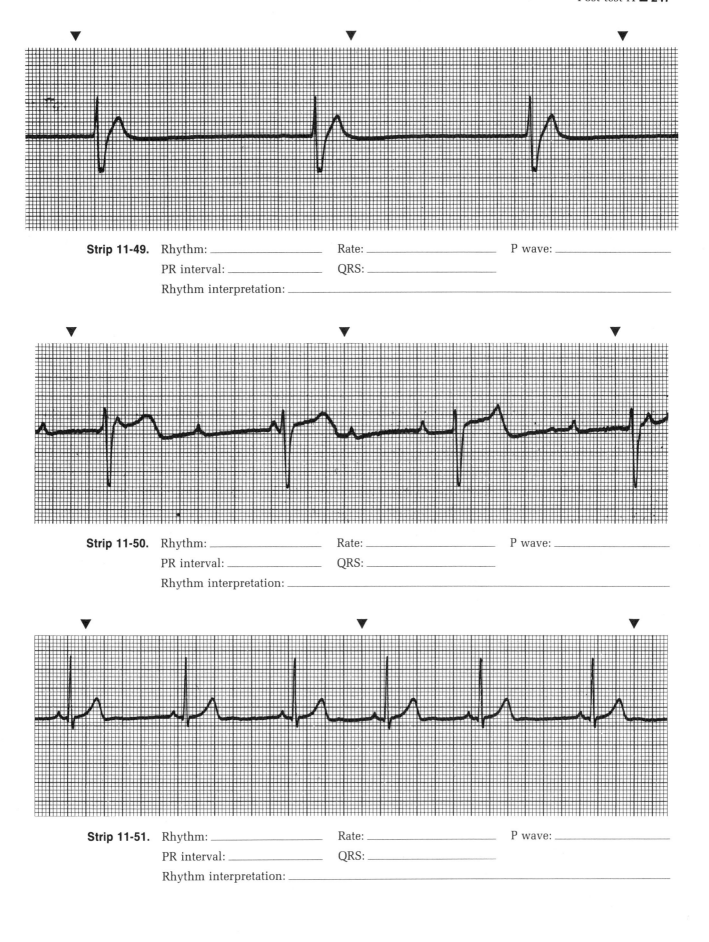

Strip 11-49. Rhythm: _____ Rate: _____ P wave: _____

PR interval: _____ QRS: _____

Rhythm interpretation: _____

Strip 11-50. Rhythm: _____ Rate: _____ P wave: _____

PR interval: _____ QRS: _____

Rhythm interpretation: _____

Strip 11-51. Rhythm: _____ Rate: _____ P wave: _____

PR interval: _____ QRS: _____

Rhythm interpretation: _____

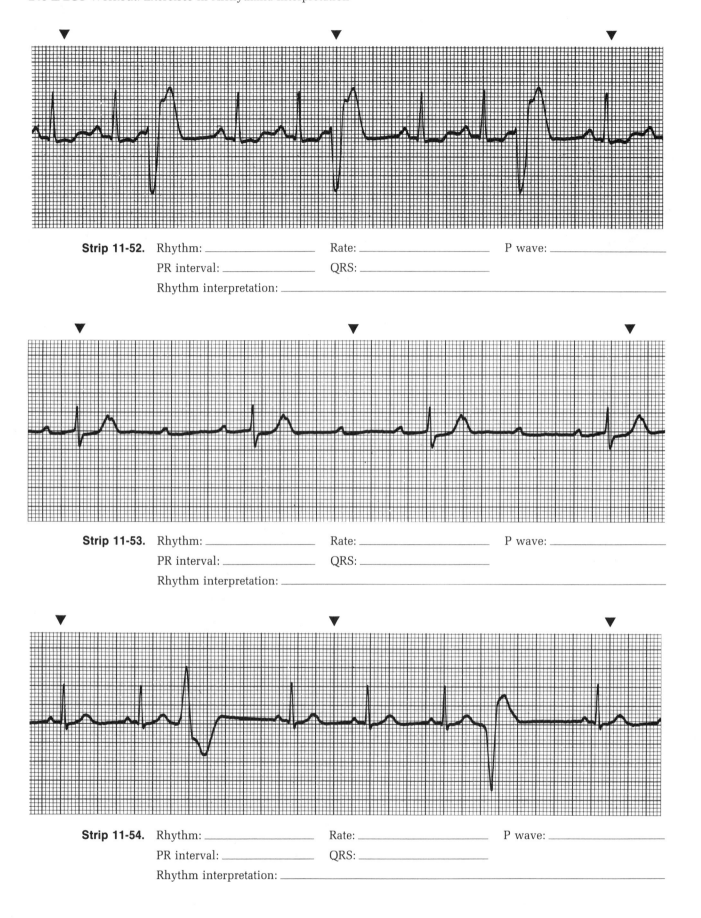

Strip 11-52. Rhythm: _____ Rate: _____ P wave: _____

PR interval: _____ QRS: _____

Rhythm interpretation: _____

Strip 11-53. Rhythm: _____ Rate: _____ P wave: _____

PR interval: _____ QRS: _____

Rhythm interpretation: _____

Strip 11-54. Rhythm: _____ Rate: _____ P wave: _____

PR interval: _____ QRS: _____

Rhythm interpretation: _____

Post-test B

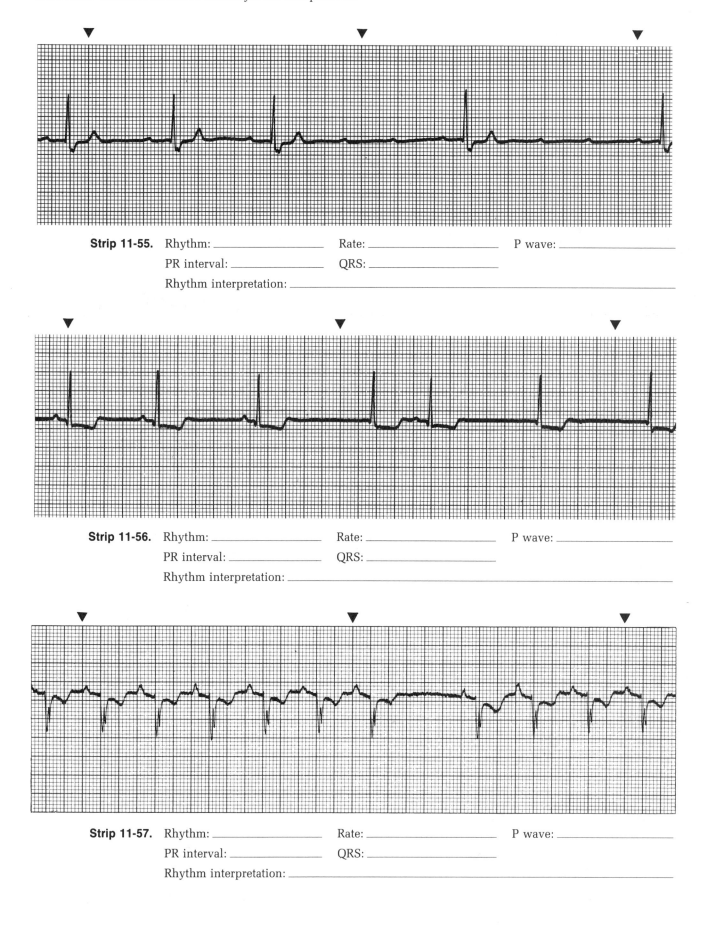

Strip 11-55. Rhythm: _____ Rate: _____ P wave: _____

PR interval: _____ QRS: _____

Rhythm interpretation: _____

Strip 11-56. Rhythm: _____ Rate: _____ P wave: _____

PR interval: _____ QRS: _____

Rhythm interpretation: _____

Strip 11-57. Rhythm: _____ Rate: _____ P wave: _____

PR interval: _____ QRS: _____

Rhythm interpretation: _____

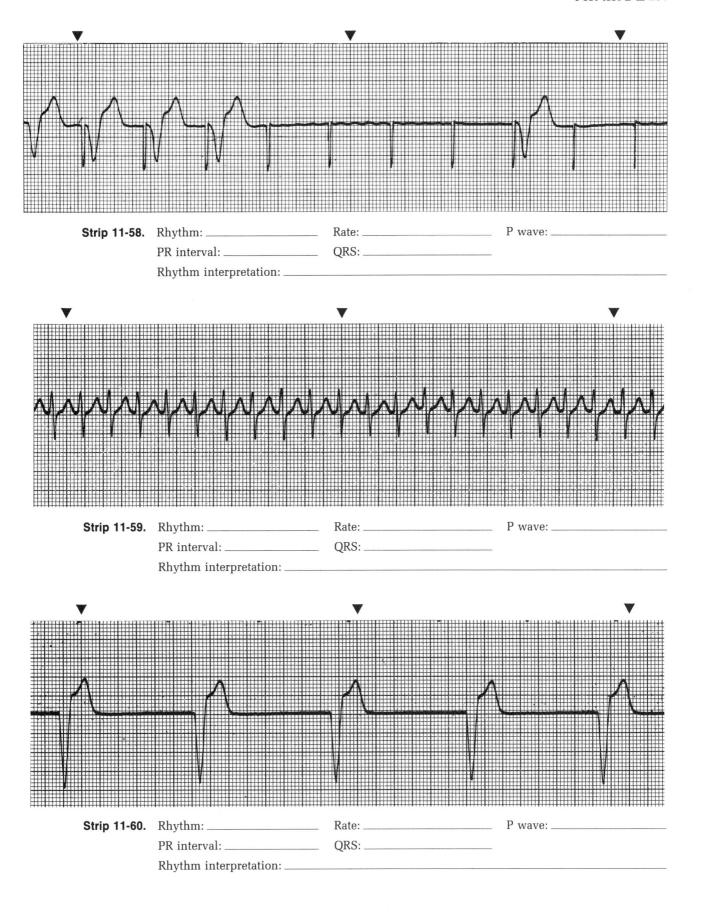

Strip 11-58. Rhythm: _____ Rate: _____ P wave: _____

PR interval: _____ QRS: _____

Rhythm interpretation: _____

Strip 11-59. Rhythm: _____ Rate: _____ P wave: _____

PR interval: _____ QRS: _____

Rhythm interpretation: _____

Strip 11-60. Rhythm: _____ Rate: _____ P wave: _____

PR interval: _____ QRS: _____

Rhythm interpretation: _____

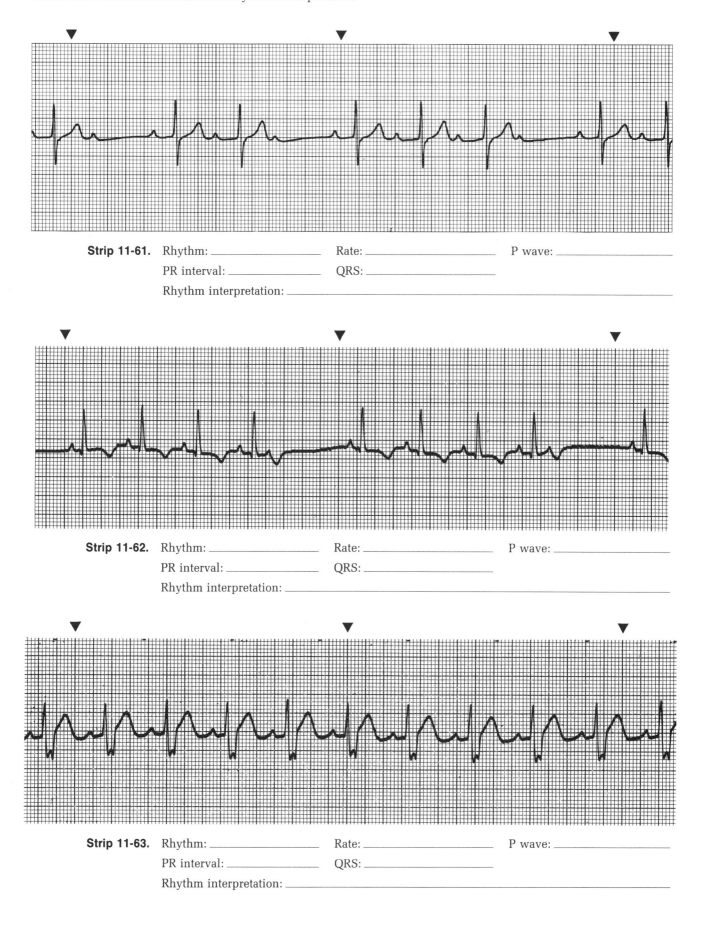

Strip 11-61. Rhythm: _____ Rate: _____ P wave: _____

PR interval: _____ QRS: _____

Rhythm interpretation: _____

Strip 11-62. Rhythm: _____ Rate: _____ P wave: _____

PR interval: _____ QRS: _____

Rhythm interpretation: _____

Strip 11-63. Rhythm: _____ Rate: _____ P wave: _____

PR interval: _____ QRS: _____

Rhythm interpretation: _____

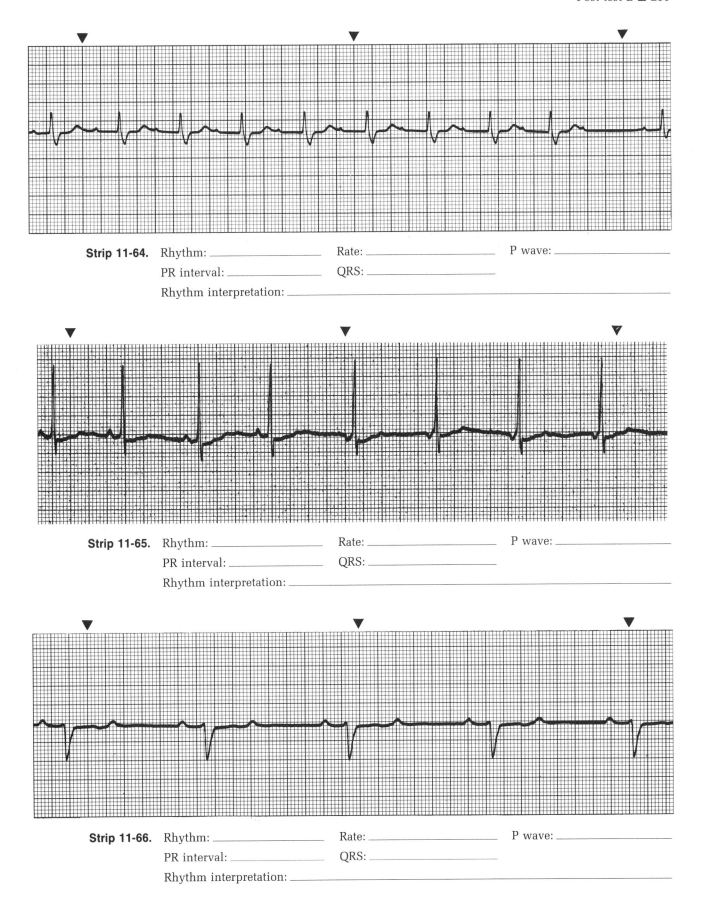

Strip 11-64. Rhythm: _____ Rate: _____ P wave: _____

PR interval: _____ QRS: _____

Rhythm interpretation: _____

Strip 11-65. Rhythm: _____ Rate: _____ P wave: _____

PR interval: _____ QRS: _____

Rhythm interpretation: _____

Strip 11-66. Rhythm: _____ Rate: _____ P wave: _____

PR interval: _____ QRS: _____

Rhythm interpretation: _____

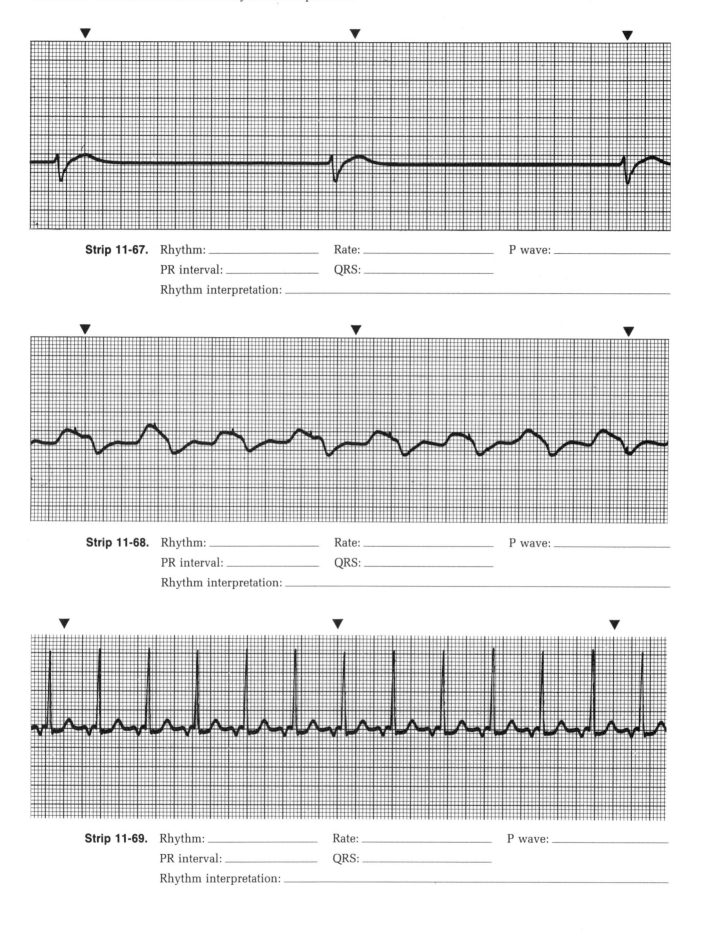

Strip 11-67. Rhythm: _____ Rate: _____ P wave: _____

PR interval: _____ QRS: _____

Rhythm interpretation: _____

Strip 11-68. Rhythm: _____ Rate: _____ P wave: _____

PR interval: _____ QRS: _____

Rhythm interpretation: _____

Strip 11-69. Rhythm: _____ Rate: _____ P wave: _____

PR interval: _____ QRS: _____

Rhythm interpretation: _____

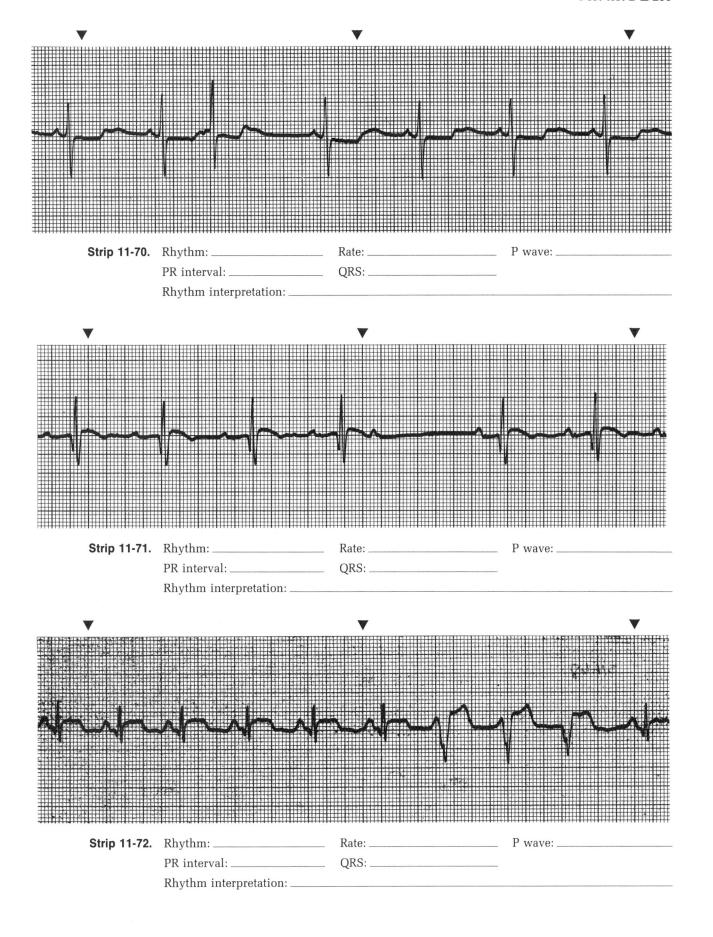

Strip 11-70. Rhythm: _____ Rate: _____ P wave: _____

PR interval: _____ QRS: _____

Rhythm interpretation: _____

Strip 11-71. Rhythm: _____ Rate: _____ P wave: _____

PR interval: _____ QRS: _____

Rhythm interpretation: _____

Strip 11-72. Rhythm: _____ Rate: _____ P wave: _____

PR interval: _____ QRS: _____

Rhythm interpretation: _____

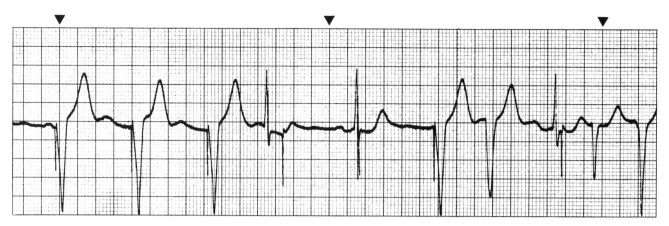

Strip 11-73.

Automatic interval rate:

Analysis:

Interpretation:

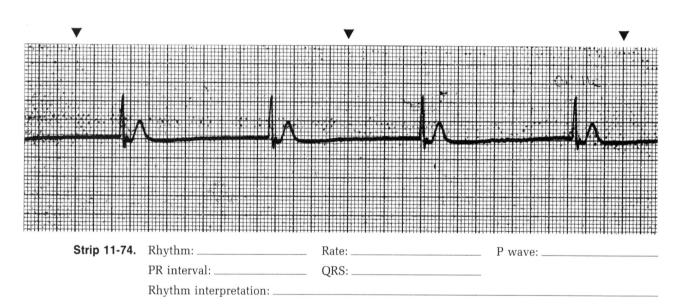

Strip 11-74. Rhythm: _____ Rate: _____ P wave: _____

PR interval: _____ QRS: _____

Rhythm interpretation: _____

Strip 11-75. Rhythm: _____ Rate: _____ P wave: _____

PR interval: _____ QRS: _____

Rhythm interpretation: _____

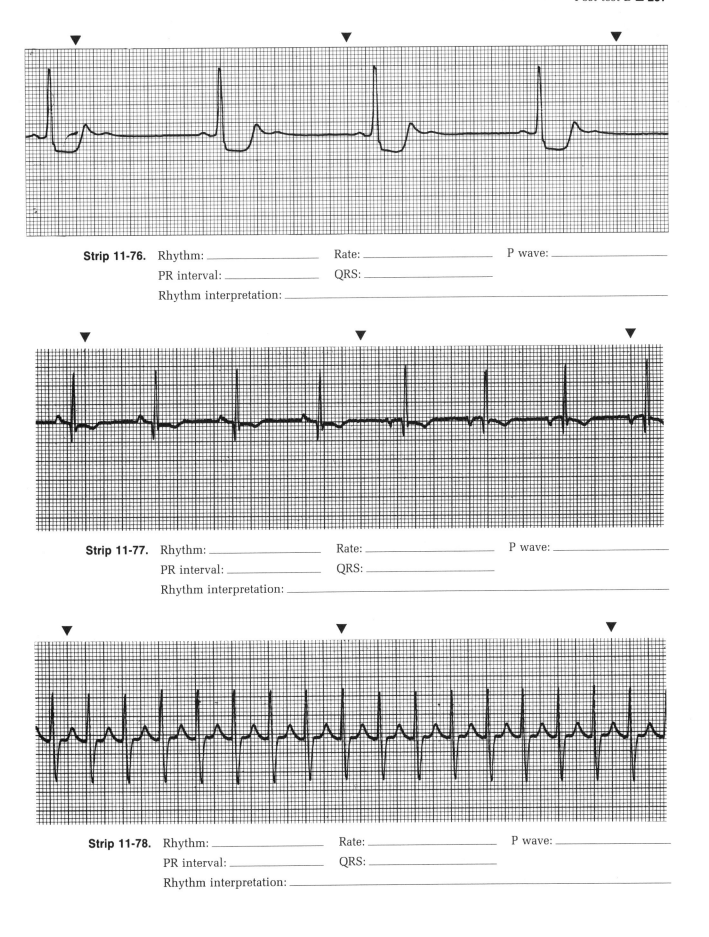

Strip 11-76. Rhythm: _____ Rate: _____ P wave: _____

PR interval: _____ QRS: _____

Rhythm interpretation: _____

Strip 11-77. Rhythm: _____ Rate: _____ P wave: _____

PR interval: _____ QRS: _____

Rhythm interpretation: _____

Strip 11-78. Rhythm: _____ Rate: _____ P wave: _____

PR interval: _____ QRS: _____

Rhythm interpretation: _____

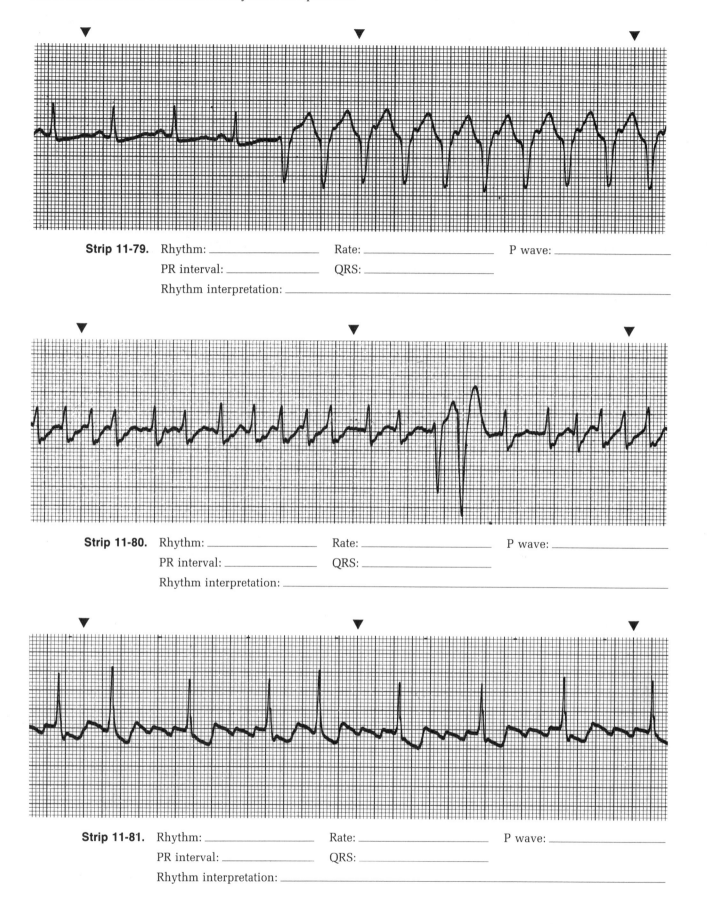

Strip 11-79. Rhythm: _____ Rate: _____ P wave: _____

PR interval: _____ QRS: _____

Rhythm interpretation: _____

Strip 11-80. Rhythm: _____ Rate: _____ P wave: _____

PR interval: _____ QRS: _____

Rhythm interpretation: _____

Strip 11-81. Rhythm: _____ Rate: _____ P wave: _____

PR interval: _____ QRS: _____

Rhythm interpretation: _____

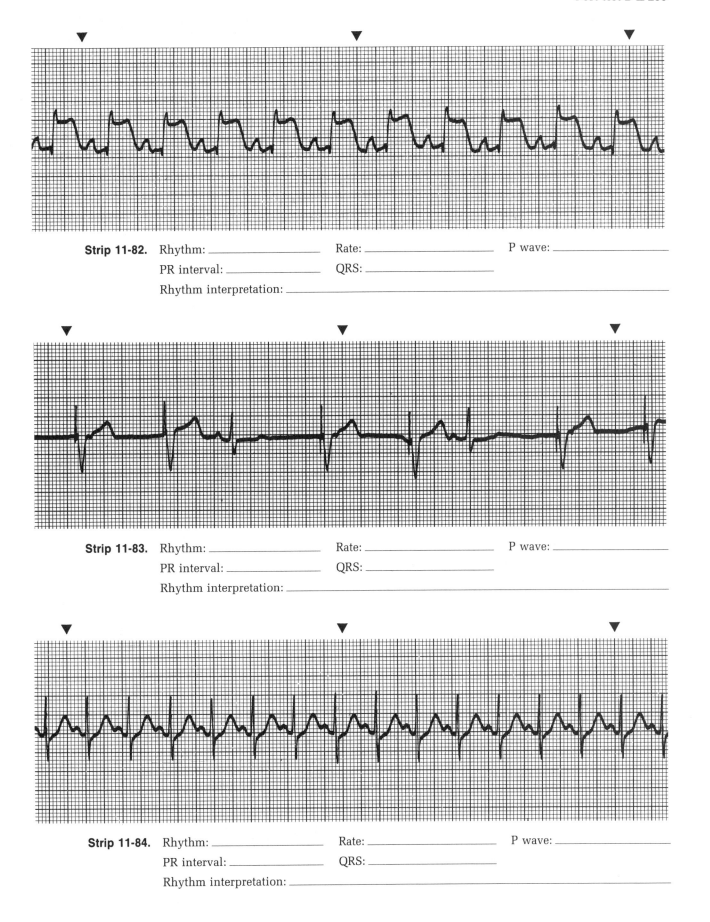

Strip 11-82. Rhythm: _____ Rate: _____ P wave: _____

PR interval: _____ QRS: _____

Rhythm interpretation: _____

Strip 11-83. Rhythm: _____ Rate: _____ P wave: _____

PR interval: _____ QRS: _____

Rhythm interpretation: _____

Strip 11-84. Rhythm: _____ Rate: _____ P wave: _____

PR interval: _____ QRS: _____

Rhythm interpretation: _____

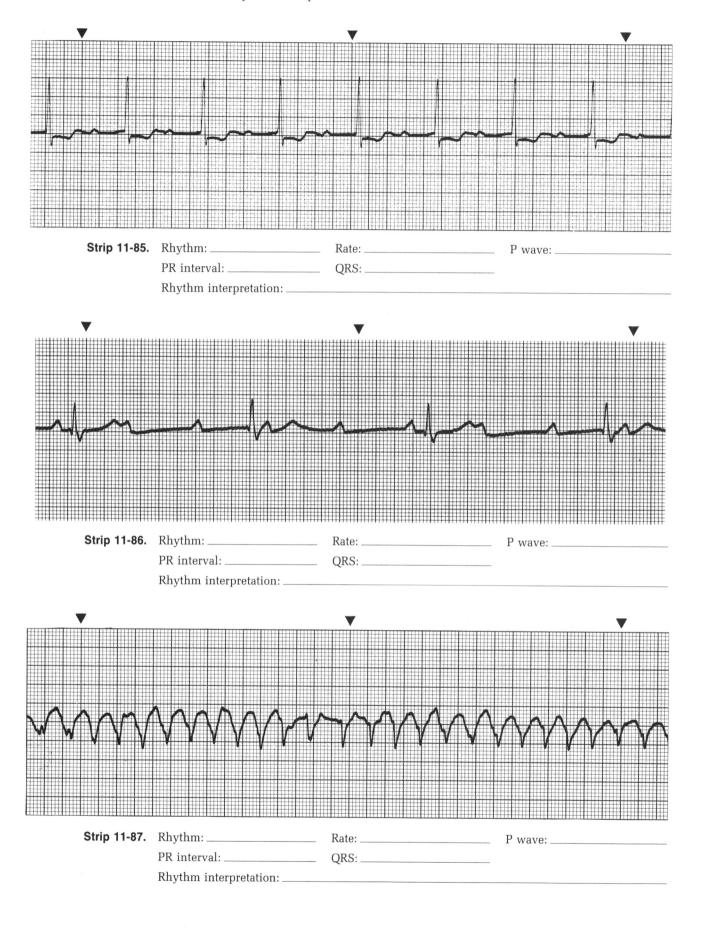

Strip 11-85. Rhythm: _____ Rate: _____ P wave: _____

PR interval: _____ QRS: _____

Rhythm interpretation: _____

Strip 11-86. Rhythm: _____ Rate: _____ P wave: _____

PR interval: _____ QRS: _____

Rhythm interpretation: _____

Strip 11-87. Rhythm: _____ Rate: _____ P wave: _____

PR interval: _____ QRS: _____

Rhythm interpretation: _____

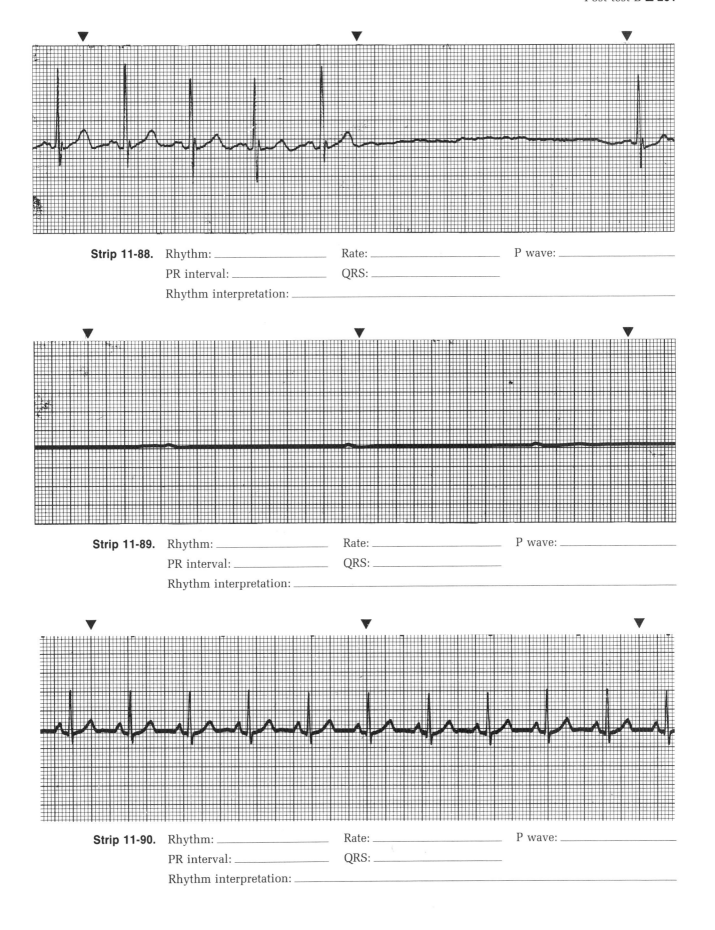

Strip 11-88. Rhythm: _____ Rate: _____ P wave: _____

PR interval: _____ QRS: _____

Rhythm interpretation: _____

Strip 11-89. Rhythm: _____ Rate: _____ P wave: _____

PR interval: _____ QRS: _____

Rhythm interpretation: _____

Strip 11-90. Rhythm: _____ Rate: _____ P wave: _____

PR interval: _____ QRS: _____

Rhythm interpretation: _____

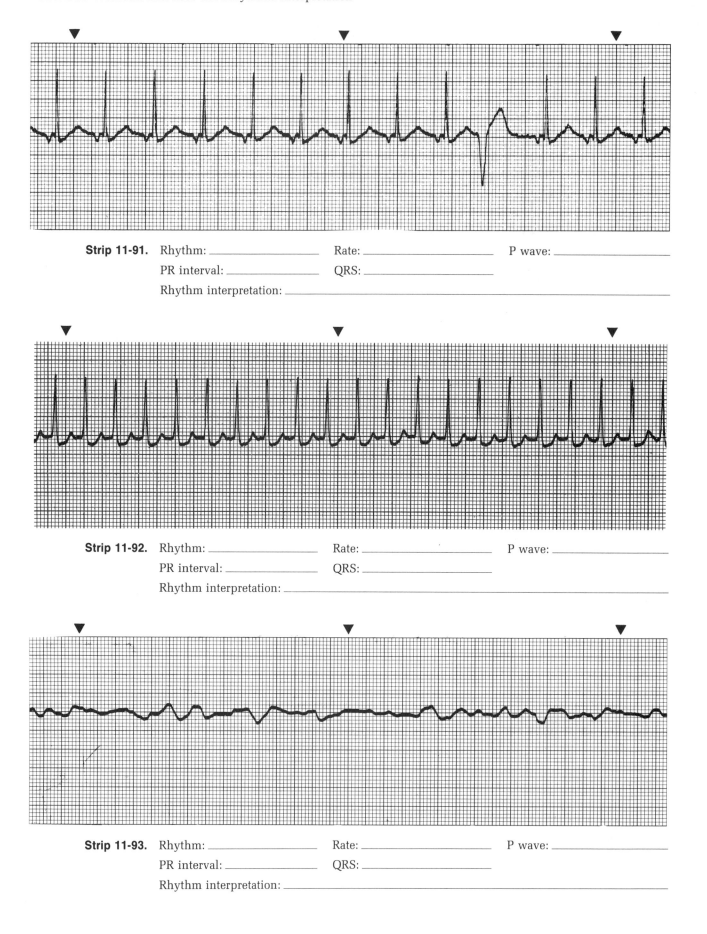

Strip 11-91. Rhythm: _____ Rate: _____ P wave: _____

PR interval: _____ QRS: _____

Rhythm interpretation: _____

Strip 11-92. Rhythm: _____ Rate: _____ P wave: _____

PR interval: _____ QRS: _____

Rhythm interpretation: _____

Strip 11-93. Rhythm: _____ Rate: _____ P wave: _____

PR interval: _____ QRS: _____

Rhythm interpretation: _____

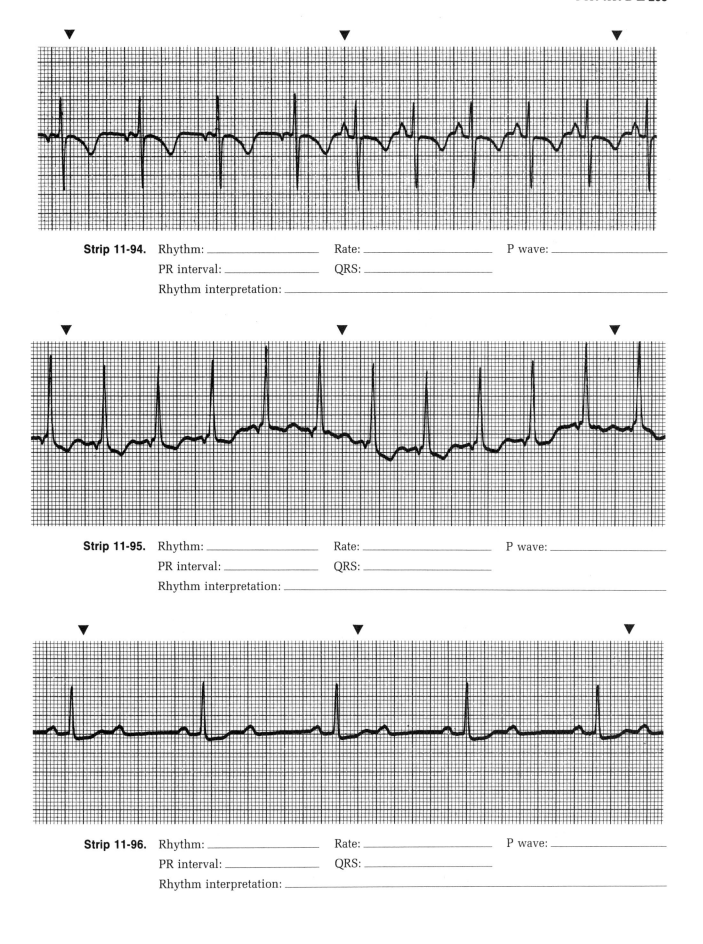

Strip 11-94. Rhythm: _____ Rate: _____ P wave: _____

PR interval: _____ QRS: _____

Rhythm interpretation: _____

Strip 11-95. Rhythm: _____ Rate: _____ P wave: _____

PR interval: _____ QRS: _____

Rhythm interpretation: _____

Strip 11-96. Rhythm: _____ Rate: _____ P wave: _____

PR interval: _____ QRS: _____

Rhythm interpretation: _____

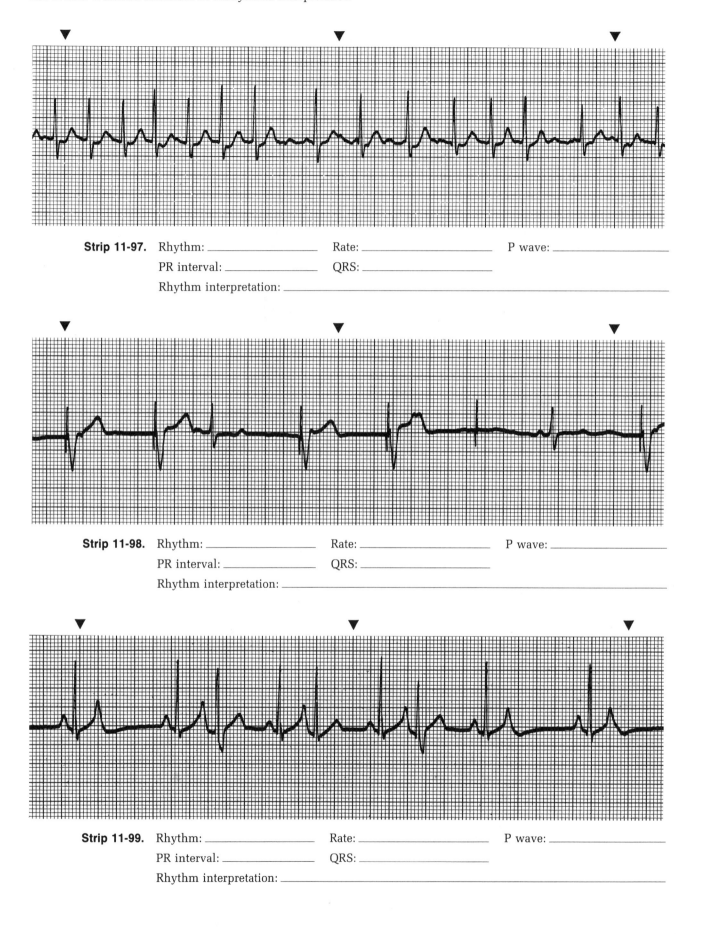

Strip 11-97. Rhythm: _____ Rate: _____ P wave: _____

PR interval: _____ QRS: _____

Rhythm interpretation: _____

Strip 11-98. Rhythm: _____ Rate: _____ P wave: _____

PR interval: _____ QRS: _____

Rhythm interpretation: _____

Strip 11-99. Rhythm: _____ Rate: _____ P wave: _____

PR interval: _____ QRS: _____

Rhythm interpretation: _____

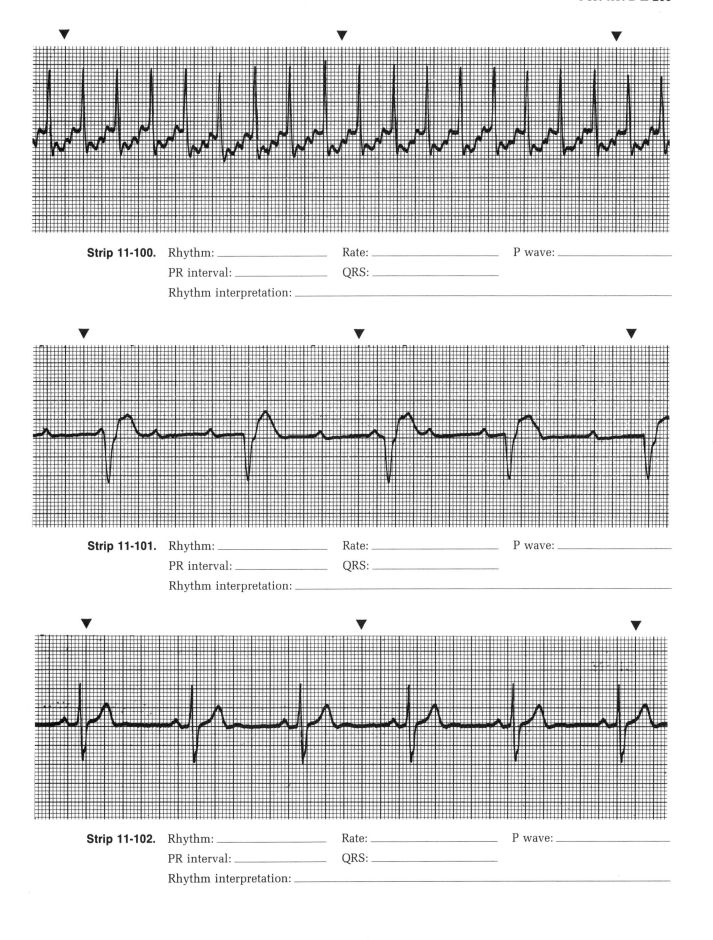

Strip 11-100. Rhythm: _____ Rate: _____ P wave: _____

PR interval: _____ QRS: _____

Rhythm interpretation: _____

Strip 11-101. Rhythm: _____ Rate: _____ P wave: _____

PR interval: _____ QRS: _____

Rhythm interpretation: _____

Strip 11-102. Rhythm: _____ Rate: _____ P wave: _____

PR interval: _____ QRS: _____

Rhythm interpretation: _____

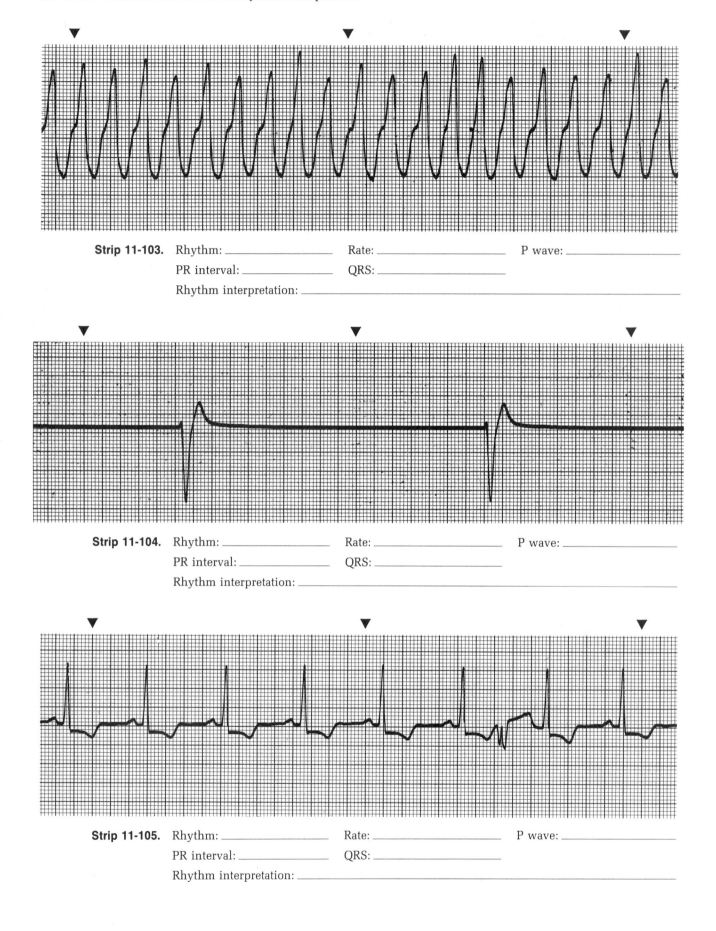

Strip 11-103. Rhythm: _____ Rate: _____ P wave: _____

PR interval: _____ QRS: _____

Rhythm interpretation: _____

Strip 11-104. Rhythm: _____ Rate: _____ P wave: _____

PR interval: _____ QRS: _____

Rhythm interpretation: _____

Strip 11-105. Rhythm: _____ Rate: _____ P wave: _____

PR interval: _____ QRS: _____

Rhythm interpretation: _____

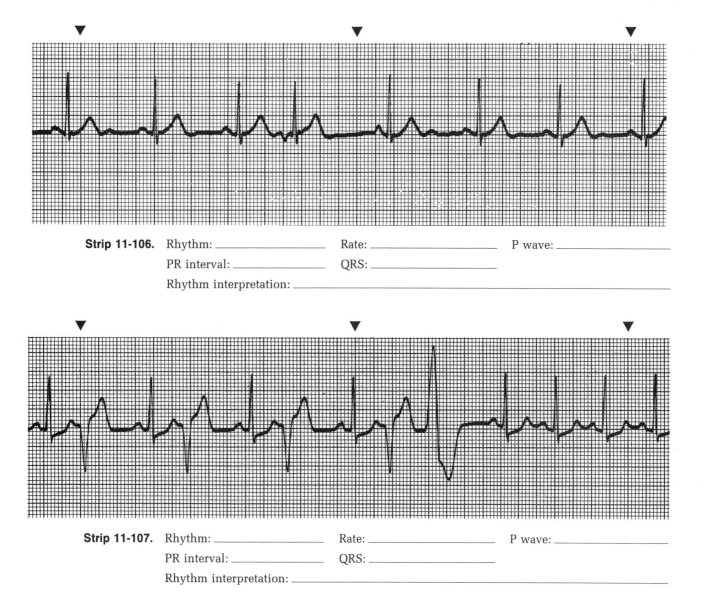

Strip 11-106. Rhythm: _____ Rate: _____ P wave: _____

PR interval: _____ QRS: _____

Rhythm interpretation: _____

Strip 11-107. Rhythm: _____ Rate: _____ P wave: _____

PR interval: _____ QRS: _____

Rhythm interpretation: _____

Appendix

Answer Keys to Chapter 3 and Chapters 5 through 11

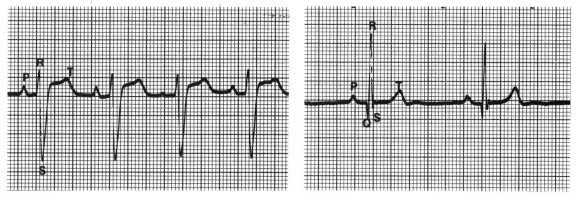

Strip 3-1.

Strip 3-2.

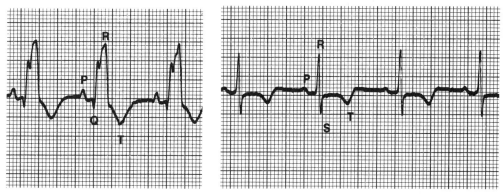

Strip 3-3.

Strip 3-4.

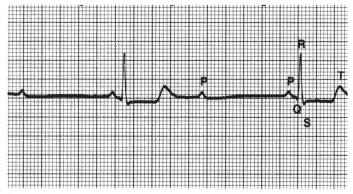

Strip 3-5.

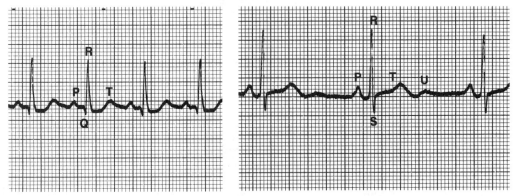

Strip 3-6.

Strip 3-7.

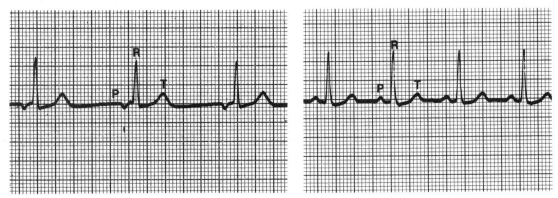

Strip 3-8.

Strip 3-9.

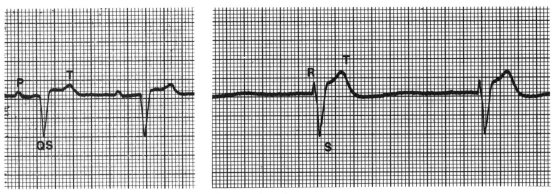

Strip 3-10.

Strip 3-11.

Strip 5-1
Rhythm: Regular
Rate: 79
P waves: Sinus
PR interval: 0.14 to 0.16 seconds
QRS: 0.06 to 0.08 seconds
Comment: An inverted T wave is present

Strip 5-2
Rhythm: Regular
Rate: 45
P waves: Sinus
PR interval: 0.14 to 0.16 seconds
QRS: 0.08 seconds

Strip 5-3
Rhythm: Regular
Rate: 88
P waves: Sinus
PR interval: 0.20 seconds
QRS: 0.08 seconds
Comment: A depressed ST segment is present

Strip 5-4
Rhythm: Irregular
Rate: 50
P waves: Sinus
PR interval: 0.16 to 0.18 seconds
QRS: 0.04 seconds

Strip 5-5
Rhythm: Regular
Rate: 100
P waves: Sinus
PR interval: 0.20 seconds
QRS: 0.08 seconds
Comment: An extremely elevated ST segment is present

Strip 5-6
Rhythm: Regular
Rate: 136
P waves: Sinus
PR interval: 0.14 to 0.16 seconds
QRS: 0.06 to 0.08 seconds

Strip 5-7
Rhythm: Regular
Rate: 68
P waves: Sinus
PR interval: 0.16 to 0.18 seconds
QRS: 0.12 to 0.14 seconds
Comment: A U wave is present

Strip 5-8
Rhythm: Irregular
Rate: 50
P waves: Sinus
PR interval: 0.12 to 0.14 seconds
QRS: 0.08 seconds
Comment: An elevated ST segment and inverted T wave are present

Strip 5-9
Rhythm: Regular
Rate: 94
P waves: Sinus
PR interval: 0.14 to 0.16 seconds
QRS: 0.06 to 0.08 seconds
Comment: A depressed ST segment is present

Strip 6-1
Rhythm: Regular
Rate: 40
P waves: Sinus
PR interval: 0.14 to 0.16 seconds
QRS: 0.08 seconds
Rhythm interpretation: Sinus bradycardia

Strip 6-2
Rhythm: Regular
Rate: 58
P waves: Sinus
PR interval: 0.18 to 0.20 seconds
QRS: 0.08 seconds
Rhythm interpretation: Sinus bradycardia; a U wave is present

Strip 6-3
Rhythm: Regular
Rate: 94
P waves: Sinus
PR interval: 0.14 to 0.16 seconds
QRS: 0.08 to 0.10 seconds
Rhythm interpretation: Normal sinus rhythm; ST depression is present

Strip 6-4
Rhythm: Regular
Rate: 107
P waves: Sinus
PR interval: 0.14 to 0.16 seconds
QRS: 0.08 to 0.10 seconds
Rhythm interpretation: Sinus tachycardia; T wave inversion is present

Strip 6-5
Rhythm: Regular
Rate: 56
P waves: Sinus
PR interval: 0.16 to 0.18 seconds
QRS: 0.04 to 0.06 seconds
Rhythm interpretation: Sinus bradycardia

Strip 6-6
Rhythm: Basic rhythm regular; irregular during pause
Rate: Basic rhythm 100
P waves: Sinus in basic rhythm; absent during pause
PR interval: 0.16 to 0.20 seconds
QRS: 0.08 to 0.10 seconds in basic rhythm
Rhythm interpretation: Normal sinus rhythm with sinus block; an inverted T wave is present

Strip 6-7
Rhythm: Regular
Rate: 45
P waves: Sinus
PR interval: 0.18 to 0.20 seconds
QRS: 0.08 seconds
Rhythm interpretation: Sinus bradycardia; T wave inversion is present

Strip 6-8
Rhythm: Irregular
Rate: 50
P waves: Sinus
PR interval: 0.14 to 0.16 seconds
QRS: 0.04 seconds
Rhythm interpretation: Sinus arrhythmia; sinus bradycardia

Strip 6-9
Rhythm: Basic rhythm regular; irregular during pause
Rate: Basic rhythm rate 60
P waves: Normal in basic rhythm; absent during pause
PR interval: 0.18 to 0.20 seconds in basic rhythm; absent during pause
QRS: 0.04 to 0.06 seconds in basic rhythm; absent during pause
Rhythm interpretation: Normal sinus rhythm with sinus arrest; a U wave is present

Strip 6-10
Rhythm: Regular
Rate: 125
P waves: Sinus
PR interval: 0.12 seconds
QRS: 0.06 to 0.08 seconds
Rhythm interpretation: Sinus tachycardia; ST segment depression is present

Strip 6-11
Rhythm: Regular
Rate: 88
P waves: Sinus
PR interval: 0.16 seconds
QRS: 0.06 to 0.08 seconds
Rhythm interpretation: Normal sinus rhythm

Strip 6-12
Rhythm: Regular
Rate: 54
P waves: Sinus
PR interval: 0.16 to 0.18 seconds
QRS: 0.08 seconds
Rhythm interpretation: Sinus bradycardia; an inverted T wave is present

Strip 6-13
Rhythm: Irregular
Rate: 60
P waves: Sinus
PR interval: 0.14 to 0.16 seconds
QRS: 0.08 to 0.10 seconds
Rhythm interpretation: Sinus arrhythmia

Strip 6-14
Rhythm: Regular
Rate: 68
P waves: Sinus
PR interval: 0.14 to 0.16 seconds
QRS: 0.08 seconds
Rhythm interpretation: Normal sinus rhythm; a U wave is present

Strip 6-15
Rhythm: Basic rhythm irregular
Rate: Basic rhythm rate 60
P waves: Sinus
PR interval: 0.16 to 0.18 seconds
QRS: 0.08 to 0.10 seconds
Rhythm interpretation: Sinus arrhythmia with sinus arrest/block; ST segment depression and T wave inversion are present

Strip 6-16
Rhythm: Regular
Rate: 115
P waves: Sinus
PR interval: 0.16 to 0.18 seconds
QRS: 0.06 to 0.08 seconds
Rhythm interpretation: Sinus tachycardia; a depressed ST segment and an inverted T wave are present

Strip 6-17
Rhythm: Regular
Rate: 58
P waves: Sinus
PR interval: 0.12 to 0.16 seconds
QRS: 0.04 seconds
Rhythm interpretation: Sinus bradycardia; T wave inversion is present

Strip 6-18
Rhythm: Irregular
Rate: 40
P waves: Sinus
PR interval: 0.16 to 0.18 seconds
QRS: 0.06 to 0.08 seconds
Rhythm interpretation: Sinus arrhythmia/sinus bradycardia; ST segment depression is present

Strip 6-19
Rhythm: Regular
Rate: 79
P waves: Sinus
PR interval: 0.16 to 0.20 seconds
QRS: 0.06 seconds
Rhythm interpretation: Normal sinus rhythm

Strip 6-20
Rhythm: Basic rhythm regular; irregular during pause
Rate: Basic rhythm rate 88
P waves: Sinus in basic rhythm; absent during pause
PR interval: 0.14 to 0.16 seconds in basic rhythm
QRS: 0.08 seconds in basic rhythm
Rhythm interpretation: Normal sinus rhythm with sinus block; a U wave is present

Strip 6-21
Rhythm: Regular
Rate: 136
P waves: Sinus
PR interval: 0.14 to 0.16 seconds
QRS: 0.08 to 0.10 seconds
Rhythm interpretation: Sinus tachycardia

Strip 6-22
Rhythm: Regular
Rate: 100
P waves: Sinus
PR interval: 0.12 seconds
QRS: 0.04 to 0.06 seconds
Rhythm interpretation: Normal sinus rhythm; an extremely elevated ST segment is present

Strip 6-23
Rhythm: Irregular
Rate: 50
P waves: Sinus
PR interval: 0.12 to 0.16 seconds
QRS: 0.06 to 0.08 seconds
Rhythm interpretation: Sinus arrhythmia; sinus bradycardia

Strip 6-24
Rhythm: Basic rhythm regular; irregular during pause
Rate: Basic rhythm rate 84
P waves: Sinus
PR interval: 0.16 seconds in basic rhythm; absent during pause
QRS: 0.08 seconds in basic rhythm; absent during pause
Rhythm interpretation: Normal sinus rhythm with sinus arrest

Strip 6-25
Rhythm: Regular
Rate: 115
P waves: Sinus
PR interval: 0.12 seconds
QRS: 0.08 to 0.10 seconds
Rhythm interpretation: Sinus tachycardia

Strip 6-26
Rhythm: Regular
Rate: 48
P waves: Sinus
PR interval: 0.14 to 0.16 seconds
QRS: 0.08 seconds
Rhythm interpretation: Sinus bradycardia; a U wave is present

Strip 6-27
Rhythm: Regular
Rate: 94
P waves: Sinus
PR interval: 0.14 to 0.16 seconds
QRS: 0.06 to 0.08 seconds
Rhythm interpretation: Normal sinus rhythm; ST segment depression is present

Strip 6-28
Rhythm: Irregular
Rate: 60
P waves: Sinus
PR interval: 0.12 to 0.16 seconds
QRS: 0.08 to 0.10 seconds
Rhythm interpretation: Sinus arrhythmia

Strip 6-29
Rhythm: Regular
Rate: 75
P waves: Sinus
PR interval: 0.16 seconds
QRS: 0.08 seconds
Rhythm interpretation: Normal sinus rhythm

Strip 6-30
Rhythm: Basic rhythm regular; irregular during pause
Rate: Basic rhythm rate 68; rate slows to 63 following pause; rate suppression can occur following a pause in the basic rhythm; after several cycles the rate returns to the basic rate
P waves: Sinus in basic rhythm; absent during pause
PR interval: 0.16 seconds in basic rhythm; absent during pause
QRS: 0.06 to 0.08 seconds in basic rhythm; absent during pause
Rhythm interpretation: Normal sinus rhythm with sinus arrest; a U wave is present

Strip 6-31
Rhythm: Regular
Rate: 56
P waves: Sinus
PR interval: 0.12 to 0.14 seconds
QRS: 0.08 to 0.10 seconds
Rhythm interpretation: Sinus bradycardia; ST segment depression and T wave inversion are present

Strip 6-32
Rhythm: Irregular
Rate: 50
P waves: Sinus
PR interval: 0.14 to 0.16 seconds
QRS: 0.06 to 0.08 seconds
Rhythm interpretation: Sinus arrhythmia; sinus bradycardia; ST segment depression is present

Strip 6-33
Rhythm: Regular
Rate: 136
P waves: Sinus
PR interval: 0.14 to 0.16 seconds
QRS: 0.04 to 0.06 seconds
Rhythm interpretation: Sinus tachycardia; ST segment depression is present

Strip 6-34
Rhythm: Regular
Rate: 88
P waves: Sinus
PR interval: 0.18 to 0.20 seconds
QRS: 0.08 seconds
Rhythm interpretation: Normal sinus rhythm; ST segment depression is present

Strip 6-35
Rhythm: Irregular
Rate: 60
P waves: Sinus
PR interval: 0.14 to 0.16 seconds
QRS: 0.08 seconds
Rhythm interpretation: Sinus arrhythmia

Strip 6-36
Rhythm: Regular
Rate: 52
P waves: Sinus
PR interval: 0.12 seconds
QRS: 0.08 seconds
Rhythm interpretation: Sinus bradycardia; ST segment elevation and T wave inversion are present

Strip 6-37
Rhythm: Basic rhythm regular; irregular during pause
Rate: Basic rhythm rate 88
P waves: Sinus
PR interval: 0.20 seconds
QRS: 0.06 to 0.08 seconds
Rhythm interpretation: Normal sinus rhythm with sinus arrest; ST segment depression is present

Strip 6-38
Rhythm: Regular
Rate: 115
P waves: Sinus
PR interval: 0.12 seconds
QRS: 0.06 to 0.08 seconds
Rhythm interpretation: Sinus tachycardia

Strip 6-39
Rhythm: Regular
Rate: 125
P waves: Sinus
PR interval: 0.12 to 0.14 seconds
QRS: 0.08 seconds
Rhythm interpretation: Sinus tachycardia; ST segment depression and T wave inversion are present

Strip 6-40
Rhythm: Regular
Rate: 47
P waves: Sinus
PR interval: 0.14 to 0.16 seconds
QRS: 0.06 to 0.08 seconds
Rhythm interpretation: Sinus bradycardia; ST segment depression is present

Strip 6-41
Rhythm: Regular
Rate: 100
P waves: Sinus
PR interval: 0.18 to 0.20 seconds
QRS: 0.08 seconds
Rhythm interpretation: Normal sinus rhythm; ST segment depression is present

Strip 6-42
Rhythm: Irregular
Rate: 40
P waves: Sinus
PR interval: 0.18 to 0.20 seconds
QRS: 0.08 seconds
Rhythm interpretation: Sinus arrhythmia with sinus bradycardia; ST segment elevation is present

Strip 6-43
Rhythm: Basic rhythm regular; irregular during pause
Rate: Basic rhythm rate 63
P waves: Sinus in basic rhythm; absent during pause
PR interval: 0.18 to 0.20 seconds in basic rhythm; absent during pause
QRS: 0.04 to 0.06 seconds in basic rhythm; absent during pause
Rhythm interpretation: Normal sinus rhythm with sinus arrest; ST segment depression is present

Strip 6-44
Rhythm: Irregular
Rate: 50
P waves: Sinus
PR interval: 0.18 to 0.20 seconds
QRS: 0.06 to 0.08 seconds
Rhythm interpretation: Sinus arrhythmia; sinus bradycardia; a U wave is present

Strip 6-45
Rhythm: Regular
Rate: 26
P waves: Sinus
PR interval: 0.14 to 0.16 seconds
QRS: 0.08 to 0.10 seconds
Rhythm interpretation: Sinus bradycardia, ST segment depression is present

Strip 6-46
Rhythm: Regular
Rate: 68
P waves: Sinus
PR interval: 0.16 seconds
QRS: 0.08 seconds
Rhythm interpretation: Normal sinus rhythm; sinus arrhythmia; a U wave is present

Strip 6-47
Rhythm: Regular
Rate: 125
P waves: Sinus
PR interval: 0.12 seconds
QRS: 0.06 to 0.08 seconds
Rhythm interpretation: Sinus tachycardia; ST segment depression and T wave inversion are present

Strip 6-48
Rhythm: Irregular
Rate: 70
P waves: Sinus
PR interval: 0.16 to 0.20 seconds
QRS: 0.04 to 0.06 seconds
Rhythm interpretation: Sinus arrhythmia; a U wave is present

Strip 6-49
Rhythm: Regular
Rate: 47
P waves: Sinus
PR interval: 0.14 to 0.16 seconds
QRS: 0.08 seconds
Rhythm interpretation: Sinus bradycardia; a U wave is present

Strip 6-50
Rhythm: Regular
Rate: 94
P waves: Sinus
PR interval: 0.16 to 0.18 seconds
QRS: 0.06 to 0.08 seconds
Rhythm interpretation: Normal sinus rhythm

Strip 6-51
Rhythm: Regular
Rate: 107
P waves: Sinus
PR interval: 0.12 to 0.14 seconds
QRS: 0.06 to 0.08 seconds
Rhythm interpretation: Sinus tachycardia

Strip 6-52
Rhythm: Basic rhythm regular; irregular during pause
Rate: Basic rhythm rate 68
P waves: Sinus in basic rhythm; absent during pause
PR interval: 0.18 to 0.20 seconds in basic rhythm; absent during pause
QRS: 0.06 to 0.08 seconds in basic rhythm; absent during pause
Rhythm interpretation: Normal sinus rhythm with sinus arrest; a U wave is present

Strip 6-53
Rhythm: Irregular
Rate: 50
P waves: Sinus
PR interval: 0.14 to 0.16 seconds
QRS: 0.06 to 0.08 seconds
Rhythm interpretation: Sinus arrhythmia; sinus bradycardia; a U wave is present

Strip 6-54
Rhythm: Regular
Rate: 42
P waves: Sinus
PR interval: 0.20 seconds
QRS: 0.08 to 0.10 seconds
Rhythm interpretation: Sinus bradycardia; ST segment elevation is present

Strip 6-55
Rhythm: Regular
Rate: 65
P waves: Sinus
PR interval: 0.16 to 0.18 seconds
QRS: 0.06 seconds
Rhythm interpretation: Normal sinus rhythm

Strip 6-56
Rhythm: Regular
Rate: 125
P waves: Sinus
PR interval: 0.16 seconds
QRS: 0.08 seconds
Rhythm interpretation: Sinus tachycardia; ST segment depression is present

Strip 6-57
Rhythm: Irregular
Rate: 50
P waves: Sinus
PR interval: 0.20 seconds
QRS: 0.06 to 0.08 seconds
Rhythm interpretation: Sinus arrhythmia; sinus bradycardia; a U wave is present

Strip 6-58
Rhythm: Regular
Rate: 68
P waves: Sinus
PR interval: 0.16 to 0.20 seconds
QRS: 0.06 to 0.08 seconds
Rhythm interpretation: Normal sinus rhythm; ST segment depression and T wave inversion are present

Strip 6-59
Rhythm: Regular
Rate: 50
P waves: Sinus
PR interval: 0.20 seconds
QRS: 0.06 to 0.08 seconds
Rhythm interpretation: Sinus bradycardia; ST segment depression and T wave inversion are present

Strip 6-60
Rhythm: Basic rhythm regular; irregular during pause
Rate: Basic rhythm rate 88
P waves: Sinus in basic rhythm; absent during pause
PR interval: 0.14 to 0.20 seconds in basic rhythm; absent during pause
QRS: 0.08 to 0.10 seconds in basic rhythm; absent during pause
Rhythm interpretation: Normal sinus rhythm with sinus block; ST segment depression is present

Strip 6-61
Rhythm: Regular
Rate: 60
P waves: Sinus
PR interval: 0.14 to 0.16 seconds
QRS: 0.08 seconds
Rhythm interpretation: Normal sinus rhythm; a U wave is present

Strip 6-62
Rhythm: Regular
Rate: 125
P waves: Sinus
PR interval: 0.12 seconds
QRS: 0.04 seconds
Rhythm interpretation: Sinus tachycardia; ST segment depression is present

Strip 6-63
Rhythm: Regular
Rate: 47
P waves: Sinus
PR interval: 0.20 seconds
QRS: 0.06 to 0.08 seconds
Rhythm interpretation: Sinus bradycardia; ST segment depression is present

Strip 6-64
Rhythm: Regular
Rate: 79
P waves: Sinus
PR interval: 0.14 to 0.16 seconds
QRS: 0.04 to 0.06 seconds
Rhythm interpretation: Normal sinus rhythm; T wave inversion is present

Strip 6-65
Rhythm: Regular
Rate: 125
P waves: Sinus
PR interval: 0.14 to 0.16 seconds
QRS: 0.08 to 0.10 seconds
Rhythm interpretation: Sinus tachycardia; ST segment depression is present

Strip 6-66
Rhythm: Regular
Rate: 100
P waves: Sinus
PR interval: 0.20 seconds
QRS: 0.08 seconds
Rhythm interpretation: Normal sinus rhythm; an extremely elevated ST segment is present

Strip 6-67
Rhythm: Regular
Rate: 44
P waves: Sinus
PR interval: 0.14 to 0.16 seconds
QRS: 0.08 seconds
Rhythm interpretation: Sinus bradycardia; a U wave is present

Strip 6-68
Rhythm: Regular
Rate: 94
P waves: Sinus
PR interval: 0.16 to 0.20 seconds
QRS: 0.06 to 0.08 seconds
Rhythm interpretation: Normal sinus rhythm; ST segment depression and a T wave inversion are present

Strip 6-69
Rhythm: Regular
Rate: 115
P waves: Sinus
PR interval: 0.14 to 0.16 seconds
QRS: 0.06 to 0.08 seconds
Rhythm interpretation: Sinus tachycardia

Strip 6-70
Rhythm: Basic rhythm regular; irregular during pause
Rate: Basic rhythm rate 56; rate slows to 50 after pause; rate suppression can occur following a pause in the basic rhythm; after several cycles the rate returns to the basic rate
P waves: Sinus in basic rhythm; absent during pause
PR interval: 0.14 to 0.16 in basic rhythm; absent during pause
QRS: 0.08 to 0.10 seconds in basic rhythm; absent during pause
Rhythm interpretation: Sinus bradycardia with sinus arrest

Strip 6-71
Rhythm: Irregular
Rate: 60
P waves: Sinus
PR interval: 0.12 to 0.16 seconds
QRS: 0.06 to 0.08 seconds
Rhythm interpretation: Sinus arrhythmia; a U wave is present

Strip 6-72
Rhythm: Regular
Rate: 72
P waves: Sinus
PR interval: 0.12 to 0.14 seconds
QRS: .04 to .06 seconds
Rhythm interpretation: Normal sinus rhythm; ST segment depression and T wave inversion are present

Strip 6-73
Rhythm: Regular
Rate: 54
P waves: Sinus
PR interval: 0.16 to 0.18 seconds
QRS: 0.08 seconds
Rhythm interpretation: Sinus bradycardia

Strip 6-74
Rhythm: Regular
Rate: 88
P waves: Sinus
PR interval: 0.16 to 0.20 seconds
QRS: 0.08 to 0.10 seconds
Rhythm interpretation: Normal sinus rhythm; ST segment depression is present

Strip 6-75
Rhythm: Regular
Rate: 94
P waves: Sinus
PR interval: 0.16 to 0.20 seconds
QRS: 0.06 to 0.08 seconds
Rhythm interpretation: Normal sinus rhythm

Strip 6-76
Rhythm: Regular
Rate: 125
P waves: Sinus
PR interval: 0.12 seconds
QRS: 0.06 to 0.08 seconds
Rhythm interpretation: Sinus tachycardia

Strip 6-77
Rhythm: Regular
Rate: 75
P waves: Sinus
PR interval: 0.16 seconds
QRS: 0.08 seconds
Rhythm interpretation: Normal sinus rhythm; ST segment elevation is present

Strip 6-78
Rhythm: Regular
Rate: 48
P waves: Sinus
PR interval: 0.12 seconds
QRS: 0.06 to 0.08 seconds
Rhythm interpretation: Sinus bradycardia

Strip 6-79
Rhythm: Basic rhythm regular; irregular during pause
Rate: Basic rhythm rate 47
P waves: Sinus in basic rhythm; absent during pause
PR interval: 0.20 in basic rhythm; absent during pause
QRS: 0.06 to 0.08 seconds in basic rhythm; absent during pause
Rhythm interpretation: Sinus bradycardia with sinus arrest

Strip 6-80
Rhythm: Regular
Rate: 84
P waves: Sinus
PR interval: 0.16 seconds
QRS: 0.04 to 0.06 seconds
Rhythm interpretation: Normal sinus rhythm; ST segment elevation and T wave inversion are present

Strip 6-81
Rhythm: Irregular
Rate: 60
P waves: Sinus
PR interval: 0.18 to 0.20 seconds
QRS: 0.06 to 0.08 seconds
Rhythm interpretation: Sinus arrhythmia; a U wave is present

Strip 6-82
Rhythm: Regular
Rate: 125
P waves: Sinus
PR interval: 0.14 to 0.16 seconds
QRS: 0.06 to 0.08 seconds
Rhythm interpretation: Sinus tachycardia

Strip 6-83
Rhythm: Basic rhythm irregular
Rate: Basic rhythm rate about 60
P waves: Sinus
PR interval: 0.20 seconds in basic rhythm; absent during pause
QRS: 0.06 to 0.08 seconds in basic rhythm; absent during pause
Rhythm interpretation: Sinus arrhythmia with sinus arrest-block; ST segment depression is present

Strip 6-84
Rhythm: Regular
Rate: 88
P waves: Sinus
PR interval: 0.12 seconds
QRS: 0.06 to 0.08 seconds
Rhythm interpretation: Normal sinus rhythm; T wave inversion is present

Strip 6-85
Rhythm: Regular
Rate: 115
P waves: Sinus
PR interval: 0.12 to 0.16 seconds
QRS: 0.08 seconds
Rhythm interpretation: Sinus tachycardia

Strip 6-86
Rhythm: Regular
Rate: 54
P waves: Sinus
PR interval: 0.12 to 0.16 seconds
QRS: 0.08 seconds
Rhythm interpretation: Sinus bradycardia; a U wave is present

Strip 6-87
Rhythm: Basic rhythm regular; irregular during pause
Rate: Basic rhythm rate 84; rate slow to 75 for one cycle following the pause—rate suppression is common following pauses in the basic rhythm
P waves: Sinus in basic rhythm; absent during pause
PR interval: 0.16 to 0.18 seconds in basic rhythm; absent during pause
QRS: 0.06 to 0.08 seconds in basic rhythm; absent during pause
Rhythm interpretation: Normal sinus rhythm with sinus arrest

Strip 6-88
Rhythm: Regular
Rate: 100
P waves: Sinus
PR interval: 0.18 to 0.20 seconds
QRS: 0.06 to 0.08 seconds
Rhythm interpretation: Normal sinus rhythm; ST segment depression is present

Strip 6-89
Rhythm: Regular
Rate: 54
P waves: Sinus
PR interval: 0.18 to 0.20 seconds
QRS: 0.06 to 0.08 seconds
Rhythm interpretation: Sinus bradycardia

Strip 6-90
Rhythm: Regular
Rate: 88
P waves: Sinus
PR interval: 0.12 seconds
QRS: 0.08 seconds
Rhythm interpretation: Normal sinus rhythm; ST segment depression is present

Strip 6-91
Rhythm: Regular
Rate: 83
P waves: Sinus
PR interval: 0.16 to 0.20 seconds
QRS: 0.04 to 0.06 seconds
Rhythm interpretation: Normal sinus rhythm; T wave inversion is present

Strip 6-92
Rhythm: Irregular
Rate: 70
P waves: Sinus
PR interval: 0.12 seconds
QRS: 0.04 to 0.06 seconds
Rhythm interpretation: Sinus arrhythmia; ST segment depression and T wave inversion are present

Strip 6-93

Rhythm: Basic rhythm regular; irregular during pause
Rate: Basic rhythm rate 65
P waves: Sinus in basic rhythm; absent during pause
PR interval: 0.20 seconds in basic rhythm; absent during pause
QRS: 0.04–0.06 seconds in basic rhythm; absent during pause
Rhythm interpretation: Normal sinus rhythm with sinus arrest

Strip 6-94

Rhythm: Regular
Rate: 150
P waves: Sinus
PR interval: 0.12 seconds
QRS: 0.04 to 0.06 seconds
Rhythm interpretation: Sinus tachycardia

Strip 6-95

Rhythm: Regular
Rate: 107
P waves: Sinus
PR interval: 0.16 to 0.20 seconds
QRS: 0.08 seconds
Rhythm interpretation: Sinus tachycardia; ST segment depression is present

Strip 7-1

Rhythm: Irregular
Rate: 70
P waves: Fibrillation waves
PR interval: Not discernible
QRS: 0.06 to 0.08 seconds
Rhythm interpretation: Atrial fibrillation; some flutter waves are noted

Strip 7-2

Rhythm: Regular
Rate: 188
P waves: Hidden in T waves
PR interval: Not measurable
QRS: 0.08 seconds
Rhythm interpretation: Paroxysmal atrial tachycardia

Strip 7-3

Rhythm: Basic rhythm regular; irregular with PAC
Rate: Basic rhythm 63
P waves: Sinus P waves with basic rhythm; premature P wave with PAC (this P wave closely resembles that of the sinus node)
PR interval: 0.16 seconds (basic rhythm)
QRS: 0.06 seconds
Rhythm interpretation: Normal sinus rhythm with one PAC; ST segment depression and T wave inversion are noted

Strip 7-4

Rhythm: Irregular
Rate: 100
P waves: Vary in size, shape, position
PR interval: 0.12 seconds
QRS: 0.06 to 0.08 seconds
Rhythm interpretation: Wandering atrial pacemaker

Strip 7-5

Rhythm: Basic rhythm regular; irregular with PAC
Rate: Basic rate 84
P waves: Sinus P waves are present; premature, abnormal P waves with a premature beat
PR interval: 0.16 seconds (basic rhythm)
QRS: 0.08 seconds
Rhythm interpretation: Sinus rhythm with a premature atrial contraction; a U wave is noted

Strip 7-6

Rhythm: Regular
Rate: 167
P waves: Pointed, abnormal
PR interval: 0.14 to 0.16 seconds
QRS: 0.06 to 0.08 seconds
Rhythm interpretation: Paroxysmal atrial tachycardia; ST segment depression is present

Strip 7-7

Rhythm: Basic rhythm regular; irregular with nonconducted PAC
Rate: Basic rhythm rate 88
P waves: Sinus P waves with basic rhythm; premature, abnormal P wave with nonconducted PAC
PR interval: 0.16 seconds
QRS: 0.06 to 0.08 seconds
Rhythm interpretation: Normal sinus rhythm with nonconducted PAC; ST segment depression is present

Strip 7-8
Rhythm: Irregular
Rate: Atrial, 320; ventricular, 80
P waves: Flutter waves are present (varying ratios)
PR: Not measurable
QRS: 0.08 seconds
Interpretation: Atrial flutter with variable block

Strip 7-9
Rhythm: Irregular
Rate: About 70
P waves: Vary in size, shape, and position
PR interval: 0.12 to 0.14 seconds
QRS: 0.06 to 0.08 seconds
Rhythm interpretation: Wandering atrial pacemaker; T wave inversion is noted

Strip 7-10
Rhythm: Irregular
Rate: Ventricular, 140
P waves: Fibrillation waves
PR interval: Not discernible
QRS: 0.06 to 0.08 seconds
Rhythm interpretation: Atrial fibrillation; ST segment depression and T wave inversion are present

Strip 7-11
Rhythm: Basic rhythm regular; irregular with PACs
Rate: Basic rate 72
P waves: Sinus P waves are present; premature, abnormal P waves with premature beats
PR interval: 0.16 seconds
QRS: 0.06 to 0.08 seconds
Rhythm interpretation: Sinus rhythm with premature atrial contractions (three on tracing); ST segment depression is present

Strip 7-12
Rhythm: Regular
Rate: Atrial, 288; ventricular, 72
P waves: Four flutter waves to each QRS
PR interval: Not measurable
QRS: 0.08 seconds
Rhythm interpretation: Atrial flutter with 4:1 block

Strip 7-13
Rhythm: Basic rhythm regular; irregular with PAC and nonconducted PACs
Rate: Basic rhythm 79
P waves: Sinus P waves with basic rhythm; premature P wave with PAC (shape resembles sinus P waves); the two nonconducted PACs (after the sixth and seventh QRS) are premature, pointed, and deform the T waves
PR interval: 0.14 to 0.16 seconds (basic rhythm)
QRS: 0.08 to 0.10 seconds
Interpretation: Normal sinus rhythm with one PAC and two nonconducted PACs; ST segment depression is present

Strip 7-14
Rhythm: Irregular
Rate: Ventricular, 110
P waves: Fibrillatory waves are present
PR interval: Not measurable
QRS: 0.06 to 0.08 seconds
Rhythm interpretation: Atrial fibrillation; some flutter waves are noted

Strip 7-15
Rhythm: Regular
Rate: 188
P waves: Not identified
PR interval: Not discernible
QRS: 0.04 to 0.06 seconds
Rhythm interpretation: Paroxysmal atrial tachycardia; ST depression is present

Strip 7-16
Rhythm: Regular
Rate: Atrial, 300; ventricular, 100
P waves: Three flutter waves before each QRS
PR interval: Not measurable
QRS: 0.08 seconds
Rhythm interpretation: Atrial flutter with 3:1 block

Strip 7-17
Rhythm: Irregular
Rate: Ventricular: 150
P waves: Fibrillation waves
PR interval: Not discernible
QRS: 0.08 seconds
Rhythm interpretation: Atrial fibrillation; ST segment depression is present

Strip 7-18
Rhythm: Irregular
Rate: Atrial, 320; ventricular, 90
P waves: Flutter waves (varying ratios)
PR interval: Not discernible
QRS: 0.04 to 0.06 seconds
Rhythm interpretation: Atrial flutter with variable block

Strip 7-19
Rhythm: Regular
Rate: 88
P waves: Varying in size and shape
PR interval: 0.12 to 0.20 seconds
QRS: 0.06 to 0.08 seconds
Rhythm interpretation: Wandering atrial pacemaker; ST segment elevation is present

Strip 7-20
Rhythm: Regular
Rate: 188
P waves: Hidden in T waves
PR interval: Not measurable
QRS: 0.04 seconds
Rhythm interpretation: Paroxysmal atrial tachycardia; ST segment depression is present

Strip 7-21
Rhythm: Basic rhythm regular; irregular with PAC
Rate: 107 (basic rhythm)
P waves: Sinus P waves are present; premature, abnormal P waves with a premature beat
PR interval: 0.12 seconds
QRS: 0.06 to 0.08 seconds
Rhythm interpretation: Sinus tachycardia with one premature atrial contraction

Strip 7-22
Rhythm: Regular
Rate: Atrial, 316; ventricular, 79
P waves: Four flutter waves to each QRS
PR interval: Not discernible
QRS: 0.06 seconds
Rhythm interpretation: Atrial flutter with 4 : 1 block

Strip 7-23
Rhythm: Basic rhythm regular; irregular with nonconducted PAC
Rate: Basic rhythm rate 72
P waves: Sinus P waves with basic rhythm; premature, abnormal P waves with nonconducted PAC
PR interval: 0.16 to 0.18 seconds
QRS: 0.06 to 0.08 seconds
Rhythm interpretation: Normal sinus rhythm with nonconducted PAC; ST segment depression is present

Strip 7-24
Rhythm: Irregular
Rate: Ventricular rate 170
P waves: Fibrillatory waves are present
PR interval: Not measurable
QRS: 0.08 seconds
Rhythm interpretation: Atrial fibrillation

Strip 7-25
Rhythm: Regular
Rate: 84
P waves: Vary in size, shape, and position
PR interval: 0.12 to 0.14 seconds
QRS: 0.06 to 0.08 seconds
Rhythm interpretation: Wandering atrial pacemaker; T wave inversion is present

Strip 7-26
Rhythm: Basic rhythm regular; irregular with PAC
Rate: Basic rhythm 79
P waves: Sinus P waves with basic rhythm; premature, abnormal P waves with PAC
PR interval: 0.16 seconds (basic rhythm)
QRS: 0.04 to 0.06 seconds
Rhythm interpretation: Normal sinus rhythm with one PAC

Strip 7-27
Rhythm: Regular
Rate: Atrial, 230; ventricular, 115
P waves: Two flutter waves to each QRS
PR interval: Not discernible
QRS: 0.08 to 0.10 seconds
Rhythm interpretation: Atrial flutter with 2:1 block

Strip 7-28
Rhythm: Basic rhythm regular; irregular with PACs
Rate: Basic rhythm 42
P waves: Sinus P waves with basic rhythm; premature, abnormal P waves with PACs
PR interval: 0.12 to 0.14 seconds (basic rhythm)
QRS: 0.08 to 0.10 seconds
Rhythm interpretation: Sinus bradycardia with four PACs

Strip 7-29
Rhythm: Regular
Rate: 188
P waves: Not identified
PR interval: Not discernible
QRS: 0.06 to 0.08 seconds
Rhythm interpretation: Paroxysmal atrial tachycardia; ST segment depression is present

Strip 7-30
Rhythm: Regular
Rate: Atrial; 300; ventricular; 150
P wave: Two flutter wave to each QRS
PR interval: Not discernible
QRS: 0.04 to 0.06 seconds
Rhythm interpretation: Atrial flutter with 2:1 block

Strip 7-31
Rhythm: Basic rhythm regular; irregular with PACs and atrial fibrillation
Rate: Basic rhythm rate 68; Atrial fibrillation rate 70
P waves: Sinus P waves are present with basic rhythm; premature, abnormal P waves with PACs; fibrillation waves with atrial fibrillation
PR interval: 0.12 to 0.14 seconds (basic rhythm)
QRS: 0.08 to 0.10 seconds
Rhythm interpretation: Normal sinus rhythm with two PACs, the second PAC leading to atrial fibrillation; ST segment depression is present

Strip 7-32
Rhythm: Basic rhythm regular; irregular with nonconducted PAC
Rate: Basic rhythm rate 88
P waves: Sinus P waves with basic rhythm; premature, abnormal P wave deforming T wave with nonconducted PAC
PR interval: 0.12 seconds (basic rhythm)
QRS: 0.06 to 0.08 seconds
Rhythm interpretation: Normal sinus rhythm with one nonconducted PAC; ST segment depression is present

Strip 7-33
Rhythm: Basic rhythm regular; irregular with PAC
Rate: Basic rate 88
P waves: Sinus P waves are present; one abnormal premature P wave with a premature beat
PR interval: 0.12 seconds (basic rhythm)
QRS: 0.08 seconds
Rhythm interpretation: Sinus rhythm with one premature atrial contraction; ST segment depression is present

Strip 7-34
Rhythm: Irregular
Rate: 50 ventricular rate
P waves: Fibrillatory waves are present
PR interval: Not measurable
QRS: 0.06 to 0.08 seconds
Rhythm interpretation: Atrial fibrillation; ST segment depression and T wave inversion are present

Strip 7-35
Rhythm: Regular
Rate: 188
P waves: Not identified
PR interval: Not discernible
QRS: 0.08 seconds
Rhythm interpretation: Paroxysmal atrial tachycardia; ST segment depression is present

Strip 7-36
Rhythm: Irregular
Rate: 50
P waves: Varying in size and shape
PR interval: 0.18 to 0.20 seconds
QRS: 0.08 to 0.10 seconds
Rhythm interpretation: Wandering atrial pacemaker

Strip 7-37
Rhythm: Irregular
Rate: Atrial, 260; ventricular, 70
P waves: Flutter waves (varying ratios)
PR interval: Not measurable
QRS: 0.08 seconds
Rhythm interpretation: Atrial flutter with variable block

Strip 7-38
Rhythm: Regular
Rate: 214
P waves: Not discernible
PR interval: Not discernible
QRS: 0.08 seconds
Rhythm interpretation: Paroxysmal atrial tachycardia; ST segment elevation is present

Strip 7-39
Rhythm: Basic rhythm regular; irregular with PACs
Rate: Basic rhythm rate 100
P waves: Sinus P waves with basic rhythm;
premature, abnormal P waves with PACs
PR interval: 0.12 seconds (basic rhythm)
QRS: 0.06 to 0.08 seconds
Rhythm interpretation: Normal sinus rhythm with
two PACs; a U wave is present

Strip 7-40
Rhythm: Irregular
Rate: Ventricular, 90
P waves: Fibrillation waves
PR interval: Not discernible
QRS: 0.08 seconds
Rhythm interpretation: Atrial fibrillation; some
flutter waves are present

Strip 7-41
Rhythm: Basic rhythm regular; irregular with
nonconducted PAC
Rate: Basic rhythm rate 79
P waves: Sinus P waves with basic rhythm;
premature, abnormal P waves with nonconducted
PAC
PR: 0.20 seconds
QRS: 0.08 seconds
Interpretation: Normal sinus rhythm with one
nonconducted PAC; a U wave is present

Strip 7-42
Rhythm: Basic rhythm regular; irregular with
nonconducted PAC
Rate: 72
P waves: Sinus P waves are present; one
premature, abnormal P wave without a QRS
PR interval: 0.16 seconds
QRS: 0.08 seconds
Rhythm interpretation: Sinus rhythm with one
nonconducted premature atrial conduction; ST
segment depression and T wave inversion are
present

Strip 7-43
Rhythm: Regular
Rate: 68
P waves: Vary in size, shape, and position
PR interval: 0.12 seconds
QRS: 0.04 to 0.06 seconds
Rhythm interpretation: Wandering atrial
pacemaker; ST segment depression is present

Strip 7-44
Rhythm: Regular
Rate: Atrial, 300; ventricular, 150
P waves: Three flutter waves to each QRS not
measurable
PR interval: Not measurable
QRS: 0.04 to 0.06 seconds
Rhythm interpretation: Atrial flutter with 3:1
block

Strip 7-45
Rhythm: Regular
Rate: 188
P waves: Hidden in T waves
PR interval: Not measurable
QRS: 0.04 to 0.06 seconds
Rhythm interpretation: Paroxysmal atrial
tachycardia; ST segment depression is present

Strip 7-46
Rhythm: Basic rhythm regular; irregular with PAC
Rate: Basic rate 100
P waves: Sinus P waves present; abnormal,
premature P wave present with PAC
PR interval: 0.12 to 0.14 seconds (basic rhythm)
QRS: 0.04 to 0.06 seconds
Rhythm interpretation: Sinus rhythm with one
premature atrial contraction; ST segment
depression is present.

Strip 7-47
Rhythm: Basic rhythm regular; irregular with
nonconducted PAC
Rate: Basic rhythm rate 84
P waves: Sinus P waves present; premature,
abnormal P wave with PAC
PR interval: 0.14 to 0.16 (basic rhythm)
QRS: 0.06 to 0.08 seconds (basic rhythm)
Rhythm interpretation: Normal sinus rhythm with
one PAC; ST segment depression is present

Strip 7-48
Rhythm: Irregular
Rate: Ventricular rate: 50
P waves: Fibrillatory waves present
PR interval: Not measurable
QRS: 0.04 to 0.06 seconds
Rhythm interpretation: Atrial fibrillation

Strip 7-49

Rhythm: Irregular
Rate: Atrial, 280; ventricular, 50
P waves: Flutter waves present (varying ratios)
PR interval: Not measurable
QRS: 0.06 to 0.08 seconds
Rhythm interpretation: Atrial flutter with variable block

Strip 7-50

Rhythm: Irregular
Rate: Atrial, 300; ventricular, 100
P waves: Flutter waves (varying ratios)
PR interval: Not discernible
Rhythm interpretation: Atrial flutter with variable block

Strip 7-51

Rhythm: Regular
Rate: 150
P waves: Hidden in T waves
PR interval: Not measurable
QRS: 0.08 to 0.10 seconds
Rhythm interpretation: Paroxysmal atrial tachycardia

Strip 7-52

Rhythm: Basic rhythm regular; irregular with PAC
Rate: 94
P waves: Sinus P waves present; two premature abnormal P waves with premature beats
PR interval: 0.12 seconds (basic rhythm)
QRS: 0.08 seconds
Rhythm interpretation: Normal sinus rhythm with two premature atrial contractions

Strip 7-53

Rhythm: Irregular
Rate: Ventricular rate, 130
P waves: Fibrillatory waves present
PR interval: Not measurable
QRS: 0.06 to 0.08 seconds
Rhythm interpretation: Atrial fibrillation; ST segment depression is present

Strip 7-54

Rhythm: Basic rhythm regular; irregular with nonconducted PACs
Rate: Basic rate 125
P waves: Sinus P waves present; premature, abnormal P waves with premature beats
PR interval: 0.12 seconds (basic rhythm)
QRS: 0.06 to 0.08 seconds
Rhythm interpretation: Sinus tachycardia with premature atrial contractions (two in tracing); ST segment depression is present

Strip 7-55

Rhythm: Irregular
Rate: Ventricular, 50
P waves: Fibrillation waves
PR interval: Not discernible
QRS: 0.08 to 0.10 seconds
Rhythm interpretation: Atrial fibrillation

Strip 7-56

Rhythm: Basic rhythm regular; irregular with PAC
Rate: Basic rate 125
P waves: Sinus P waves present; one premature, abnormal P wave with a premature beat
PR interval: 0.12 seconds (basic rhythm)
QRS: 0.06 to 0.08 seconds
Rhythm interpretation: Sinus tachycardia with one premature atrial contraction; ST segment depression is present

Strip 7-57

Rhythm: Regular
Rate: Atrial, 428; ventricular, 107
P waves: Four flutter waves to each QRS
PR interval: Not measurable
QRS: 0.04 to 0.06 seconds
Rhythm interpretation: Atrial flutter with 4:1 block

Strip 7-58

Rhythm: Basic rhythm regular; irregular with PAC
Rate: Basic rate 72
P waves: Sinus P waves present; one abnormal, premature P wave with a premature beat
PR interval: 0.16 (basic rhythm)
QRS: 0.10 seconds
Rhythm interpretation: Normal sinus rhythm with one premature atrial contraction

Strip 7-59

Rhythm: Irregular
Rate: 70
P waves: Vary in size, shape, and position
PR interval: 0.14 to 0.16 seconds
QRS: 0.06 to 0.08 seconds
Rhythm interpretation: Wandering atrial pacemaker; T wave inversion is present

Strip 7-60

Rhythm: Irregular
Rate: Atrial, 300; ventricular, 80
P waves: Flutter waves are present (varying ratios)
PR: Not measurable
QRS: 0.08 to 0.10 seconds
Interpretation: Atrial flutter with variable block

Strip 7-61
Rhythm: Regular to irregular
Rate: 88, progressing to 140
P waves: Sinus P waves and fibrillation waves
PR interval: 0.12 seconds (basic rhythm)
QRS: 0.08 seconds
Rhythm interpretation: Normal sinus rhythm converting to atrial fibrillation; ST segment depression is present

Strip 7-62
Rhythm: Basic rhythm regular; irregular with PACs
Rate: Basic rate 88
P waves: Sinus P waves present; premature, abnormal P waves present with premature beats
PR interval: 0.12 to 0.14 seconds (basic rhythm)
QRS: 0.08 seconds
Rhythm interpretation: Normal sinus rhythm with a single premature atrial contraction and paired premature atrial contractions; ST segment depression is present

Strip 7-63
Rhythm: Irregular
Rate: Ventricular rate, 80
P waves: Fibrillatory waves present
PR interval: Not measurable
QRS: 0.04 to 0.06 seconds
Rhythm interpretation: Atrial fibrillation; ST segment depression is present

Strip 7-64
Rhythm: Regular
Rate: 214
P waves: Not identified
PR interval: Not discernible
QRS: 0.04 to 0.06 seconds
Rhythm interpretation: Paroxysmal atrial tachycardia; ST segment depression is present

Strip 7-65
Rhythm: Basic rhythm regular; irregular with PACs
Rate: Basic rhythm rate 65
P waves: Sinus P waves with basic rhythm; premature, abnormal P waves with PACs
PR interval: 0.16 to 0.20 seconds (basic rhythm)
QRS: 0.08 to 0.10 seconds
Rhythm interpretation: Normal sinus rhythm with three PACs (conducted with a long PR interval of 0.24 seconds); ST segment depression is present

Strip 7-66
Rhythm: Basic rhythm regular; irregular with nonconducted PAC
Rate: Basic rate 100
P waves: Sinus P waves present; one premature, abnormal P wave not followed by a QRS complex
PR interval: 0.12 seconds
QRS: 0.08 seconds
Rhythm interpretation: Normal sinus rhythm with one nonconducted, premature, atrial contraction

Strip 7-67
Rhythm: Basic rhythm regular; irregular with PACs
Rate: Basic rate 88
P waves: Sinus P waves present; premature, abnormal P waves with premature beats
PR interval: 0.14 to 0.16 seconds (basic rhythm)
QRS: 0.04 to 0.06 seconds
Rhythm interpretation: Normal sinus rhythm with three premature atrial contractions

Strip 7-68
Rhythm: Regular
Rate: 214
P waves: Not identified
PR interval: Not discernible
QRS: 0.04 seconds
Rhythm interpretation: Paroxysmal atrial tachycardia; ST segment depression is present

Strip 7-69
Rhythm: Regular
Rate: Atrial, 272; ventricular, 136
P waves: Two flutter waves to each QRS
PR interval: Not discernible
QRS: 0.04 to 0.06 seconds
Rhythm interpretation: Atrial flutter with 2:1 block

Strip 7-70
Rhythm: Irregular
Rate: Ventricular rate, 130
P waves: Fibrillatory waves; some flutter waves are seen
PR interval: Not measurable
QRS: 0.04 seconds
Rhythm interpretation: Atrial fibrillation; some flutter waves are noted; ST segment depression is present

Strip 7-71
Rhythm: Basic rhythm regular; irregular with PACs
Rate: Basic rhythm rate 88
P waves: Sinus P waves with basic rhythm; premature, abnormal P waves with PACs
PR interval: 0.14 to 0.16 seconds (basic rhythm)
QRS: 0.06 to 0.08 seconds
Rhythm interpretation: Normal sinus rhythm with paired PACs

Strip 7-72
Rhythm: Regular
Rate: 54
P waves: Varying in size and shape
PR interval: 0.12 seconds
QRS: 0.08 to 0.10 seconds
Rhythm interpretation: Wandering atrial pacemaker; ST segment depression is present

Strip 7-73
Rhythm: Irregular
Rate: Atrial, about 370; ventricular, 50
P waves: Flutter waves before each QRS (varying ratios)
PR interval: Not measurable
QRS: 0.08 seconds
Rhythm interpretation: Atrial flutter with variable block

Strip 7-74
Rhythm: Basic rhythm regular; irregular with PAC
Rate: Basic rhythm rate 65
P waves: Sinus P waves with basic rhythm; premature, abnormal P wave with PAC
PR interval: 0.12 seconds (basic rhythm)
QRS: 0.06 to 0.08 seconds
Rhythm interpretation: Normal sinus rhythm with PAC; a U wave is present

Strip 7-75
Rhythm: Regular
Rate: 150
P waves: Hidden in T waves
PR interval: Not measurable
QRS: 0.06 to 0.08 seconds
Rhythm interpretation: Paroxysmal atrial tachycardia

Strip 7-76
Rhythm: Irregular
Rate: Ventricular rate, 80
P waves: Fibrillatory waves
PR interval: Not measurable
QRS: 0.04 seconds
Rhythm interpretation: Atrial fibrillation; ST segment depression and T wave inversion are present

Strip 7-77
Rhythm: Regular
Rate: 88
P waves: Vary in size, shape, position
PR interval: 0.12 to 0.14 seconds
QRS: 0.06 to 0.08 seconds
Rhythm interpretation: Wandering atrial pacemaker; T wave inversion is present

Strip 7-78
Rhythm: Irregular
Rate: 50
P waves: Vary in size, shape, and position
PR interval: 0.12 to 0.16 seconds
QRS: 0.08 seconds
Rhythm interpretation: Wandering atrial pacemaker; ST segment depression is present

Strip 7-79
Rhythm: Regular
Rate: Atrial, 450; ventricular, 150
P waves: Three flutter waves to each QRS
PR interval: Not measurable
QRS: 0.04 seconds
Rhythm interpretation: Atrial flutter with 3:1 block

Strip 7-80
Rhythm: Basic rhythm regular; irregular with PACs
Rate: Basic rhythm rate 47
P waves: Sinus P waves with basic rhythm; premature, abnormal P waves with PACs
PR interval: 0.12–0.14 seconds (basic rhythm)
QRS: 0.06 to 0.08 seconds
Rhythm interpretation: Sinus bradycardia with three PACs (occurring in bigeminal pattern)

Strip 7-81
Rhythm: Regular
Rate: 68
P waves: Vary in size, shape, and position
PR interval: 0.12 to 0.16 seconds
QRS: 0.08 seconds
Rhythm interpretation: Wandering atrial pacemaker; a U wave is present

Strip 7-82
Rhythm: Irregular
Rate: Ventricular, 100; atrial, 290
P waves: Flutter waves before each QRS (varying ratios)
PR interval: Not discernible
QRS: 0.08 seconds
Rhythm interpretation: Atrial flutter with variable block

Strip 7-83
Rhythm: Regular
Rate: 214
P waves: Not identified
PR interval: Not discernible
QRS: 0.04 to 0.06 seconds
Rhythm interpretation: Paroxysmal atrial tachycardia; ST segment depression is present

Strip 7-84
Rhythm: Irregular
Rate: 40
P waves: Fibrillatory waves present
PR interval: Not measurable
QRS: 0.06 to 0.08 seconds
Rhythm interpretation: Atrial fibrillation

Strip 7-85
Rhythm: Regular
Rate: 65
P waves: Varying in size and shape
PR interval: 0.14 to 0.18 seconds
QRS: 0.04 to 0.08 seconds
Rhythm interpretation: Wandering atrial pacemaker; ST segment depression is present

Strip 7-86
Rhythm: Basic rhythm regular; irregular with PACs
Rate: Basic rhythm rate 65
P waves: Sinus P waves with basic rhythm; premature, abnormal P waves with PACs
PR interval: 0.16 to 0.20 seconds (basic rhythm)
QRS: 0.08 seconds
Rhythm interpretation: Normal sinus rhythm with two PACs; ST segment depression is present

Strip 7-87
Rhythm: Regular
Rate: Atrial, 300; vetricular, 75
P waves: Four flutter waves to each QRS
PR interval: Not measurable
QRS: 0.10 seconds
Rhythm interpretation: Atrial flutter with 4:1 block

Strip 7-88
Rhythm: Irregular
Rate: Ventricular rate, 40
P waves: Fibrillatory waves present
PR interval: Not measurable
QRS: 0.04 to 0.06 seconds
Rhythm interpretation: Atrial fibrillation; ST segment depression is present

Strip 7-89
Rhythm: Basic rhythm regular; irregular with PAC
Rate: Basic rhythm rate 72
P waves: Sinus P waves with basic rhythm; premature, abnormal P waves with PAC
PR interval: 0.12 seconds
QRS: 0.08 seconds
Rhythm interpretation: Normal sinus rhythm with one PAC; a U wave is present

Strip 7-90
Rhythm: Regular
Rate: 100
P waves: Varying in size and shape
PR interval: 0.12 to 0.16 seconds
QRS: 0.08 seconds
Rhythm interpretation: Wandering atrial pacemaker; ST segment depression is present.

Strip 7-91
Rhythm: Basic rhythm regular; irregular with PAC
Rate: Basic rhythm 63
P waves: Sinus P waves with basic rhythm; premature, abnormal P waves with PAC
PR interval: 0.14 to 0.16 seconds
QRS: 0.04 to 0.06 seconds
Rhythm interpretation: Normal sinus rhythm with one PAC; a U wave is present

Strip 7-92
Rhythm: Regular
Rate: Atrial, 235; ventricular, 47
P waves: Five flutter waves to each QRS
PR interval: Not discernible
QRS: 0.08 seconds
Rhythm interpretation: Atrial flutter with 5:1 block; T wave inversion is present

Strip 8-1
Rhythm: Basic rhythm regular; irregular with PJC
Rate: Basic rhythm 58
P waves: Sinus P waves with basic rhythm; premature, inverted P wave with PJC
PR: 0.14 to 0.16 seconds (basic rhythm); 0.08 seconds (PJC)
QRS: 0.06 seconds (basic rhythm and PJC)
Rhythm interpretation: Sinus bradycardia with one PJC; a U wave is noted

Strip 8-2
Rhythm: Regular
Rate: 60
P waves: Sinus P waves present
PR interval: 0.24
QRS: 0.06 to 0.08 seconds
Rhythm interpretation: Normal sinus rhythm with first-degress AV block; ST segment elevation and T wave inversion are present

Strip 8-3
Rhythm: Regular
Rate: Atrial, 104; verticular, 52
P waves: Two sinus P waves to each QRS complex
PR interval: 0.20 and constant
QRS: 0.12
Rhythm interpretation: Second-degree AV block Mohitz II. Clinical correlation is suggested to diagnose Mobitz II when 2:1 conduction is present; ST segment elevation is present

Strip 8-4
Rhythm: Basic rhythm regular; irregular with junctional beat
Rate: Basic rhythm rate 58
P waves: Sinus P waves with basic rhythm; hidden P wave with junctional beat
PR interval: 0.16 to 0.18 seconds (basic rhythm)
QRS: 0.08 to 0.10 seconds (basic rhythm and junctional beat)
Rhythm interpretation: Sinus bradycardia with junctional escape beat following a pause in the basic rhythm, ST segment depression is present

Strip 8-5
Rhythm: Regular
Rate: 115
P waves: Inverted
PR interval: 0.08 seconds
QRS: 0.04 seconds
Rhythm interpretation: Junctional tachycardia

Strip 8-6
Rhythm: Regular
Rate: 45
P waves: Sinus P waves present
PR interval: 0.24 to 0.26 seconds
QRS: 0.06 to 0.08 seconds
Rhythm interpretation: Sinus bradycardia with first-degree AV block; ST segment depression is present

Strip 8-7
Rhythm: Regular
Rate: 65
P waves: Inverted before each QRS
PR interval: 0.08 seconds
QRS: 0.06 to 0.08 seconds
Rhythm interpretation: Accelerated junctional rhythm; ST segment elevation and T wave inversion are present

Strip 8-8
Rhythm: Irregular ventricular rhythm; regular atrial rhythm
Rate: Atrial, 75; ventricular, 70
P waves: Sinus P waves present; one P wave without QRS
PR interval: Progresses from 0.28 to 0.36 seconds
QRS: 0.04 to 0.08 seconds
Rhythm interpretation: Second-degree AV block, Mobitz I; ST segment depression and T wave inversion are present

Strip 8-9
Rhythm: Regular
Rate: 47
P waves: Hidden in QRS
PR interval: Not measurable
QRS: 0.08 seconds
Rhythm interpretation: Junctional rhythm; ST segment depression is present

Strip 8-10
Rhythm: Regular
Rate: Atrial, 84; ventricular, 42
P waves: Two sinus P waves to each QRS
PR interval: 0.28 seconds (remains constant)
QRS: 0.12 seconds
Rhythm interpretation: Second-degree AV block, Mobitz II; Clinical correlation is suggested to diagnose Mobitz II when 2:1 conduction is present; ST segment depression is present

Strip 8-11
Rhythm: Regular
Rate: Atrial, 60; ventricular, 38
P waves: Sinus P waves present, not relating to QRS complexes; hidden in QRS complexes and T waves
PR interval: Varies greatly
QRS: 0.12 to 0.16 seconds
Rhythm interpretation: Third-degree AV block

Strip 8-12
Rhythm: Regular
Rate: 79
P waves: Hidden in QRS
PR interval: Not discernible
QRS: 0.06 to 0.08 seconds
Rhythm interpretation: Accelerated junctional rhythm; T wave inversion is present

Strip 8-13
Rhythm: Regular
Rate: 84
P waves: Sinus P waves present
PR interval: 0.24 to 0.28 seconds
QRS: 0.08 seconds
Rhythm interpretation: Sinus rhythm with first-degree AV block

Strip 8-14
Rhythm: Basic rhythm regular; irregular with PJC
Rate: Basic rhythm rate 136
P waves: Sinus P waves with basic rhythm; hidden P wave with PJC
PR interval: 0.12 to 0.14 seconds
QRS: 0.06 seconds
Rhythm interpretation: Sinus tachycardia with PJC

Strip 8-15
Rhythm: Regular
Rate: 94
P waves: Sinus
PR interval: 0.28 seconds
QRS: 0.04 to 0.06 seconds
Rhythm interpretation: Sinus rhythm with first-degree AV block; ST segment depression is present

Strip 8-16
Rhythm: Basic rhythm regular; irregular with pause and junctional beats
Rate: Basic rhythm rate 47
P waves: sinus P wave with basic rhythm; hidden P waves with junctional beats
PR interval: 0.16 to 0.20 seconds
QRS: 0.06 seconds
Rhythm interpretation: Sinus bradycardia with two junctional escape beats following a pause in the basic rhythm

Strip 8-17
Rhythm: Regular
Rate: atrial, 108; ventricular, 54
P waves: Two P waves to each QRS complex
PR interval: 0.20 and constant
QRS: 0.08 to 0.10 seconds
Rhythm interpretation: Second-degree AV block Mobitz II. Clinical correlation is suggested to diagnose Mobitz II when 2:1 conduction is present; ST segment elevation and T wave inversion are present

Strip 8-18
Rhythm: Irregular ventricular rhythm; regular atrial rhythm
Rate: Atrial, 65; ventricular, 50
P waves: Sinus P waves present; one P wave without QRS
PR interval: Progresses from 0.20 to 0.48 seconds
QRS: 0.04 seconds
Rhythm interpretation: Second-degree AV block, Mobitz I

Strip 8-19
Rhythm: Regular
Rate: 125
P waves: Inverted before each QRS
PR interval: 0.08 to 0.10 seconds
QRS: 0.06 seconds
Rhythm interpretation: Junctional tachycardia

Strip 8-20
Rhythm: Regular
Rate: Atrial, 84; ventricular, 28
P waves: Sinus P waves not relating to the QRS complexes; hidden in QRS complexes and waves
PR interval: Varies greatly
QRS: 0.24 seconds
Rhythm interpretation: Third-degree AV block

Strip 8-21
Rhythm: Basic rhythm regular; irregular with PJC
Rate: Basic rhythm rate 60
P waves: Sinus P waves with basic rhythm; premature, inverted P wave with PJC
PR interval: 0.12 to 0.14 seconds (basic rhythm); 0.08 seconds (PJC)
QRS: 0.08 seconds (basic rhythm and PJC)
Rhythm interpretation: Normal sinus rhythm with one PJC

Strip 8-22
Rhythm: Regular
Rate: Atrial, 100; ventricular, 50
P waves: Two sinus P waves before each QRS complex
PR interval: 0.16 and constant
QRS: 0.08 seconds
Rhythm interpretation: Second-degree AV Block, Mobitz II. Clinical correlation is suggested to diagnose Mobitz II when 2:1 conduction is present

Strip 8-23
Rhythm: Regular
Rate: 65
P waves: Inverted before each QRS
PR interval: 0.08 seconds
QRS: 0.04 to 0.06 seconds
Rhythm interpretation: Accelerated junctional rhythm; ST segment elevation is present

Strip 8-24
Rhythm: Irregular ventricular rhythm; regular atrial rhythm
Rate: Atrial, 68; ventricular, 60
P waves: Sinus P waves present; one without a QRS
PR interval: Progresses from 0.28 to 0.36 seconds
QRS: 0.08 seconds
Rhythm interpretation: Second-degree AV block, Mobitz I; a U wave is present

Strip 8-25
Rhythm: Regular
Rate: 75
P waves: Sinus P waves
PR interval: 0.28
QRS: 0.08 seconds
Rhythm interpretation: Sinus rhythm with first-degree AV block

Strip 8-26
Rhythm: Basic rhythm regular; irregular with PJCs
Rate: Basic rhythm rate 100
P waves: Sinus P waves with basic rhythm; premature, inverted P waves with PJCs
PR interval: 0.20 seconds (basic rhythm); 0.06 seconds (PJC)
QRS: 0.06 to 0.08 seconds (basic rhythm and PJC)
Rhythm interpretation: Normal sinus rhythm with paired PJCs; ST segment depression is present

Strip 8-27
Rhythm: Regular
Rate: 42
P waves: Hidden in QRS complexes
PR interval: Not measurable
QRS: 0.04 to 0.06 seconds
Rhythm interpretation: Junctional rhythm; ST segment depression is present

Strip 8-28
Rhythm: Basic rhythm regular; irregular with nonconducted PAC
Rate: Basic rhythm rate 56
P waves: Sinus P waves with basic rhythm; premature, abnormal P wave without QRS
PR interval: 0.28 seconds
QRS: 0.08 seconds
Rhythm interpretation: Sinus bradycardia with first-degree AV block and nonconducted PAC; ST segment depression is present

Strip 8-29
Rhythm: Irregular ventricular rhythm; regular atrial rhythm
Rate: Atrial, 79; ventricular, 50
P waves: Sinus P waves present; three P waves without QRS
PR interval: Progresses from 0.16 to 0.28 seconds
QRS: 0.06 to 0.08 seconds
Rhythm interpretation: Second-degree AV block, Mobitz I

Strip 8-30
Rhythm: Regular
Rate: Atrial, 84; ventricular, 39
P waves: Sinus P waves not relating to the QRS complexes; hidden in QRS and T waves
PR interval: Varies greatly
QRS: 0.08 seconds
Rhythm interpretation: Third-degree AV block; ST segment depression and T wave inversion are present

Strip 8-31
Rhythm: Regular
Rate: Atrial, 84; ventricular, 28
P waves: Three sinus P waves to each QRS
PR interval: 0.28 to 0.32 (remains constant)
QRS: 0.08 seconds
Rhythm interpretation: Second-degree AV block, Mobitz II

Strip 8-32
Rhythm: Regular
Rate: Atrial, 79; ventricular, 60
P waves: Sinus P waves present; P waves bear no relationship to QRS; hidden in QRS and T waves
PR interval: Varies greatly
QRS: 0.08 seconds
Rhythm interpretation: Third-degree AV block; extremely elevated ST segment is noted

Strip 8-33
Rhythm: Basic rhythm regular; irregular with PAC
Rate: Basic rhythm rate 100
P waves: Inverted before QRS in basic rhythm; upright and premature with PAC
PR interval: 0.08 seconds (basic rhythm); 0.12 seconds (PAC)
QRS: 0.08 seconds (basic rhythm and PAC)
Rhythm interpretation: Accelerated junctional rhythm with one PAC; ST segment depression is present

Strip 8-34
Rhythm: Irregular ventricular rhythm; regular atrial rhythm
Rate: Atrial, 75; ventricular, 50
P waves: Sinus P waves present; two P waves without QRS
PR interval: Progresses from 0.28 to 0.40 seconds
QRS: 0.08 to 0.10 seconds
Rhythm interpretation: Second-degree AV block, Mobitz I

Strip 8-35
Rhythm: Regular
Rate: 72
P waves: Sinus P waves present
PR interval: 0.36 seconds
QRS: 0.04 to 0.06 seconds
Rhythm interpretation: Sinus rhythm with first-degree AV block

Strip 8-36
Rhythm: Regular
Rate: 41
P waves: Inverted after QRS
PR interval: 0.04 to 0.06 seconds
QRS: 0.06 to 0.08 seconds
Rhythm interpretation: Junctional rhythm

Strip 8-37
Rhythm: Basic rhythm regular; irregular with PJC
Rate: Basic rhythm rate 58
P waves: Sinus P waves with basic rhythm; premature, inverted P waves with PJCs
PR interval: 0.16 seconds (basic rhythm); 0.08 to 0.10 seconds (PJC)
QRS: 0.08 seconds (basic rhythm and PJC)
Rhythm interpretation: Sinus bradycardia with two PJCs; a U wave is present

Strip 8-38
Rhythm: Regular
Rate: Atrial, 96; ventricular, 32
P waves: Three sinus P waves to each QRS (one hidden in T wave)
PR interval: 0.12 to 0.14 seconds (remain constant)
QRS: 0.12 seconds
Rhythm interpretation: Second-degree AV block, Mobitz II

Strip 8-39
Rhythm: Regular
Rate: Atrial, 52; ventricular, 26
P waves: Two sinus P waves present before each QRS complex
PR interval: 0.22 (remains constant)
QRS: 0.12 seconds
Rhythm interpretation: Second-degree AV block, Mobitz II. Clinical correlation is suggested to diagnose Mobitz II when 2:1 conduction is present

Strip 8-40
Rhythm: Regular ventricular rhythm; irregular atrial rhythm
Rate: Atrial, 90; ventricular, 30
P waves: Sinus P waves present; bear no relationship to QRS, hidden in QRS and T waves
PR interval: Varies greatly
QRS: 0.12 seconds
Rhythm interpretation: Third-degree AV block

Strip 8-41
Rhythm: Regular
Rate: 68
P waves: Inverted before each QRS
PR interval: 0.08 seconds
QRS: 0.08 seconds
Rhythm interpretation: Accelerated junctional rhythm

Strip 8-42
Rhythm: Regular
Rate: Atrial, 104; ventricular, 52
P waves: Two sinus P waves to each QRS complex
PR interval: 0.24 and constant
QRS: 0.06 to 0.08 seconds
Rhythm interpretation: Second-degree AV block, Mobitz II. Clinical correlation is suggested to diagnose Mobitz II when 2:1 conduction is present ST segment elevation and T wave inversion are present

Strip 8-43
Rhythm: First rhythm irregular; second rhythm regular
Rate: First rhythm about 80; second rhythm 42
P waves: Fibrillatory waves in first rhythm; hidden P waves in second rhythm
PR interval: Not measurable in either rhythm
QRS: 0.06 seconds
Rhythm interpretation: Atrial fibrillation to junctional rhythm; ST segment depression is present

Strip 8-44
Rhythm: Basic rhythm regular; irregular with premature beats
Rate: Basic rhythm rate 60
P waves: Sinus P waves with basic rhythm; premature, abnormal P waves with premature beats
PR interval: 0.12 to 0.16 seconds (basic rhythm); 0.12 seconds (PAC); 0.08 sec (PJC)
QRS: 0.06 to 0.08 seconds
Rhythm interpretation: Normal sinus rhythm with one PAC and one PJC; ST segment depression and T wave inversion are present

Strip 8-45
Rhythm: Regular
Rate: Atrial, 84; ventricular, 38
P waves: Sinus P waves present; P waves bear no relationship to QRS; hidden in QRS and T waves
QRS: 0.08 to 0.10 seconds
Rhythm interpretation: Third-degree AV block; ST segment depression is present

Strip 8-46
Rhythm: Irregular
Rate: 40
P waves: Sinus P waves are present
PR interval: 0.28 seconds
QRS: 0.08 to 0.10 seconds
Rhythm interpretation: Sinus arrhythmia with first-degree AV block; a U wave is present

Strip 8-47
Rhythm: Irregular ventricular rhythm; regular atrial rhythm
Rate: Atrial, 88; ventricular, 70
P waves: Sinus P waves present
PR interval: 0.24, lengthening to 0.32
QRS: 0.06 to 0.08 seconds
Rhythm interpretation: Second-degree AV block, Mobitz I

Strip 8-48
Rhythm: Regular
Rate: Atrial, 108; ventricular, 54
P waves: Two sinus P waves before each QRS complex
PR interval: 0.18 to 0.20 seconds (remains constant)
QRS: 0.08 seconds
Rhythm interpretation: Second-degree AV block Mobitz II. Clinical correlation is suggested to diagnose Mobitz II when 2:1 conduction is present. ST segment elevation and T wave inversion are present

Strip 8-49
Rhythm: Irregular
Rate: 40
P waves: Inverted before each QRS
PR interval: 0.04 to 0.06 seconds
QRS: 0.08 to 0.10 seconds
Rhythm interpretation: Junctional rhythm; ST segment depression is present

Strip 8-50
Rhythm: Basic rhythm regular; irregular with escape beat
Rate: Basic rhythm rate 84; rate slows to 75 after escape beat; rate suppression can occur following premature or escape beats; after several cycles rate will return to basic rate
P waves: Sinus P waves present; P wave hidden with escape beat
PR interval: 0.14 to 0.16 seconds
QRS: 0.06 to 0.08 seconds
Rhythm interpretation: Normal sinus rhythm with junctional escape beat following a pause in the basic rhythm; a U wave is present

Strip 8-51
Rhythm: Regular ventricular rhythm; irregular atrial rhythm
Rate: Atrial, 70; ventricular, 25
P waves: Sinus P waves present; bear no relationship to QRS
PR interval: Varies greatly
QRS: 0.12 seconds
Rhythm interpretation: Third-degree AV block

Strip 8-52
Rhythm: Regular
Rate: 63
P waves: Hidden in QRS
PR interval: Not measurable
QRS: 0.08 seconds
Rhythm interpretation: Accelerated junctional rhythm

Strip 8-53
Rhythm: Regular
Rate: Atrial, 76; ventricular, 38
P waves: Two sinus P waves before each QRS complex
PR interval: 0.28 and constant
QRS: 0.12 seconds
Rhythm interpretation: Second-degree AV block, Mobitz II. Clinical correlation is suggested to diagnose Mobitz II when 2:1 conduction is present

Strip 8-54
Rhythm: Regular
Rate: 94
P waves: Inverted before QRS
PR interval: 0.08 seconds
QRS: 0.06 to 0.08 seconds
Rhythm interpretation: Accelerated junctional rhythm

Strip 8-55
Rhythm: Basic rhythm regular; irregular with PJCs
Rate: Basic rate 84
P waves: Sinus P waves present; P waves hidden with PJCs
PR interval: 0.12 seconds
QRS: 0.06 to 0.08 seconds
Rhythm interpretation: Sinus rhythm with three premature junctional contractions; ST segment depression is present

Strip 8-56
Rhythm: Both rhythms regular
Rate: 72 (first rhythm) about 150 (second rhythm)
P waves: Sinus P waves (first rhythm) inverted P waves (second rhythm)
PR interval: 0.12 seconds (first rhythm); 0.08 to 0.10 seconds (second rhythm)
QRS: 0.08 seconds
Rhythm interpretation: Normal sinus rhythm changing to junctional tachycardia; ST segment depression is present

Strip 8-57
Rhythm: Regular
Rate: 84
P waves: Sinus P waves present
PR interval: 0.30 to 0.32 seconds
QRS: 0.04 seconds
Rhythm interpretation: Normal sinus rhythm with first-degree AV block; ST segment elevation is present

Strip 8-58
Rhythm: Regular
Rate: Atrial, 75; ventricular, 30
P waves: Sinus P waves present; bear no relationship to QRS
PR interval: Varies greatly
QRS: 0.12 to 0.14 seconds
Rhythm interpretation: Third-degree AV block

Strip 8-59
Rhythm: Regular
Rate: Atrial, 93; ventricular, 31
P waves: 3 sinus P waves to each QRS
PR interval: 0.32 to 0.36 seconds
QRS: 0.08 seconds
Rhythm interpretation: Second-degree AV block, Mobitz II; ST segment depression is present

Strip 8-60
Rhythm: Basic rhythm regular; irregular with premature beats
Rate: Basic rhythm rate 60
P waves: Sinus P waves present with basic rhythm; premature, abnormal P waves with premature beats
PR interval: 0.12 seconds (basic rhythm); 0.12 seconds (PAC); 0.08 to 0.10 seconds (PJCs)
QRS: 0.08 seconds
Rhythm interpretation: Normal sinus rhythm with one PAC and paired PJCs

Strip 8-61
Rhythm: Regular
Rate: 47
P waves: Hidden in QRS
PR interval: Not measurable
QRS: 0.10 seconds
Rhythm interpretation: Junctional rhythm

Strip 8-62
Rhythm: Irregular
Rate: 60
P waves: Sinus P waves present
PR interval: 0.28 to 0.32 seconds
QRS: 0.08 seconds
Rhythm interpretation: Sinus arrhythmia with
first-degree AV block; T wave inversion is present

Strip 8-63
Rhythm: Irregular ventricular rhythm; regular atrial
rhythm
Rate: Atrial, 79; ventricular, 50
P waves: Sinus P waves are present
PR interval: Progresses from 0.24 to 0.32 seconds
QRS: 0.08 seconds
Rhythm interpretation: Second-degree AV block,
Mobitz I

Strip 8-64
Rhythm: Regular
Rate: Atrial, 72; ventricular, 31
P waves: Sinus P waves present; bear no
relationship to QRS; hidden in QRS complexes and
T waves
PR interval: Varies greatly
QRS: 0.12 seconds
Rhythm interpretation: Third-degree AV block

Strip 8-65
Rhythm: Regular
Rate: Atrial, 90; ventricular, 45
P waves: Two sinus P waves to each QRS
PR interval: 0.24 to 0.26 seconds (remains
constant)
QRS: 0.12 seconds
Rhythm interpretation: Second-degree AV block,
Mobitz II; clinical correlation is suggested to
diagnose Mobitz II when 2:1 conduction is present;
ST segment elevation is present

Strip 8-66
Rhythm: Regular
Rate: 79
P waves: Absent
PR interval: Not measurable
QRS: 0.08 to 0.10 seconds
Rhythm interpretation: Accelerated junctional
rhythm; ST segment depression is present

Strip 8-67
Rhythm: Basic rhythm regular, irregular with
nonconducted PAC
Rate: Basic rhythm rate 54
P waves: Sinus P waves present; premature,
abnormal P wave without a QRS complex
PR interval: 0.24 to 0.28 seconds
QRS: 0.04 to 0.06 seconds
Rhythm interpretation: Sinus bradycardia;
first-degree AV block; nonconducted premature
atrial contraction; T wave inversion is present

Strip 8-68
Rhythm: Basic rhythm regular; irregular with
premature beats
Rate: Basic rhythm rate 72
P waves: Sinus P waves with basic rhythm;
premature, abnormal P waves with premature beats
PR interval: 0.14 to 0.16 seconds (basic rhythm);
0.12 seconds (PACs); 0.10 seconds (PJCs)
QRS: 0.06 to 0.08 seconds
Rhythm interpretation: Normal sinus rhythm with
two PACs and one PJC; a U wave is present

Strip 8-69
Rhythm: Basic rhythm regular; irregular with
premature beats
Rate: Basic rhythm rate 52
P waves: Hidden with basic rhythm; premature,
abnormal with premature beats
PR interval: Not measurable in basic rhythm; 0.16
(PACs)
QRS: 0.06 to 0.08 seconds
Rhythm interpretation: Junctional rhythm with two
PACs; ST segment depression is present

Strip 8-70
Rhythm: Irregular ventricular rhythm; regular atrial
rhythm
Rate: Atrial, 88; ventricular, 70
P waves: Sinus P waves present
PR interval: Progressses from 0.24 to 0.28 seconds
QRS: 0.08 seconds
Rhythm interpretation: Second-degree AV block
Mobitz I

Strip 8-71
Rhythm: Regular
Rate: Atrial, 80; ventricular, 40
P waves: Two sinus P waves to each QRS
PR interval: 0.24 seconds (remain constant)
QRS: 0.04 to 0.06 seconds
Rhythm interpretation: Second-degree AV Block,
Mobitz II; clinical correlation is suggested to
diagnose Mobitz II when 2:1 conduction is present;
ST segment depression is present

Strip 8-72
Rhythm: Regular
Rate: Atrial, 94; ventricular, 40
P waves: Sinus P waves are present; bear no relationship to QRS; hidden in QRS complexes and T waves
PR interval: Varies greatly
QRS: 0.10 seconds
Rhythm interpretation: Third-degree AV block

Strip 8-73
Rhythm: Regular
Rate: 84
P waves: Hidden in QRS complexes
PR interval: Not measurable
QRS: 0.06 seconds
Rhythm interpretation: Accelerated junctional rhythm; ST segment depression and T wave inversion are present

Strip 8-74
Rhythm: Irregular ventricular rhythm; regular atrial rhythm
Rate: Atrial, 84; ventricular, 50
P waves: Sinus P waves present
PR interval: 0.20, lengthening to 0.24
QRS: 0.08 seconds
Rhythm interpretation: Second-degree AV block; Mobitz I; ST segment elevation and T wave inversion are present

Strip 8-75
Rhythm: Basic rhythm regular; irregular with escape beat
Rate: Basic rhythm rate 58
P waves: Sinus P waves with basic rhythm; hidden P wave with escape beat
PR interval: 0.16 to 0.18 seconds
QRS: 0.08 to 0.10 seconds
Rhythm interpretation: Sinus bradycardia with junctional escape beat following a pause in the basic rhythm

Strip 8-76
Rhythm: Irregular
Rate: 50
P waves: after QRS
PR interval: 0.04 seconds
QRS: 0.08 to 0.10 seconds
Rhythm interpretation: Junctional rhythm

Strip 8-77
Rhythm: Regular
Rate: Atrial, 94; ventricular, 44
P waves: Sinus P waves are present; P waves bear no relationship to QRS; found hidden in QRS complexes and T waves
PR interval: Varies greatly
QRS: 0.12 to 0.14 seconds
Rhythm interpretation: Third-degree AV block; ST segment elevation is present

Strip 8-78
Rhythm: Basic rhythm regular; irregular with PJC
Rate: Basic rhythm rate 84 (rate slows to 75 following premature beat; rate suppression can occur for several cycles following premature beats)
P waves: Sinus P waves with basic rhythm; inverted P wave with PJC
PR interval: 0.12 to 0.16 seconds (basic rhythm); 0.08 seconds (PJC)
QRS: 0.06 to 0.08 seconds
Rhythm interpretation: Normal sinus rhythm with one PJC: ST segment depression is present

Strip 8-79
Rhythm: Regular
Rate: Atrial, 80; ventricular, 40
P waves: Two P waves to each QRS
PR interval: 0.12 to 0.16 seconds (remain constant)
QRS: 0.08 seconds
Rhythm interpretation: Second-degree AV block, Mobitz II; clinical correlation is suggested to diagnose Mobitz II when 2:1 conduction is present

Strip 8-80
Rhythm: Basic rhythm regular; irregular with nonconducted PAC
Rate: Basic rhythm rate 72
P waves: Sinus P waves with basic rhythm; premature, abnormal P wave without QRS
PR interval: 0.24 seconds
QRS: 0.06 to 0.08 seconds
Rhythm interpretation: Normal sinus rhythm with first-degree AV block and one nonconducted PAC; ST segment depression is present

Strip 8-81
Rhythm: Regular
Rate: 88
P waves: Inverted before each QRS
PR interval: 0.08 seconds
QRS: 0.08 seconds
Rhythm interpretation: Accelerated junctional rhythm

Strip 8-82
Rhythm: Irregular ventricular rhythm; regular atrial rhythm
Rate: Atrial, 65; ventricular, 50
P waves: Sinus P waves are present
PR interval: Progresses from 0.26 to 0.40 seconds
QRS: 0.06 to 0.08 seconds
Rhythm interpretation: Second-degree AV block, Mobitz I; ST depression is present

Strip 8-83
Rhythm: Both rhythms regular
Rate: 79 (first rhythm); 107 (second rhythm)
P waves: Sinus P waves (first rhythm) inverted P waves (second rhythm)
PR interval: 0.12 to 0.14 seconds (first rhythm) 0.08 to 0.10 seconds (second rhythm)
QRS: 0.08 seconds
Rhythm interpretation: Normal sinus rhythm changing to junctional tachycardia

Strip 8-84
Rhythm: First rhythm regular; second rhythm regular; both rhythms interrupted by PJC
Rate: First rhythm (72); second rhythm (63)
P waves: First rhythm (sinus P waves); second rhythm (inverted); PJC (inverted)
PR interval: First rhythm (0.12 to 0.14 seconds); second rhythm (0.08 seconds); PJC (0.08 second)
QRS: 0.06 to 0.08 seconds
Rhythm interpretation: Normal sinus rhythm with PJC changing to accelerated junctional rhythm

Strip 8-85
Rhythm: Regular
Rate: Atrial, 79; ventricular, 31
P waves: Sinus P waves present; bear no relationship to QRS; hidden in QRS complexes and T waves
PR interval: Varies greatly
QRS: 0.12 seconds
Rhythm interpretation: Third-degree AV block

Strip 8-86
Rhythm: Regular
Rate: 60
P waves: Sinus P waves present
PR interval: 0.24 seconds
QRS: 0.08 seconds
Rhythm interpretation: Normal sinus rhythm with first-degree AV block; ST segment depression and T wave inversion are present

Strip 8-87
Rhythm: Irregular atrial rhythm; regular ventricular rhythm
Rate: Atrial, 50; ventricular, 33
P waves: Sinus P waves not relating to the QRS complexes
PR interval: Varies greatly
QRS: 0.08 to 0.10 seconds
Rhythm interpretation: Third-degree AV block; ST segment depression and T wave inversion are present

Strip 8-88
Rhythm: Basic rhythm regular; irregular with premature and escape beats
Rate: Basic rate is 60
P waves: Sinus P waves with basic rhythm; pointed P wave with atrial beat and inverted P wave with junctional beats
PR interval: 0.12 seconds (basic rhythm); 0.14 seconds (atrial beat); 0.08 seconds (junctional beats)
QRS: 0.06 to 0.08 seconds
Rhythm interpretation: Normal sinus rhythm with one PJC and one atrial escape beat and one junctional escape beat

Strip 8-89
Rhythm: Irregular ventricular rhythm; regular atrial rhythm
Rate: Atrial, 65; ventricular, 50
P waves: Sinus P waves present
PR interval: Progresses from 0.32 to 0.44 seconds
QRS: 0.08 seconds
Rhythm interpretation: Second-degree AV block, Mobitz I

Strip 8-90
Rhythm: Regular
Rate: 107
P waves: Inverted before each QRS
PR interval: 0.08 to 0.10 seconds
QRS: 0.06 seconds
Rhythm interpretation: Junctional tachycardia

Strip 8-91
Rhythm: Regular
Rate: 88
P waves: Sinus P waves are present
PR interval: 0.28 seconds
QRS: 0.08 seconds
Rhythm interpretation: Normal sinus rhythm with first-degree AV block

Strip 8-92
Rhythm: Irregular
Rate: Atrial, 75; ventricular, 30
P waves: Sinus P waves present (two to three P waves before each QRS)
PR interval: 0.16 seconds (remains constant)
QRS: 0.12 seconds
Rhythm interpretation: Second-degree AV block, Mobitz II; ST segment depression is present

Strip 8-93
Rhythm: Irregular with escape beat
Rate: Basic rhythm 33
P waves: Sinus P waves present with basic rhythm; hidden P wave with escape beat
PR interval: 0.12 seconds
QRS: 0.06 to 0.08 seconds
Rhythm interpretation: Sinus bradycardia with a junctional escape beat following a pause in the basic rhythm

Strip 8-94
Rhythm: Regular with basic rhythm; irregular with PJCs
Rate: Basic rhythm rate 72
P waves: Sinus P waves with basic rhythm; inverted P waves with PJCs
PR interval: 0.14 seconds (basic rhythm); 0.08 seconds (PJCs)
QRS: 0.08 seconds
Rhythm interpretation: Normal sinus rhythm with 2 PJCs

Strip 8-95
Rhythm: Regular
Rate: Atrial, 90; ventricular, 45
P waves: Two sinus P waves before each QRS complex
PR interval: 0.16 seconds
QRS: 0.12 seconds
Rhythm interpretation: Second-degree AV block Mobitz II. Clinical correlation is suggested to diagnose Mobitz II when 2:1 conduction is present. T wave inversion is present

Strip 8-96
Rhythm: Irregular
Rate: First rhythm cannot be determined; second rhythm is about 30
P waves: One sinus P wave present, one premature, abnormal P wave with a premature beat
PR interval: 0.12 with sinus beat 0.12 seconds (PAC)
QRS: 0.08 to 0.10 seconds
Rhythm interpretation: Sinus beat followed by a premature atrial contraction and a junctional escape rhythm; ST segment depression is present

Strip 8-97
Rhythm: Regular
Rate: 68
P waves: Hidden in QRS complexes
PR interval: Not measurable
QRS: 0.06 to 0.08 seconds
Rhythm interpretation: Accelerated junctional rhythm

Strip 8-98
Rhythm: Regular
Rate: Atrial, 84; ventricular, 42
P waves: Two sinus P waves to each QRS complex
PR interval: 0.20 and constant
QRS: 0.06 to 0.08 seconds
Rhythm interpretation: Second-degree AV block, Mobitz II. Clinical correlation is suggested to diagnose Mobitz II when 2:1 conduction is present

Strip 8-99
Rhythm: Basic rhythm regular; irregular with PJC
Rate: Basic rhythm rate 84
P waves: Sinus P waves with basic rhythm; inverted P wave with PJC
PR interval: 0.12 seconds (basic rhythm); 0.08 seconds (PJC)
QRS: 0.06 to 0.08 seconds
Rhythm interpretation: Normal sinus rhythm with one PJC

Strip 9-1
Rhythm: Regular
Rate: First rhythm cannot be determined (only one complex); rate of second rhythm is 250
P waves: One sinus P wave is present
PR interval: 0.16
QRS: 0.06 to 0.08 seconds (sinus beat); 0.12 seconds (wide beats)
Rhythm interpretation: Sinus beat changing to ventricular tachycardia

Strip 9-2
Rhythm: Regular
Rate: 88
P waves: Sinus P waves are present
PR interval: 0.16 to 0.18 seconds
QRS: 0.12 to 0.14 seconds
Rhythm interpretation: Normal sinus rhythm with bundle branch block

Strip 9-3
Rhythm: Basic rhythm regular; irregular with PVCs
Rate: Basic rhythm rate 75
P waves: Sinus P waves with basic rhythm; no P waves associated with PVCs; sinus P waves can be seen after the PVCs
PR interval: 0.18 to 0.20 seconds
QRS: 0.08 seconds (basic rhythm); 0.12 seconds (PVCs)
Rhythm interpretation: Normal sinus rhythm with two unifocal PVCs

Strip 9-4
Rhythm: Regular
Rate: 30
P waves: Absent
PR interval: Not measurable owing to absence of P wave
QRS: 0.12 seconds
Rhythm interpretation: Idioventricular rhythm

Strip 9-5
Rhythm: 0
Rate: Chaotic
P waves: Chaotic wave deflection of varying height, size, and shape
PR interval: 0
QRS: Absent
Rhythm interpretation: Ventricular fibrillation

Strip 9-6
Rhythm: Basic rhythm regular; irregular with PVCs
Rate: Basic rhythm 100
P waves: Sinus P waves present with basic rhythm
PR interval: 0.14 to 0.16 seconds (basic rhythm)
QRS: 0.08 seconds (basic rhythm); 0.12 seconds (PVCs)
Rhythm interpretation: Normal sinus rhythm with unifocal PVCs in a bigeminal pattern

Strip 9-7
Rhythm: First rhythm (cannot be determined for sure; only one cardiac cycle); second rhythm irregular
Rate: First rhythm 54; second rhythm 80
P waves: Sinus P waves present with basic rhythm
PR interval: 0.16 seconds (basic rhythm)
QRS: 0.08 seconds (basic rhythm); 0.12 seconds (ventricular beats)
Rhythm interpretation: Sinus bradycardia changing to accelerated idioventricular rhythm; ST segment depression is present

Strip 9-8
Rhythm: Cannot be determined for sure (only two complexes)
Rate: About 12
P waves: Absent
PR interval: Not measurable owing to absence of P waves
QRS: 0.16 seconds
Rhythm interpretation: Secondary ventricular standstill

Strip 9-9
Rhythm: Ventricular rhythm regular; atrial rhythm slightly irregular
Rate: Atrial, about 36; ventricular, 38
P waves: Sinus P waves present; bear no relationship to QRS
PR interval: Varies
QRS: 0.12 seconds
Rhythm interpretation: Third-degree AV block changing to primary ventricular standstill, ST segment elevation is present

Strip 9-10
Rhythm: Basic rhythm regular; irregular with PVCs
Rate: Basic rhythm rate 79
P waves: Sinus P waves present with basic rhythm
PR interval: 0.16 seconds
QRS: 0.06 seconds (basic rhythm); 0.14 to 0.16 seconds (PVCs)
Rhythm interpretation: Normal sinus rhythm with paired unifocal PVCs

Strip 9-11
Rhythm: Regular
Rate: 42
P waves: Absent
PR interval: Not measurable owing to absence of P wave
QRS: 0.12 to 0.14 seconds
Rhythm interpretation: Idioventricular rhythm

Strip 9-12
Rhythm: Cannot be determined for sure; only 1 cardiac cycle
Rate: About 16
P waves: Absent
PR interval: Not measurable
QRS: 0.12 seconds
Rhythm interpretation: Secondary ventricular standstill

Strip 9-13
Rhythm: Regular
Rate: 250
P waves: None identified
PR interval: Not measurable
QRS: 0.20 seconds
Rhythm interpretation: Ventricular tachycardia

Strip 9-14
Rhythm: Basic rhythm cannot be determined for sure; only isolated sinus beats; second rhythm is regular
Rate: Basic rhythm cannot be determined; only isolated sinus complexes; second rhythm rate is 150
P waves: Sinus P waves with sinus complexes
PR interval: 0.16 seconds (sinus beats)
QRS: 0.08 seconds (sinus beats); 0.12 seconds (ventricular beats)
Rhythm interpretation: Isolated sinus beats with paired PVCs, a burst of ventricular tachycardia and two PVCs occurring in a bigeminal pattern

Strip 9-15
Rhythm: Basic rhythm irregular
Rate: 60 (basic rhythm)
P waves: Fibrillation waves present
PR interval: Not measurable
QRS: 0.06 to 0.08 seconds (basic rhythm); 0.12 seconds (PVCs)
Rhythm interpretation: Atrial fibrillation with unifocal PVCs in a bigeminal pattern; ST segment depression is present

Strip 9-16
Rhythm: Chaotic
Rate: 0
P waves: Absent; wave deflections are irregular and vary in height, size, and shape
PR interval: Not measurable
QRS: Absent
Rhythm interpretation: Ventricular fibrillation

Strip 9-17
Rhythm: Chaotic
Rate: 0
P waves: Wave deflections are chaotic and vary in height, size, and shape
PR interval: Not measurable
QRS: Absent
Rhythm interpretation: Ventricular fibrillation followed by electrical shock and return to ventricular fibrillation

Strip 9-18
Rhythm: Regular
Rate: 72
P waves: Sinus P waves are present
PR interval: 0.16 seconds
QRS: 0.12 seconds
Rhythm interpretation: Normal sinus rhythm with bundle branch block

Strip 9-19
Rhythm: Cannot be determined certainly (only one cardiac cycle)
Rate: About 14
P waves: Absent
PR interval: Not discernible
QRS: 0.32 seconds
Rhythm interpretation: Secondary ventricular standstill

Strip 9-20
Rhythm: Regular atrial rhythm
Rate: Atrial, 136; ventricular, 0 (no QRS complexes)
P waves: Sinus P waves are present
PR interval: Not measurable
QRS: Absent
Rhythm interpretation: Primary ventricular standstill

Strip 9-21
Rhythm: Irregular
Rate: 40
P waves: Absent
PR interval: Not measurable
QRS: 0.16 seconds
Rhythm interpretation: Idioventricular rhythm

Strip 9-22
Rhythm: Chaotic
Rate: 0
P waves: Absent; wave deflections are irregular and chaotic and vary in height, size, and shape
PR interval: Not discernible
QRS: Absent
Rhythm interpretation: Ventricular fibrillation

Strip 9-23
Rhythm: Regular
Rate: 100
P waves: Absent
PR interval: Not measurable
QRS: 0.12 seconds
Rhythm interpretation: Accelerated idioventricular rhythm

Strip 9-24
Rhythm: Irregular
Rate: 60
P waves: Fibrillation waves present
PR interval: Not measurable
QRS: 0.12 seconds
Rhythm interpretation: Atrial fibrillation with bundle branch block; ST segment depression and T wave inversion are present

Strip 9-25
Rhythm: Regular
Rate: 188
P waves: Not identified
PR interval: Not discernible
QRS: 0.16 seconds
Rhythm interpretation: Ventricular tachycardia; ST segment evaluation is present

Strip 9-26
Rhythm: Slightly irregular
Rate: About 23
P waves: Absent
PR interval: Not measurable
QRS: 0.20 seconds
Rhythm interpretation: Secondary ventricular standstill

Strip 9-27
Rhythm: Regular
Rate: 43
P waves: Absent
PR interval: Not measurable
QRS: 0.16 to 0.18 seconds
Rhythm interpretation: Idioventricular rhythm

Strip 9-28
Rhythm: Atrial is irregular
Rate: Atrial, 30; ventricular, 0 (no QRS complexes)
P waves: Sinus P waves present
PR interval: Not measurable
QRS: Absent
Rhythm interpretation: Primary ventricular standstill

Strip 9-29
Rhythm: First rhythm regular; second rhythm regular
Rate: First rhythm 75; second rhythm 94
P waves: First rhythm (sinus P waves); second rhythm (no P waves)
PR interval: 0.14 to 0.16 seconds (first rhythm)
QRS: 0.08 seconds (first rhythm); 0.12 seconds (second rhythm)
Rhythm interpretation: Normal sinus rhythm changing to accelerated idioventricular rhythm

Strip 9-30
Rhythm: Chaotic
Rate: 0
P waves: Absent; wave deflections are irregular and vary in height, size, and shape
PR interval: Not measurable
QRS: Absent
Rhythm interpretation: Ventricular fibrillation

Strip 9-31
Rhythm: Basic rhythm regular; irregular with PVCs
Rate: Basic rhythm rate 115
P waves: Sinus P waves with basic rhythm
PR interval: 0.14 to 0.16 seconds
QRS: 0.04 to 0.06 seconds (basic rhythm), 0.12 seconds (PVCs)
Rhythm interpretation: Sinus tachycardia with two unifocal PVCs

Strip 9-32
Rhythm: Basic rhythm regular; irregular with PVCs
Rate: Basic rate 63
P waves: Sinus P waves with basic rhythm
PR interval: 0.16 to 0.18 seconds
QRS: 0.06 to 0.08 seconds (basic rhythm); 0.12 seconds (PVCs)
Rhythm interpretation: Normal sinus rhythm with multifocal PVCs

Strip 9-33
Rhythm: Cannot be determined for sure (only one complete cardiac cycle present)
Rate: 56 (basic rate)
P waves: Sinus P waves with basic rhythm
PR interval: 0.16 seconds
QRS: 0.04 seconds (basic rhythm); 0.12 seconds (escape beats)
Rhythm interpretation: Sinus bradycardia with two ventricular escape beats

Strip 9-34
Rhythm: First rhythm (irregular); second rhythm (regular)
Rate: First rhythm 180; second rhythm 214
P waves: First rhythm (fibrillation waves); second rhythm (none identified)
PR interval: Not measurable either rhythm
QRS: First rhythm (0.06 to 0.08 seconds); second rhythm (0.12 seconds)
Rhythm interpretation: Atrial fibrillation changing to ventricular tachycardia; ST segment depression is seen with the atrial fibrillation

Strip 9-35
Rhythm: Chaotic
Rate: 0
P waves: Absent; wave deflections vary in height, size, and shape
PR interval: Not measurable
QRS: Absent
Rhythm interpretation: Ventricular fibrillation

Strip 9-36
Rhythm: Irregular
Rate: About 30
P waves: Absent
PR interval: Not measurable
QRS: 0.12 seconds
Rhythm interpretation: Idioventricular rhythm; ST segment elevation is present

Strip 9-37
Rhythm: Cannot be determined for sure (only one cardiac cycle)
Rate: About 14
P waves: Absent
PR interval: Not discernible
QRS: 0.12 seconds
Rhythm interpretation: Secondary ventricular standstill

Strip 9-38
Rhythm: Regular atrial rhythm
Rate: Atrial: 75; ventricular; 0 (no QRS complexes)
P waves: Sinus P waves present
PR interval: Not measurable
QRS: Absent
Rhythm interpretation: Primary ventricular standstill

Strip 9-39
Rhythm: Basic rhythm regular
Rate: Basic rhythm rate 115
P waves: Inverted before each QRS in basic rhythm
PR interval: 0.08 seconds (basic rhythm)
QRS: 0.06 to 0.08 seconds (basic rhythm); 0.16 seconds (PVC)
Rhythm interpretation: Junctional tachycardia with one PVC

Strip 9-40
Rhythm: Regular atrial rhythm
Rate: Atrial, 30; ventricular, 0 (no QRS complexes)
P waves: Sinus P waves present
PR interval: Not measurable
QRS: Absent
Rhythm interpretation: Primary ventricular standstill

Strip 9-41
Rhythm: Basic rhythm regular; irregular with PVCs
Rate: Basic rhythm rate 65
P waves: Sinus P waves present with basic rhythm
PR interval: 0.16 seconds
QRS: 0.06 to 0.08 seconds (basic rhythm); 0.12 seconds (PVC)
Rhythm interpretation: Normal sinus rhythm with two unifocal PVCs; ST segment depression is present

Strip 9-42
Rhythm: Basic rhythm irregular
Rate: Basic rhythm rate 100
P waves: Basic rhythm (fibrillation waves)
PR interval: Not measurable
QRS: 0.08 seconds (basic rhythm); 0.12 seconds (PVCs)
Rhythm interpretation: Atrial fibrillation with a burst of ventricular tachycardia

Strip 9-43
Rhythm: Regular
Rate: 79
P waves: Absent
PR interval: Not measurable
QRS: 0.12 seconds
Rhythm interpretation: Accelerated idioventricular rhythm

Strip 9-44
Rhythm: First rhythm (cannot be determined for sure; only one cardiac cycle present); second rhythm (regular)
Rate: First rhythm 50, second rhythm 41
P waves: Sinus P waves with first rhythm
PR interval: 0.12 seconds (first rhythm)
QRS: 0.06 to 0.08 seconds (first rhythm); 0.12 to 0.14 seconds (second rhythm)
Rhythm interpretation: Sinus bradycardia changing to idioventricular rhythm; a U wave is present

Strip 9-45
Rhythm: Regular
Rate: 79
P waves: Sinus P waves present
PR interval: 0.20
QRS: 0.12 seconds
Rhythm interpretation: Sinus rhythm with bundle branch block; T wave inversion is present

Strip 9-46
Rhythm: Basic rhythm slightly irregular; irregular with ventricular beats
Rate: Basic rhythm is about 58
P waves: Sinus P waves with basic rhythm
PR interval: 0.20 seconds
QRS: 0.06 seconds (basic rhythm); 0.16 seconds (ventricular beats)
Rhythm interpretation: Sinus bradycardia with one PVC and one ventricular escape beat; ST segment depression is present

Strip 9-47
Rhythm: Basic rhythm regular; irregular with PVC
Rate: 75 (basic rhythm)
P waves: Sinus P waves present
PR interval: 0.18 to 0.20 seconds
QRS: 0.08 seconds (sinus beats); 0.20 seconds (PVC)
Rhythm interpretation: Sinus rhythm with a premature ventricular contraction; T wave inversion is present

Strip 9-48
Rhythm: Cannot be determined for sure; only one cardiac cycle present
Rate: Less than 10
P waves: Absent
PR interval: Not measurable
QRS: 0.20 seconds
Rhythm interpretation: Secondary ventricular standstill; ST segment depression is present

Strip 9-49
Rhythm: Regular
Rate: 56
P waves: Sinus P waves present
PR interval: 0.12 to 0.16 seconds
QRS: 0.12 seconds
Rhythm interpretation: Sinus bradycardia with bundle branch block; ST segment depression is present

Strip 9-50
Rhythm: Regular
Rate: 188
P waves: Not identified
PR interval: Not measurable
QRS: 0.12 to 0.16 seconds
Rhythm interpretation: Ventricular tachycardia

Strip 9-51
Rhythm: Regular atrial rhythm; irregular ventricular rhythm
Rate: Atrial, 58; ventricular, about 40
P waves: Sinus P waves present
PR interval: Progresses from 0.30 to 0.36 seconds
QRS: 0.08 seconds (basic rhythm); 0.12 seconds (escape beat)
Rhythm interpretation: Second-degree AV block, Mobitz I with one ventricular escape beat

Strip 9-52
Rhythm: Regular
Rate: 75
P waves: Absent
PR interval: Not discernible
QRS: 0.16 seconds
Rhythm interpretation: Accelerated idioventricular rhythm

Strip 9-53
Rhythm: Slightly irregular atrial rhythm
Rate: Atrial, about 36; ventricular, 0 (no QRS complexes)
P waves: Sinus P waves present
PR interval: Not measurable
QRS: Absent
Rhythm interpretation: Primary ventricular standstill

Strip 9-54
Rhythm: Regular atrial rhythm; irregular ventricular rhythm
Rate: Atrial, 72; ventricular, 50
P waves: Sinus P waves present
PR interval: 0.16 progressing to 0.28
QRS: 0.12 seconds
Rhythm interpretation: Second-degree AV block, Mobitz I; a BBB is present

Strip 9-55
Rhythm: Regular
Rate: 41
P waves: Absent
PR interval: Not measurable
QRS: 0.16 seconds
Rhythm interpretation: Idioventricular rhythm

Strip 9-56
Rhythm: Regular
Rate: 75
P waves: Sinus P waves present
PR interval: 0.12 seconds
QRS: 0.18 to 0.20 seconds
Rhythm interpretation: Normal sinus rhythm with bundle branch block. T wave inversion is present

Strip 9-57
Rhythm: Basic rhythm regular; irregular with premature beats
Rate: Basic rhythm 94
P waves: Sinus P waves with basic rhythm; inverted P wave with PJC; no P wave with PVC
PR interval: 0.12 seconds (basic rhythm); 0.08 seconds (PJC)
QRS: 0.06 to 0.08 seconds (basic rhythm and PJC); 0.12 seconds (PVC)
Rhythm interpretation: Normal sinus rhythm with one PJC and one PVC; ST segment depression and T wave inversion are present

Strip 9-58
Rhythm: Cannot be determined for sure; only one cardiac cycle
Rate: About 22
P waves: Absent
PR interval: Not measurable
QRS: 0.16 seconds
Rhythm interpretation: Secondary ventricular standstill; ST segment depression is present

Strip 9-59
Rhythm: Chaotic
Rate: 0
P waves: Absent; wave deflections are irregular and chaotic and vary in height, size, and shape
PR interval: Not discernible
QRS: Absent
Rhythm interpretation: Ventricular fibrillation

Strip 9-60
Rhythm: Regular atrial rhythm; irregular ventricular rhythm
Rate: Atrial, 115; ventricular, 30
P waves: Sinus P waves present; bear no relationship to QRS and can be found hidden in QRS complexes and T waves
PR interval: Varies greatly
QRS: 0.12 seconds
Rhythm interpretation: Third-degree AV block changing to primary ventricular standstill; ST segment depression is present

Strip 9-61
Rhythm: Regular (first rhythm); regular (second rhythm)
Rate: 100 (first rhythm); 100 (second rhythm)
P waves: Sinus P waves with first rhythm; no P waves with second rhythm
PR interval: 0.14 to 0.16 seconds (first rhythm)
QRS: 0.06 to 0.08 seconds (first rhythm); 0.12 seconds (second rhythm)
Rhythm interpretation: Normal sinus rhythm changing to accelerated idioventricular rhythm

Strip 9-62
Rhythm: Regular
Rate: 40
P waves: Absent
PR interval: Not measurable
QRS: 0.16 seconds
Rhythm interpretation: Idioventricular rhythm

Strip 9-63
Rhythm: Regular
Rate: 250
P waves: None identified
PR interval: Not measurable
QRS: 0.16 seconds
Rhythm interpretation: Ventricular tachycardia
followed by electrical shock and return to
ventricular tachycardia

Strip 9-64
Rhythm: Regular
Rate: 88
P waves: Sinus P waves present
PR interval: 0.20 seconds
QRS: 0.12 seconds
Rhythm interpretation: Normal sinus rhythm with
bundle branch block

Strip 9-65
Rhythm: Basic rhythm regular; irregular with PVC
Rate: Basic rhythm rate 84
P waves: Sinus P waves with basic rhythm
PR interval: 0.16 to 0.18 seconds
QRS: 0.12 seconds (basic rhythm); 0.12 seconds
(PVC)
Rhythm interpretation: Normal sinus rhythm with
bundle branch block and one PVC; ST segment
depression is present

Strip 9-66
Rhythm: Basic rhythm regular
Rate: Basic rhythm rate 84
P waves: Sinus P waves present
PR interval: 0.24 seconds
QRS: 0.08 seconds
Rhythm interpretation: Normal sinus rhythm with
first-degree AV block changing to primary
ventricular standstill

Strip 9-67
Rhythm: Chaotic
Rate: None
P waves: None; wave deflections are irregular and
chaotic and vary in height, size, and shape
PR interval: Not discernible
QRS: None
Rhythm interpretation: Ventricular fibrillation

Strip 9-68
Rhythm: Regular
Rate: 214
P waves: Not identified
PR interval: Not discernible
QRS: 0.16 to 0.18 seconds
Rhythm interpretation: Ventricular tachycardia

Strip 9-69
Rhythm: Chaotic
Rate: 0
P waves: Absent; wave deflections are irregular and
chaotic and vary in height, size, and shape
PR interval: Not discernible
QRS: Absent
Rhythm interpretation: Ventricular fibrillation

Strip 9-70
Rhythm: Regular
Rate: 40
P waves: Absent
PR interval: Not measurable
QRS: 0.16 seconds
Rhythm interpretation: Idioventricular rhythm

Strip 9-71
Rhythm: Regular
Rate: 100
P waves: Absent
PR interval: Not measurable
QRS: 0.12 seconds
Rhythm interpretation: Accelerated idioventricular
rhythm

Strip 9-72
Rhythm: Cannot be determined for sure; only one
cardiac cycle
Rate: About 13
P waves: Absent
PR interval: Not measurable
QRS: 0.16 to 0.20 seconds
Rhythm interpretation: Secondary ventricular
standstill; ST segment depression is present

Strip 9-73
Rhythm: Regular
Rate: 188
P waves: Not identified
PR interval: Not measurable
QRS: About 0.24 seconds
Rhythm interpretation: Ventricular tachycardia
followed by electrical shock and return to
ventricular tachycardia

Strip 9-74
Rhythm: Basic rhythm regular; irregular with PVC
Rate: Basic rhythm rate 100
P waves: Sinus P waves with basic rhythm
PR interval: 0.14 to 0.16 seconds
QRS: 0.08 seconds (basic rhythm); 0.12 seconds
(PVC)
Rhythm interpretation: Normal sinus rhythm with
one PVC

Strip 9-75
Rhythm: Basic rhythm regular; irregular with pause
Rate: Basic rhythm rate 56
P waves: Sinus P waves present
PR interval: 0.20 seconds
QRS: 0.12 to 0.14 seconds
Rhythm interpretation: Sinus bradycardia with bundle branch block and sinus block

Strip 9-76
Rhythm: Regular atrial rhythm
Rate: Atrial, 68; ventricular, 0 (no QRS complexes)
P waves: Sinus P waves present
PR interval: Not measurable
QRS: Absent
Rhythm interpretation: Primary ventricular standstill

Strip 9-77
Rhythm: Regular
Rate: 41
P waves: Absent
PR interval: Not measurable
QRS: 0.12 seconds
Rhythm interpretation: Idioventricular rhythm

Strip 9-78
Rhythm: Cannot be determined; only one cardiac cycle
Rate: About 13
P waves: Absent
PR interval: Not measurable
QRS: 0.22 seconds
Rhythm interpretation: Secondary ventricular standstill

Strip 9-79
Rhythm: 0
Rate: 0
P waves: Absent; wave deflections are chaotic and vary in height, size, and shape
PR interval: Not measurable
QRS: Absent
Rhythm interpretation: Ventricular fibrillation changing to asystole

Strip 9-80
Rhythm: First rhythm regular; second rhythm regular
Rate: 94 (first rhythm); 75 (second rhythm)
P waves: Sinus P waves present with first rhythm
PR interval: 0.16 seconds
QRS: 0.12 seconds (first rhythm); 0.12 seconds (second rhythm)
Rhythm interpretation: Normal sinus rhythm with bundle branch block changing to accelerated idioventricular rhythm and back to NSR; T wave inversion is present

Strip 9-81
Rhythm: Regular atrial rhythm; ventricular rhythm cannot be determined for sure (only one cardiac cycle)
Rate: About 41
P waves: Sinus P waves present; bear no relationship to QRS
PR interval: Varies greatly
QRS: 0.12 seconds
Rhythm interpretation: Third-degree AV block changing to primary ventricular standstill

Strip 9-82
Rhythm: Regular
Rate: 72
P waves: Sinus P waves are present
PR interval: 0.16 seconds
QRS: 0.12 seconds
Rhythm interpretation: Normal sinus rhythm with bundle branch block

Strip 9-83
Rhythm: First rhythm regular; second rhythm irregular, chaotic
Rate: 214 (first rhythm)
P waves: None identified
PR interval: Not measurable
QRS: 0.16 to 0.18 seconds (first rhythm)
Rhythm interpretation: Ventricular tachycardia changing to ventricular fibrillation

Strip 9-84
Rhythm: Regular
Rate: 32
P waves: Absent
PR interval: Not measurable
QRS: 0.20 seconds
Rhythm interpretation: Idioventricular rhythm

Strip 9-85
Rhythm: Basic rhythm regular; irregular with PVC
Rate: Basic rhythm rate 56
P waves: Sinus P waves with basic rhythm
PR interval: 0.14 to 0.16 seconds
QRS: 0.08 seconds (basic rhythm); 0.12 seconds (PVC)
Rhythm interpretation: Sinus bradycardia with one PVC

Strip 9-86
Rhythm: Cannot be determined for sure; only one cardiac cycle
Rate: About 14
P waves: Absent
PR interval: Not measurable
QRS: 0.24 to 0.28 seconds
Rhythm interpretation: Secondary ventricular standstill

Strip 9-87
Rhythm: First rhythm regular; second rhythm irregular
Rate: 68 (first rhythm); about 80 (second rhythm)
P waves: Sinus P waves with first rhythm
PR interval: 0.12 to 0.14 seconds
QRS: 0.08 seconds (first rhythm); 0.12 seconds (second rhythm)
Rhythm interpretation: Normal sinus rhythm changing to accelerated idioventricular rhythm

Strip 9-88
Rhythm: Regular
Rate: 167
P waves: Not identified
PR interval: Not measurable
QRS: 0.16 to 0.20 seconds
Rhythm interpretation: Ventricular tachycardia (Torsades de pointes)

Strip 9-89
Rhythm: Regular
Rate: 100
P waves: Sinus P waves present
PR interval: 0.16
QRS: 0.16 seconds
Rhythm interpretation: Normal sinus rhythm with bundle branch block; ST segment elevation is present

Strip 9-90
Rhythm: Regular atrial rhythm
Rate: Atrial, 72; ventricular, 0 (no QRS complexes)
P waves: Sinus P waves present
PR interval: Not measurable
QRS: Absent
Rhythm interpretation: Primary ventricular standstill

Strip 9-91
Rhythm: Regular
Rate: About 22
P waves: Absent
PR interval: Not discernible
QRS: 0.14 seconds
Rhythm interpretation: Secondary ventricular standstill

Strip 9-92
Rhythm: Chaotic
Rate: 0
P waves: Absent; wave deflections are irregular and chaotic and vary in height, size, and shape
PR interval: Not discernible
QRS: Absent
Rhythm interpretation: Ventricular fibrillation

Strip 9-93
Rhythm: Regular
Rate: About 29
P waves: Absent
PR interval: Not measurable
QRS: 0.16 seconds
Rhythm interpretation: Idioventricular rhythm

Strip 9-94
Rhythm: Regular
Rate: 79
P waves: Sinus P waves present
PR interval: 0.18 to 0.20 seconds
QRS: 0.12 seconds
Rhythm interpretation: Normal sinus rhythm with bundle branch block

Strip 9-95
Rhythm: Basic rhythm regular
Rate: Basic rhythm rate 68
P waves: Sinus P waves with basic rhythm
PR interval: 0.16 to 0.18 seconds
QRS: 0.06 to 0.08 seconds
Rhythm interpretation: Normal sinus rhythm with one interpolated PVC. Interpolated PVCs are sandwiched between two sinus beats and have no compensatory pause. ST segment depression and T wave inversion are present

Strip 9-96
Rhythm: Basic rhythm regular; irregular with PVCs
Rate: Basic rhythm rate 72
P waves: Sinus P waves are present with basic
rhythm
PR interval: 0.12 to 0.14 seconds
QRS: 0.08 seconds (basic rhythm); 0.14 to 0.16
seconds (PVCs)
Rhythm interpretation: Normal sinus rhythm with
PVCs in a trigeminal pattern

Strip 10-1
Automatic interval rate: 72
Analysis: The first four beats are paced beats
followed by one patient beat and three paced beats
Interpretation: Normal pacemaker function

Strip 10-2
Automatic interval rate: 84
Analysis: The first three beats are paced beats,
followed by two patient beats, a pacer spike
occuring too early, a patient beat, a fusion beat,
and two paced beats
Interpretation: Undersensing malfunction

Strip 10-3
Automatic interval rate: 72
Analysis: All beats are pacemaker-induced
Interpretation: Pacemaker rhythm

Strip 10-4
Automatic interval rate: 72
Analysis: The first two beats are paced beats,
followed by two spikes that occur on time but do
not capture, and four paced beats
Interpretation: Loss of capture malfunction

Strip 10-5
Automatic interval rate: 72
Analysis: No patient beats are seen; no paced beats
are seen
Interpretation: Loss of capture in the presence of
asystole

Strip 10-6
Automatic interval rate: 50
Analysis: The first two beats are patient beats
followed by four paced beats
Interpretation: Normal pacemaker function

Strip 10-7
Automatic interval rate: 50
Analysis: The first two beats are pacemaker
induced, followed by a pseudofusion beat, two
patient beats, and one paced beat
Interpretation: Normal pacemaker function

Strip 10-8
Automatic interval rate: 72
Analysis: All beats are pacemaker-induced
Interpretation: Pacemaker rhythm

Strip 10-9
Automatic interval rate: 63
Analysis: The first two beats are paced beats
followed by a pseudofusion beat (spike on top of R
wave), a paced beat, a loss of capture spike, a
paced beat, and a patient beat
Interpretation: Loss of capture

Strip 10-10
Automatic interval rate: 88
Analysis: The first eight beats are paced beats.
When the pacemaker is turned off, the underlying
patient rhythm is atrial fibrillation with a slow
ventricular response (about 20)
Interpretation: This strip shows an indication for
permanent pacemaker implantation if the
underlying rhythm does not resolve

Strip 10-11
Automatic interval rate: 75
Analysis: The first four beats are paced beats
followed by a PVC, a paced beat that occurs too
early, a paced beat, a PVC, a spike that occurs too
early, and two paced beats
Interpretation: Undersensing malfunction; this strip
shows a sensing malfunction with capture (sixth
QRS) and without capture (spike after eighth QRS)

Strip 10-12
Automatic interval rate: 72
Analysis: The first five beats are patient beats,
followed by two paced beats, two patient beats,
one paced beat, and one patient beat. The
underlying rhythm is atrial fibrillation
Interpretation: Normal pacemaker function

Strip 10-13
Automatic interval rate: 68
Analysis: All beats are pacemaker-induced
Interpretation: Pacemaker rhythm

Strip 10-14
Automatic interval rate: 72
Analysis: The first three beats are paced beats
followed by two patient beats, and two paced
beats, one patient beat, and one paced beat
Interpretation: Normal pacemaker function

Strip 10-15
Automatic interval rate: 84
Analysis: The first three beats are paced beats; when the pacemaker is turned off the underlying rhythm is primary ventricular standstill. Two paced beats are seen when the pacemaker is turned back on
Interpretation: This strip shows an indication for permanent pacemaker implantation if the underlying rhythm does not resolve

Strip 10-16
Automatic interval rate: 72
Analysis: The first five beats are paced beats followed by a spike that occurs on time but doesn't capture. The last two beats are paced beats
Interpretation: Loss of capture

Strip 10-17
Automatic interval rate: 72
Analysis: First two beats are paced followed by a fusion beat, two patient beats, a pacer spike that occurs too early, a patient beat, a pacer spike that occurs too early, two patient beats, and one paced beat
Interpretation: Undersensing

Strip 10-18
Automatic interval rate: 72
Analysis: The first two beats are patient beats followed by a spike that occurs on time but doesn't capture, a patient beat, and five paced beats
Interpretation: Loss of capture

Strip 10-19
Automatic interval rate: 63
Analysis: The first two beats are paced beats followed by one patient beat, two paced beats, one patient beat, and one paced beat
Interpretation: Normal pacemaker function

Strip 10-20
Automatic interval rate: 72
Analysis: The first four beats are paced beats followed by one patient beat, one fusion beat, and three paced beats
Interpretation: Normal pacemaker function

Strip 10-21
Automatic interval rate: 72
Analysis: All beats are pacemaker-induced
Interpretation: Pacemaker rhythm

Strip 10-22
Automatic interval rate: Cannot be determined (only one paced beat)
Analysis: One paced beat with rhythm changing to ventricular tachycardia
Interpretation: One paced beat changing to ventricular tachycardia (Torsades de pointes)

Strip 10-23
Automatic interval rate: 72
Analysis: The first two beats are paced beats followed by one patient beat, a fusion beat, and five paced beats
Interpretation: Normal pacemaker function

Strip 10-24
Automatic interval rate: 72
Analysis: The first beat is paced followed by one loss of capture spike, one patient beat, one loss of capture spike, one patient beat, one paced beat, one loss of capture spike, one patient beat, one loss of capture spike, and one patient beat
Interpretation: Frequent loss of capture malfunction

Strip 10-25
Automatic interval rate: 72
Analysis: No patient beats are seen; all QRS complexes are pacemaker-induced
Interpretation: Pacemaker rhythm

Strip 10-26
Automatic interval rate: 72
Analysis: The first two beats are paced beats followed by one PVC, two paced beats, one pseudofusion beat, one patient beat, and two paced beats
Interpretation: Normal pacemaker function

Strip 10-27
Automatic interval rate: 84
Analysis: The first two beats are paced beats followed by two loss of capture spikes, one paced beat, two loss of capture spikes, two paced beats, and one loss of capture spike
Interpretation: Frequent loss of capture malfunction

Strip 10-28
Automatic interval rate: 72
Analysis: The first three beats are paced beats followed by one patient beat, two paced beats, one pseudofusion beat (spike superimposed on R wave), and two paced beats
Interpretation: Normal pacemaker function

Strip 10-29

Automatic interval rate: 72
Analysis: The first two beats are paced beats followed by three patient beats (second a PVC), and three paced beats
Interpretation: Normal pacemaker function; underlying rhythm is atrial fibrillation

Strip 10-30

Automatic interval rate: 65
Analysis: The first two beats are patient beats followed by three pseudofusion beats, and four patient beats
Interpretation: Normal pacemaker function

Strip 10-31

Automatic interval rate: Cannot be determined for sure since there aren't two consecutively paced beats present
Analysis: Strip shows six patient beats and 5 loss-of-capture spikes. No paced beats are seen
Interpretation: Complete loss of capture

Strip 10-32

Automatic interval rate: 72
Analysis: The first beat is paced followed by one patient beat, one fusion beat, two patient beats (second a PVC), one paced beat that occurs too early, two paced beats, one patient beat (PVC), one paced beat occuring too early, one patient beat (PVC), and a spike occuring too early
Interpretation: Frequent undersensing malfunction; this strip shows a sensing malfunction with capture (sixth and tenth QRS) and without capture (spike after 11th QRS)

Strip 10-33

Automatic interval rate: 72
Analysis: The first four beats are paced beats followed by two patient beats and three paced beats
Interpretation: Normal pacemaker function

Strip 10-34

Automatic interval rate: 68
Analysis: The first beat is a paced beat followed by a loss of-capture spike, one patient beat, one loss-of-capture spike, one patient beat, one paced beat, one loss-of-capture spike, one patient beat, one loss-of-capture spike, and one patient beat
Interpretation: Frequent loss of capture malfunction

Strip 10-35

Automatic interval rate: 56
Analysis: The first two beats are paced beats followed by one patient beat, one paced beat, one patient beat, one paced beat that occurs too early, two paced beats, and one patient beat
Interpretation: Undersensing malfunction

Strip 11-1

Rhythm: Regular
Rate: 107
P waves: Sinus P waves are present
PR interval: 0.12 seconds
QRS: 0.06 to 0.08 seconds
Rhythm interpretation: Sinus tachycardia

Strip 11-2

Rhythm: Regular
Rate: 58
P waves: Sinus P waves are present
PR interval: 0.12 to 0.14 seconds
QRS: 0.12 seconds
Rhythm interpretation: Sinus bradycardia with bundle branch block; ST segment depression is present

Strip 11-3

Rhythm: Regular
Rate: 21
P waves: Two sinus P waves to each QRS
PR interval: 0.32 to 0.36 seconds (remain constant)
QRS: 0.12 seconds
Second-degree AV block, Mobitz II; clinical correlation is suggested to diagnose Mobitz II when 2 : 1 conduction is present

Strip 11-4

Rhythm: Irregular
Rate: 90
P waves: Fibrillatory waves are present—some flutter waves are seen mixed with the fibrillatory waves
PR interval: Not measurable
QRS: 0.04 seconds
Rhythm interpretation: Atrial fibrillation; ST segment depression is present

Strip 11-5

Rhythm: Regular
Rate: 48
P waves: Hidden in QRS
PR interval: Not measurable
QRS: 0.08 seconds
Rhythm interpretation: Junctional rhythm; ST segment depression is present

Strip 11-6
Rhythm: Regular
Rate: 188
P waves: Not discernible
PR interval: Not discernible
QRS: 0.08 seconds
Rhythm interpretation: Atrial tachycardia; ST
segment depression is present

Strip 11-7
Automatic interval rate: 72
Analysis: The first two beats are paced beats,
followed by a patient beat, three paced beats, a
patient beat, and two paced beats
Rhythm interpretation: Normal pacemaker function

Strip 11-8
Rhythm: Regular
Rate: Atrial, 88; ventricular, 38
P waves: Sinus P waves present; bear no
relationship to QRS; can be found hidden in T
waves and in QRS
PR interval: Varies greatly
QRS: 0.12 seconds
Rhythm interpretation: Third-degree AV block; ST
segment depression is present

Strip 11-9
Rhythm: Regular
Rate: 188
P waves: Not discernible
PR interval: Not discernible
QRS: 0.16 to 0.20 seconds
Rhythm interpretation: Ventricular tachycardia

Strip 11-10
Rhythm: Regular
Rate: 42
P waves: Absent
PR interval: Not measurable
QRS: 0.16 seconds
Rhythm interpretation: Idioventricular rhythm

Strip 11-11
Rhythm: Basic rhythm regular; irregular with PVC
Rate: Basic rhythm rate 79
P waves: Sinus P waves with basic rhythm
PR interval: 0.14 to 0.16 seconds
QRS: 0.06 to 0.08 seconds (basic rhythm); 0.12
seconds (PVC)
Rhythm interpretation: Normal sinus rhythm with
one PVC; ST segment depression and T wave
inversion are present

Strip 11-12
Rhythm: Regular
Rate: 68
P waves: Inverted before each QRS
PR interval: 0.08 seconds
QRS: 0.06 to 0.08 seconds
Rhythm interpretation: Accelerated junctional
rhythm

Strip 11-13
Rhythm: Regular
Rate: Atrial, 450; ventricular, 150
P waves: Three flutter waves to each QRS
PR interval: Not measurable
QRS: 0.04 seconds
Rhythm interpretation: Atrial flutter with 3:1
block

Strip 11-14
Rhythm: Regular
Rate: 65
P waves: Sinus P waves are present
PR interval: 0.12 seconds
QRS: 0.06 to 0.08 seconds
Rhythm interpretation: Normal sinus rhythm; ST
segment depression is present

Strip 11-15
Rhythm: Regular
Rate: 94
P waves: Absent
PR interval: Not measurable
QRS: 0.12 seconds
Rhythm interpretation: Accelerated idioventricular
rhythm

Strip 11-16
Rhythm: Basic rhythm regular; irregular with
nonconducted PAC
Rate: Basic rhythm 75
P waves: Sinus P waves present with basic rhythm;
one premature, abnormal P wave without QRS
PR interval: 0.24 to 0.28 seconds
QRS: 0.06 to 0.08 seconds
Rhythm interpretation: Normal sinus rhythm with
first-degree AV block and one nonconducted PAC

Strip 11-17
Rhythm: Regular
Rate: 115
P waves: Sinus P waves are present
PR interval: 0.14 to 0.16 seconds
QRS: 0.06 seconds
Rhythm interpretation: Sinus tachycardia

Strip 11-18
Rhythm: Regular
Rate: 52
P waves: Sinus P waves are present
PR interval: 0.18 to 0.20 seconds
QRS: 0.06 to 0.08 seconds
Rhythm interpretation: Sinus bradycardia; a U wave is present

Strip 11-19
Rhythm: Basic rhythm regular; irregular with PJCs
Rate: Basic rhythm rate 88
P waves: Sinus P waves with basic rhythm; inverted P waves with PJCs
PR interval: 0.16 seconds (basic rhythm); 0.08 to 0.10 seconds (PJCs)
QRS: 0.04 seconds
Rhythm interpretation: Normal sinus rhythm with two PJCs; ST segment depression is present

Strip 11-20
Rhythm: Regular
Rate: 63
P waves: Vary in size, shape, and position
PR interval: 0.12 to 0.14 seconds
QRS: 0.06 to 0.08 seconds
Rhythm interpretation: Wandering atrial pacemaker; ST segment depression is present

Strip 11-21
Rhythm: Chaotic
Rate: 0 (no QRS complexes)
P waves: No P waves; wave deflections are chaotic, irregular and vary in height, size, and shape
PR interval: Not measurable
QRS: Absent
Rhythm interpretation: Ventricular fibrillation

Strip 11-22
Rhythm: Regular
Rate: 107
P waves: Inverted before each QRS
PR interval: 0.08 seconds
QRS: 0.04 to 0.06 seconds
Rhythm interpretation: Junctional tachycardia

Strip 11-23
Rhythm: Irregular atrial rhythm
Rate: Atrial, 40; ventricular, 0
P waves: Sinus P waves are present
PR interval: Not measurable
QRS: Absent
Rhythm interpretation: Primary ventricular standstill

Strip 11-24
Rhythm: Regular
Rate: 94
P waves: Sinus P waves present
PR interval: 0.26 to 0.28 seconds
QRS: 0.04 to 0.06 seconds
Rhythm interpretation: Normal sinus rhythm with first-degree AV block; ST segment depression is present

Strip 11-25
Rhythm: Regular
Rate: 188
P waves: Not discernible
PR interval: Unmeasurable
QRS: 0.16 to 0.20 seconds
Rhythm interpretation: Ventricular tachycardia; ST segment elevation is present

Strip 11-26
Rhythm: Regular atrial rhythm; irregular ventricular rhythm
Rate: Atrial, 72; ventricular, 60
P waves: Sinus P waves present
PR interval: 0.24 progressing to 0.32
QRS: 0.12 seconds
Rhythm interpretation: Normal sinus rhythm with second-degree AV block, Mobitz I and bundle branch block

Strip 11-27
Rhythm: Regular
Rate: 68
P waves: Sinus P waves are present
PR interval: 0.12 seconds
QRS: 0.06 to 0.08 seconds
Rhythm interpretation: Normal sinus rhythm; ST segment depression is present

Strip 11-28
Rhythm: Basic rhythm regular; irregular with pause
Rate: Basic rhythm 72 (rate slows to 63 during first cycle following pause; rate suppression can occur for several cycles following an interruption in the basic rhythm)
P waves: Sinus P waves are present
PR interval: 0.16 to 0.18 seconds
QRS: 0.04 to 0.06 seconds
Rhythm interpretation: Normal sinus rhythm with sinus arrest

Strip 11-29

Rhythm: Basic rhythm regular, irregular with PAC
Rate: Basic rhythm rate 60
P waves: Sinus P waves present with basic rhythm; one premature, abnormal P wave with PAC
PR interval: 0.18 to 0.20 seconds (basic rhythm); 0.20 seconds (PAC)
QRS: 0.04 to 0.06 seconds
Rhythm interpretation: Normal sinus rhythm with one PAC; ST segment depression and T wave inversion is present

Strip 11-30

Rhythm: Basic rhythm regular; irregular with PVCs
Rate: Basic rhythm rate 72
P waves: Sinus P waves are present
PR interval: 0.12 to 0.14 seconds
QRS: 0.12 seconds (basic rhythm and PVCs)
Rhythm interpretation: Normal sinus rhythm with bundle branch block and paired PVCs; a U wave is present

Strip 11-31

Rhythm: Regular
Rate: Atrial, 290; ventricular, 58
P waves: Five flutter waves to each QRS
PR interval: Unmeasurable
QRS: 0.06 to 0.08 seconds
Rhythm interpretation: Atrial flutter with 5:1 block

Strip 11-32

Rhythm: Basic rhythm regular; irregular with escape beat
Rate: About 84
P waves: Sinus P waves are present; hidden P wave with escape beat
PR interval: 0.14 to 0.16 seconds
QRS: 0.08 seconds
Rhythm interpretation: Normal sinus rhythm with one junctional escape beat; ST segment depression and a U wave are present

Strip 11-33

Rhythm: First rhythm cannot be determined (one sinus beat); second rhythm regular
Rate: 31 (second rhythm)
P waves: Sinus P wave with sinus beat
PR interval: 0.16 (sinus beat)
QRS: 0.08 to 0.10 seconds (sinus beat); 0.12 seconds (second rhythm)
Rhythm interpretation: Sinus beat changing to idioventricular rhythm

Strip 11-34

Automatic interval rate: 63
Analysis: The first three beats are paced beats followed by loss of capture, patient beat, and two paced beats
Interpretation: Loss of capture
Rhythm interpretation: Loss of capture

Strip 11-35

Rhythm: Cannot be determined for sure (only one cardiac cycle)
Rate: About 13
P waves: Absent
PR interval: Not measurable
QRS: 0.16 seconds
Rhythm interpretation: Secondary ventricular standstill

Strip 11-36

Rhythm: Chaotic
Rate: 0
P waves: Absent; wave deflections are chaotic, irregular and vary in size, shape, and height
PR interval: Not measurable
QRS: Absent
Rhythm interpretation: Ventricular fibrillation followed by electrical shock and return to ventricular fibrillation

Strip 11-37

Rhythm: Regular
Rate: 52
P waves: Sinus P waves are present
PR interval: 0.18 to 0.20 seconds
QRS: 0.06 to 0.08 seconds
Rhythm interpretation: Sinus bradycardia; a U wave is present

Strip 11-38

Rhythm: Basic rhythm regular; irregular with PAC
Rate: Basic rhythm rate 75
P waves: Sinus P waves present (basic rhythm); premature, abnormal P wave with PAC
PR interval: 0.16 seconds (basic rhythm); 0.12 seconds (PAC)
QRS: 0.06 to 0.08 seconds
Rhythm interpretation: Normal sinus rhythm with one PAC; a U wave is present

Strip 11-39
Rhythm: Irregular
Rate: 60
P waves: Fibrillatory waves are present
PR interval: not measurable
QRS: 0.12 seconds
Rhythm interpretation: Atrial fibrillation with bundle branch block; ST segment depression and T wave inversion are present

Strip 11-40
Automatic interval rate: 68
Analysis: All beats are paced
Interpretation: Paced rhythm

Strip 11-41
Rhythm: Regular atrial rhythm
Rate: Atrial, 68; ventricular, 0
P waves: Sinus P waves present
PR interval: Not measurable
QRS: Absent
Rhythm interpretation: Primary ventricular standstill

Strip 11-42
Rhythm: Basic rhythm irregular
Rate: Basic rhythm rate 60
P waves: Fibrillation waves present
PR interval: Not measurable
QRS: 0.08 seconds (basic rhythm); 0.12 to 0.16 seconds (PVCs)
Rhythm interpretation: Atrial fibrillation with paired PVCs; ST segment depression is present

Strip 11-43
Rhythm: Basic rhythm regular; irregular with PAC
Rate: Basic rhythm 65
P waves: Sinus P waves present; one premature, abnormal P wave with a premature beat
PR interval: 0.16 seconds
QRS: 0.08 to 0.10 seconds
Rhythm interpretation: Normal sinus rhythm with one premature atrial contraction

Strip 11-44
Rhythm: Regular
Rate: 47
P waves: Sinus P waves present
PR interval: 0.14 to 0.16 seconds
QRS: 0.06 to 0.08 seconds
Rhythm interpretation: Sinus bradycardia

Strip 11-45
Rhythm: Irregular to regular
Rate: Approximately 120 changing to a paced rate of 72
P waves: Fibrillation waves present in the first half of the tracing
PR interval: Unmeasurable
QRS: 0.06 to 0.08 seconds; 0.12 (paced beats)
Rhythm interpretation: Atrial fibrillation, changing to a pacemaker rhythm; ST segment depression is present

Strip 11-46
Automatic interval rate: 72
Analysis: First four beats are paced beats, followed by one patient beat, sensing malfunction, patient beat, a fusion beat, and two paced beats
Rhythm interpretation: Sensing malfunction

Strip 11-47
Rhythm: Regular
Rate: 42
P waves: Hidden in QRS
PR interval: Not measurable
QRS: 0.08 to 0.10 seconds
Rhythm interpretation: Junctional rhythm

Strip 11-48
Rhythm: Regular
Rate: 48
P waves: Absent
PR interval: Not measurable
QRS: 0.12 seconds
Rhythm interpretation: Idioventricular rhythm; ST segment elevation is present

Strip 11-49
Rhythm: Regular
Rate: About 26
P waves: Absent
PR interval: Not measurable
QRS: 0.14 to 0.16 seconds
Rhythm interpretation: Secondary ventricular standstill

Strip 11-50
Rhythm: Irregular atrial and ventricular rhythm
Rate: Atrial, 70; ventricular, 30
P waves: Sinus P waves are present; P waves bear no relationship to QRS; can be found hidden in QRS and T waves
PR interval: Varies greatly
QRS: 0.12 seconds
Rhythm interpretation: Third-degree AV block